T0227036

3D Imaging Technologies for Facial Plastic Surgery

Guest Editor

JOHN PALLANCH, MD, MS

FACIAL PLASTIC SURGERY CLINICS OF NORTH AMERICA

www.facialplastic.theclinics.com

November 2011 • Volume 19 • Number 4

SAUNDERS an imprint of ELSEVIER, Inc.

W.B. SAUNDERS COMPANY
A Division of Elsevier Inc.

1600 John F. Kennedy Blvd., Suite 1800, Philadelphia, PA 19103-2899

http://www.theclinics.com

FACIAL PLASTIC SURGERY CLINICS OF NORTH AMERICA Volume 19, Number 4
November 2011 ISSN 1064-7406, ISBN 978-1-4557-0445-3

Editor: Joanne Husovski

Facial Plastic Surgery Clinics of North America (ISSN 1064-7406) is published quarterly by Elsevier Inc., 360 Park Avenue South, New York, NY 10010-1710. Months of issue are February, May, August, and November. Business and Editorial Offices: 1600 John F. Kennedy Blvd., Suite 1800, Philadelphia, PA 19103-2899. Periodicals postage paid at New York, NY, and additional mailing offices. Subscription prices are $329.00 per year (US individuals), $459.00 per year (US institutions), $375.00 per year (Canadian individuals), $550.00 per year (Canadian institutions), $449.00 per year (foreign individuals), $550.00 per year (foreign institutions), $156.00 per year (US students), and $217.00 per year (foreign students). Foreign air speed delivery is included in all *Clinics* subscription prices. All prices are subject to change without notice. POSTMASTER: Send address changes to *Facial Plastic Surgery Clinics*, Elsevier Health Sciences Division, Subscription Customer Service, 3251 Riverport Lane, Maryland Heights, MO 63043. **Customer service: 1-800-654-2452 (US and Canada); 1-314-447-8871 (outside US and Canada); Fax: 314-447-8029; E-mail:journalscustomerservice-usa@elsevier.com (for print support); journalsonline support-usa@elsevier.com (for online support).**

Reprints. For copies of 100 or more of articles in this publication, please contact the Commercial Reprints Department, Elsevier Inc., 360 Park Avenue South, New York, NY 10010-1710. Tel.: 212-633-3812; Fax: 212-462-1935; E-mail: reprints@elsevier.com.

Facial Plastic Surgery Clinics of North America is covered in *MEDLINE/PubMed* (*Index Medicus*).

Contributors

CONSULTING EDITOR

J. REGAN THOMAS, MD, FACS
Professor and Chairman, Department
of Otolaryngology, University of Illinois at
Chicago, Chicago, Illinois

GUEST EDITOR

JOHN PALLANCH, MD, MS
Division Chair of Rhinology, ENT Department,
Mayo Clinic, Rochester, Minnesota

GUEST FOREWORD

RICHARD A. ROBB, PhD
Scheller Professor in Medical Research;
Professor of Biophysics and Computer
Science, Director, Mayo Biomedical Imaging
Resource Lab, Mayo Clinic College of
Medicine, Rochester, Minnesota

AUTHORS

S.H. AMIN, MD
Chief Resident, Kaiser Northern California
Otolaryngology Residency Program, Oakland,
California

GIUSEPPE GIOVANNI BARBARINO, PhD
Institute of Mechanical Systems, ETH-Swiss
Federal Institute of Technology, Zurich,
Switzerland

R. BRYAN BELL, DDS, MD, FACS
Clinical Associate Professor, Department
of Oral and Maxillofacial Surgery, Oregon
Health and Science University; Medical
Director, Oral, Head and Neck Cancer
Program, Providence Cancer Center,
Providence Portland Medical Center;
Attending Surgeon, Trauma Service/Oral
and Maxillofacial Surgery Service,
Legacy Emanuel Medical Center,
Portland, Oregon

PATRICK J. BYRNE, MD
Associate Professor, Division Director of
Facial Plastic and Reconstructive Surgery,
Department of Otolaryngology–Head and Neck
Surgery, Johns Hopkins School of Medicine,
Baltimore, Maryland

MAXIMILIAN CATENACCI, MD
Skindermolaser, Roma, Italy

C. CINGI, MD
Department of Otorhinolaryngology, Faculty
of Medicine, Osmangazi University,
Eskisehir, Turkey

MATTEO TRETTI CLEMENTONI, MD
Istituto Dermatologico Europeo, Milano, Italy

TATIANA K. DIXON, MD
Resident, Department of Otolaryngology–Head
and Neck Surgery, University of Illinois at
Chicago, Chicago, Illinois

KELLY S. DUNCAN, BA
Executive Vice President, Sales, Marketing &
Business Development, 3dMD, Atlanta,
Georgia

MANFRED FREY, MD
Division of Plastic and Reconstructive Surgery,
Department of Surgery, Medical University
of Vienna, Vienna, Austria

MARK J. GLASGOLD, MD
Robert Wood Johnson Medical School,
University of Medicine and Dentistry of
New Jersey, New Brunswick, New Jersey

ROBERT A. GLASGOLD, MD
Robert Wood Johnson Medical School,
University of Medicine and Dentistry of
New Jersey, New Brunswick, New Jersey

D.C. HATCHER, DC, DDS, MSc, MRCD(c)
Clinical Professor, University of Southern
Nevada; Adjunct Associate Clinical Professor,
University of Pacific; Private Practice at
Diagnostic Digital Imaging, Sacramento,
California

PETER A. HILGER, MD
Division of Facial Plastic and Reconstructive
Surgery, Department of Otolaryngology–Head
and Neck Surgery, University of Minnesota,
Minneapolis, Minnesota

DAVID L. HIRSCH, DDS, MD, FACS
Attending Physician, Division of Oral and
Maxillofacial Surgery, Department of Plastic
and Reconstructive Surgery, New York
University Langone Medical Center,
New York, New York

ALINA HOLD, MD
Division of Plastic and Reconstructive Surgery,
Department of Surgery, Medical University
of Vienna, Vienna, Austria

ROMAN KANTOR, PhD
Miravex Ltd, Trinity Research and Innovation,
O'Reilly Institute, Trinity College Dublin, Dublin,
Ireland

**CHUNG HOW KAU, BDS, MScD, MBA,
PhD, MOrth, FDS, FFD, FAMS**
Chairman and King James IV Professor,
Department of Orthodontics, University of
Alabama at Birmingham, School of Dentistry,
Birmingham, Alabama

J. KIM, MD
Clinical Fellow, Division of Facial Plastic
Surgery and Reconstructive Surgery,
University of California Davis Health System,
University of California Davis Medical Group,
Sacramento, California

HUGO B. KITZINGER, MD
Division of Plastic and Reconstructive Surgery,
Department of Surgery, Medical University of
Vienna, Vienna, Austria

CHRISTOPHER LANE
President, 3dMD, Atlanta, Georgia

ROSALIA LAVAGNO, MD
Istituto Dermatologico Europeo, Milano, Italy

JAMIE LEVINE, MD, FACS
Attending Physician, Department of Plastic
and Reconstructive Surgery, New York
University Langone Medical Center,
New York, New York

GUIDO MARIOTTO, PhD
Miravex Ltd, Trinity Research and Innovation,
O'Reilly Institute, Trinity College Dublin,
Dublin, Ireland

MICHAEL R. MARKIEWICZ, DDS, MPH, MD
Resident in Training, Department of Oral and
Maxillofacial Surgery, Oregon Health and
Science University, Portland, Oregon

EDOARDO MAZZA, PhD
Professor, Institute of Mechanical Systems,
ETH-Swiss Federal Institute of Technology,
Zurich, Switzerland; Mechanics for Modeling
and Simulation, EMPA– Materials Science
and Technology, Dübendorf, Switzerland

KATE MCCARN, MD
Division of Facial Plastic and Reconstructive
Surgery, Department of Otolaryngology–Head
and Neck Surgery, University of Minnesota,
Minneapolis, Minnesota

JASON D. MEIER, MD
University of Florida, Jacksonville, Florida

MARIA MICHAELIDOU, MD
Division of Plastic and Reconstructive Surgery,
Department of Surgery, Medical University
of Vienna, Vienna, Austria

F. OGHAN, MD
Department of Otorhinolaryngology, Faculty
of Medicine, Dumlupinar University, Kutahya,
Turkey

DAVID OTTERBURN, MD
Former Fellow in Microvascular Reconstructive
Surgery, Department of Plastic and
Reconstructive Surgery, New York University
Langone Medical Center, New York, New York

JOHN PALLANCH, MD, MS
Division Chair of Rhinology, ENT Department,
Mayo Clinic, Rochester, Minnesota

ASHISH PATEL, DDS, MD
Resident, Division of Oral and Maxillofacial
Surgery, New York University Langone
Medical Center, New York, New York

EVA PLACHETA, MD
Division of Plastic and Reconstructive Surgery,
Department of Surgery, Medical University
of Vienna, Vienna, Austria

IGOR PONA, MD
Division of Plastic and Reconstructive Surgery,
Department of Surgery, Medical University
of Vienna, Vienna, Austria

PIERRE SAADEH, MD, FACS
Attending Physician, Department of Plastic
and Reconstructive Surgery, New York
University Langone Medical Center,
New York, New York

STEPHEN A. SCHENDEL, MD, DDS
Professor Emeritus of Surgery, Stanford
University Medical Center, Stanford,
California

IGOR SHVETS, PhD
Professor, School of Physics, Trinity College
Dublin, Dublin, Ireland

BABAR SULTAN, MD
Resident, Department of Otolaryngology–Head
and Neck Surgery, Johns Hopkins School of
Medicine, Baltimore, Maryland

JONATHAN M. SYKES, MD
Professor and Director of Facial Plastic Surgery
and Reconstructive Surgery, University of
California Davis Health System, University
of California Davis Medical Group,
Sacramento, California

DEAN M. TORIUMI, MD
Professor and Head, Division of Facial
Plastic and Reconstructive Surgery,
Department of Otolaryngology–Head and
Neck Surgery, University of Illinois at
Chicago, Chicago, Illinois

CHIEH-HAN JOHN TZOU, MD
Division of Plastic and Reconstructive Surgery,
Department of Surgery, Medical University
of Vienna, Vienna, Austria

This page intentionally left blank

Contents

in whom the nasal surgical guide was used intraoperatively for reconstruction of full-thickness, complex nasal defects. This effort highlights the multidisciplinary approach involving a surgeon and anaplastologist integrated with the latest technology to provide patients with the best possible outcomes.

The authors present an overview of 3D computer-aided design and computer-aided modeling tools available to the facial plastic surgeon. They describe the role of 3D tools in all phases of computer-aided surgery including: data acquisition, planning, surgery, and assessment. Applications of these tools include obtaining 3D measurements, using mirror imaging to reconstruct missing areas of the head and neck, and 3D sizing or segmentation of bone and soft tissue. They review clinical outcomes obtained from studies reviewing 3D tools. These systems have potential value for education, reducing operating room time, and improving clinical outcomes.

Cases in subdisciplines of craniomaxillofacial surgery—corrective jaw surgery, maxillofacial trauma, temporomandibular joint/skull base, jaw reconstruction, and post-ablative reconstruction—illustrate the ease of use, cost effectiveness, and superior results that can be achieved when using computer-assisted design and 3D volumetric analysis in preoperative surgical planning. This article discusses the materials and methods needed to plan cases, illustrates implementation of guides and implants, and describes postoperative analysis in relation to the virtually planned surgery.

3D TO ASSESS CHANGES RESULTING FROM SURGERY

This article describes the equipment and software used to create facial 3D imaging and discusses the validation and reliability of the objective assessments done using this equipment. By overlaying preoperative and postoperative 3D images, it is possible to assess the surgical changes in 3D. Methods are described to assess the 3D changes from the rhinoplasty techniques of nasal dorsal augmentation, increasing tip projection, narrowing the nose, and nasal lengthening.

The authors present quantitative and objective 3D data from their studies showing long-term results with facial volume augmentation. The first study analyzes fat grafting of the midface and the second study presents augmentation of the tear trough with hyaluronic filler. Surgeons using 3D quantitative analysis can learn the duration of results and the optimal amount to inject, as well as showing patients results that are not demonstrable with standard, 2D photography.

Facial Plastic Surgery Clinics
of North America

THE CLINICS ARE NOW AVAILABLE ONLINE!

Access your subscription at:
www.theclinics.com

This page intentionally left blank

Glossary

Anaplastologist: specialist in the prosthetic rehabilitation of absent or disfigured aesthetically critical portions of the body, such as the ear and nose

ATM: articulation temporomandibular

CAD/CAM: computer-aided design/computer-aided modeling

CBCT: cone beam computed tomography

DICOM: Digital Imaging and Communications in Medicine

DISCRETIZATION: Converting continuous models into discrete parts in a new model to make suitable for numerical evaluation

FE: finite element

FE model: finite element model

FFOF: free fibular osteocutaneous flap

HYBRID STEREOPHOTOGRAMMETRY: a combination of both active and passive methods of stereophotogrammetry (see articles by Tzou and Schendel)

IFM 3D: 3D image fusion management; database management (done with software) of the different 3D images for each patient for different kinds of imaging and different dates of image acquisition

IPL: intense pulsed light; noncoherent light from 500 to 1200 nm used with a cutoff filter for selective photohemolysis

PACS: picture archiving communication systems

PMS: patient management software

PSAR: patient-specific anatomic reconstruction; an anatomically accurate record in which all the 3D images of the patient are superimposed into one valid 3D structure, including combination with biomechanical properties

PSAR: (as per Lane and Schendel) patient-specific anatomic reconstruction; the PSAR is an anatomically accurate record in which all the 3D images of the patient (ie, computed tomography/CBCT, magnetic resonance imaging, facial surface images, teeth) are superimposed into one valid 3D structure and combined with the relevant biomechanical properties

RMS: root mean square

SLMs: stereolithographic models

Facial Plast Surg Clin N Am 19 (2011) xiii
doi:10.1016/j.fsc.2011.07.015

This page intentionally left blank

Introduction to 3D Imaging Technologies for the Facial Plastic Surgeon

John Pallanch, MD, MS

KEYWORDS

- Facial plastic surgery • 3D imaging • Facial anatomy
- 3D image analysis

An introduction to 3D tools in the field of facial plastic surgery in 2011 should start with a look at where we would like to be: What does the optimal facial plastic surgery 3D image dream machine look like? How close are we to having that?

The dream device would use a method of 3D imaging that would be quickly acquired, be consistently repeatable, and have no safety concerns for the patient. The imaging would yield sub-sub-millimeter 3D data, including skin surface and tone, underlying soft tissue and muscles, bone, and teeth. It would capture and store the patient's 3D image, including all of their anthropometric data. The patient model could be viewed three-dimensionally from any angle and with any anatomic parts variably transparent. Through entering a few demographics, the facial appearance of the patient at various ages or weights could be displayed. The surgeon would be able to perform virtual surgery, and the healed results, incorporating the behavior of all underlying and surrounding tissues, would morph into view before the planning surgeon's eyes. The results of surgery could be displayed for any selected period after the procedure. Although the results would have no more certainty than a weather prediction, the percentage probabilities of the displayed results would be given. Alternative surgical approaches could be attempted and the surgeon would be alerted as to which had the greatest risk. For discussion with the patient, it could demonstrate from any angle possible changes that might be accomplished with surgery and those that are

not possible. The surgeon, in conjunction with the patient, could select the approach that might accomplish the goals in the safest and most predictable manor. It would then store the preoperative plan for viewing in the operating room.

All of this would be accomplished on a platform that would be economically accessible for wide distribution and have an optimized user interface.

I believe that most surgeons would agree that such a tool would be useful. I was anxious to find out, as I requested the 3D articles for this review of the current state of the art for 3D imaging, how close we have come to this dream scenario. The articles that follow show the great strides that have been made. How close are we? As the authors have reported, many of the prerequisites for development of the tool described have already been attained. However, most of the authors, although giving examples of the implementation of components of this vision, have also talked about the many unattained applications to be realized in the future.

3D tools for surgery allow 3D analysis of images in a way that is meaningful to surgeons for increased insight and understanding of a patient's anatomy. What is meant by 3D analysis of images? There are actually many facets to what 3D analysis can do. Put simply, it is a way to see more than one plane at the same time in the same image, although this does not always mean having a stereoscopic view. When we close one eye we do not see in 3D. But if we move around an object while looking with one eye we take in more data than a single

Division Chair of Rhinology, ENT Department, Mayo Clinic, 200 First Street SW, Rochester, MN 55901, USA
E-mail address: Pallanch.John@mayo.edu

Facial Plast Surg Clin N Am 19 (2011) xv–xvi
doi:10.1016/j.fsc.2011.07.001

plane. When we look in a mirror, we are looking at a flat surface but are receiving 3D information. When facial data is collected in an instant using a 3D stereophotogrammetric camera, information is stored that tells more than just the skin tones present in a single plane. 3D analysis tools allow viewing the image data from various points in space to see the changing contours and tones of a surface. When a CT is performed, data are collected, forming a cloud of data points in a cube or cylinder. 3D tools can be used to show internal anatomy in cut volumes and shaded surfaces, or even to navigate virtual endoscopic pathways through this volume of data, therefore providing an added dimension in understanding of the pre-surgical map of a patient's anatomy. It means new surgical tools that allow things to be accomplished that could not previously. The articles in this issue describe these 3D tools and others that have proven to be useful in facial plastic surgery. Other applications continue to be discovered.

HOW DID WE GET TO WHERE WE ARE IN THE FIELD OF 3D IMAGE ANALYSIS AND VISUALIZATION?

It is on the shoulders of giants in 3D image analysis like Dr Richard Robb that current 3D developers stand. Dr Robb and his team developed 3D tools, always working a step ahead of what the computer hardware and software were capable of accomplishing. As computer technology and speed advanced exponentially, so did their ability to realize their vision. At a time when conventional acquisition of a single CT slice took 60 seconds, they were able to acquire and render CT data to show a beating heart. But the software tools to take multiple beams of CT data and create a 3D object had to be created from scratch. Many of the tools they developed are now in common use in this field, including in their own Analyze software (Analyze 10.0, Mayo Biomedical Imaging Resource, Rochester, MN, USA). A single example of their multitude of contributions is the 3D icon that is seen in displays showing the orientation of the view. These tools laid the groundwork for what is seen today in the 3D renderings that have been a common part of, for example, most facial trauma practices.

Some themes prevail throughout these articles. One is the inadequacy of measurements or analysis done in 2D. Comparing image analysis in 3D with that performed in two dimensions is analogous to comparing the impact of viewing a sculpture with viewing a drawing of the same subject. Everything surgeons do is in 3D, resulting in 3D changes in tissue. Whether the surgery is reconstructive or purely aesthetic, being able to plan in 3D or execute with 3D guides using premanufactured 3D templates or prostheses, or even image guidance, can be invaluable. It also can make surgeons more efficient, surgery safer, and anesthesia shorter.

Another prevailing theme is the desire of facial plastic surgeons to have an optimal method to objectively assess their results and help discover what surgical techniques are most beneficial for different types of pathology or patients. This vision raises the question of whether improved methods of analysis will bring us closer to understanding what makes a face "attractive." Dr Richard Jacobson, who has extensive experience with 3D analysis of imaging data, including from cone beam imaging, has noted that the "average" or "normal" features that are present in people are not necessarily what makes them be considered beautiful or striking (Jacobson Richard, personal communication, 2011). Whether 3D analysis allows better portrayal of the elements of appearance that result in a given individual's favorable aesthetic attributes remains to be reported.

We are in the early stages of many future articles objectifying the difference that 3D technology can make in outcomes, such as surgeon satisfaction, patient satisfaction, operative results, operative time, and costs. Several of the articles summarize the current state of outcomes studies in this field.

What lies ahead? We have all seen the exponential changes in personal computing. We have far greater computing capability in our cell phone than was used to land men on the moon. Inexpensive home computers have more 3D graphics processing capability than workstations of a few years ago. These advancements should all be favorable for accelerating the arrival of the dream machine in its ultimate form. If a fraction of the resources that are needed to create a single video game or movie special effect were dedicated to refining and expanding 3D image analysis tools, we would have the dream machine today. I hope you enjoy reading these articles and seeing where we are today in the field of 3D imaging technologies for facial plastic surgery.

Foreword

3D Imaging Technologies for Facial Plastic Surgery is a wonderful compilation of relevant and timely articles in the field of facial plastic surgery using 3D imaging systems and techniques. Synergism among articles is high with regard to covering the spectrum of the evolution and use of these technologies in the practice of facial plastic surgery.

The discipline of modern medical imaging is really quite young, having its landmark launch in the early 1970s with the development of CT scanning. With that advent, imaging became fully digital and 3D. This heralded the beginning of a rich future for imaging in the health care industry that computers and electronic imaging would facilitate and advance. Computers are so embedded in medical imaging that we have almost lost sight of them as the enabling technology, which has made multimodality, multidimensional, multifaceted medical imaging possible to do and impossible to be without. The roots of this swift, remarkable revolution remain important. An understanding of the principles, tenets, and concepts underlying modern medical imaging is critically necessary to realize its full potential. This timely compendium will contribute to that realization.

Craniofacial surgeons were early adopters of 3D medical imaging and facilitated its translation into routine clinical practice. In the early 1970s, as soon as CT scanners became commercially available, their first and almost immediate application was in the hands of neuroradiologists and craniofacial surgeons. A majority of the early clinical publications regarding 3D CT imaging emanated from these two disciplines. This researcher became involved in the 1970s and 1980s with craniofacial surgeons in developing techniques to use 3D CT scans for preoperative planning of complex facial reconstruction procedures. In those early years, only skeletal anatomy was used in preoperative planning. The current, now routine inclusion of soft tissue imaging, modeling, and manipulation not only facilitates more comprehensive preoperative treatment planning, but also yields faithful predictions of surgical outcomes. Now, multiple imaging modalities, such as magnetic resonance imaging and surface scanning lasers, are combined and integrated ("fused") with CT imaging to provide powerful capabilities in facial plastic surgery only dreamed about in the early days of 3D imaging. Articles found in this review of the current state of 3D imaging attest to the exciting evolution of image fusion, interactive sculpting, analytic assessments of structure to function relationships, all in three dimensions, and even four dimensions (dynamic imaging systems can capture motion, biomechanical properties, and progression of tissue changes over time). 3D imaging has now cut a wide swath in acceptance and utilization by a number of disciplines in surgery and medicine, but valid claims to the earliest and most routine applications of this technology remain the purview of craniofacial plastic surgeons. The term "3D" as a modifier of the imaging technologies used is no longer necessary, so prevalent and routine has it become in modern practice.

The preceding explains the significance and timeliness of this review. It provides a cogent, neither overly simplified nor excessively complex, overview of the field. Indeed, there is something for everyone in the field contained in this publication. Students, trainees, young scientists, and practitioners, whether junior or experienced, can readily gain knowledge and useful insights. Such empowerment will inevitably lead to advancing the state of the art, as well as of the science, in 3D facial plastic surgery. It is reasonable to assume that the diligent reader who studies and peruses this information will be able to implement more productively the principles and technologies outlined. And the readers, who dive aggressively into the supporting material in the articles, including the references to both prior and current work, will find themselves in danger of becoming experts in the field, so comprehensive and relevant and up to date is the content presented. What interns and residents and junior surgical faculty can gain from this publication, senior faculty and practicing professionals can use as an expedient window to modern applications or as a refresher. I congratulate Dr John Pallanch, Guest Editor, who has pulled together this marvelous review, and believe that he, along with all the contributing authors, should be proud of this work and derive satisfaction from its publication.

Richard A. Robb, PhD
Mayo Clinic College of Medicine
Rochester, MN 55905, USA

E-mail address:
robb.richard@mayo.edu

Facial Plast Surg Clin N Am 19 (2011) xvii
doi:10.1016/j.fsc.2011.07.016
1064-7406/11/$ – see front matter

This page intentionally left blank

3D and the Next Dimension for Facial Plastic Surgery

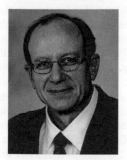

John Pallanch, MD, MS
Guest Editor

The 2011 observations that I make in this preface will likely be dated very quickly. We are at an active and vital yet emerging time in 3D tools. We, as consumers (and as surgeons), are living in exciting technological times where change is the norm and widespread adaptation, of platforms that had previously not caught on, has happened because of critical refinements. Networked cell phones with intuitive touch screens and e-readers are two examples.

3D media using stereo vision has been around almost as long as photography. Those of us who had "View-Masters" as children enjoyed seeing storybook characters in 3D. We've all seen antique 3D viewers (including for temporal bone sections) and the posters of a bespectacled 1950's audience viewing a 3D movie. Twenty-five years ago we (some of us) played 3D video games with our children using shuttered glasses with a much slower frame rate and lower resolution that didn't quite catch on. To have 3D cinema and media move to the mainstream took a critical point in technology and skill by the motion picture industry and a higher quality of artistic material and execution for widespread audience appeal. Dr Richard Robb in his "Biomedical Imaging, Visualization, and Analysis"[1] quotes Albert Einstein, "After a certain high level of technical skill is achieved, science and art tend to coalesce in esthetics, plasticity, and form."[2]

3D has arrived as never before. As consumers we can take pictures or videos with 3D cameras and view them on the large screen in 3D using 3D glasses. We can watch movies in 3D at home and play video games in 3D. Cameras and accelerometers in our video games and cell phones detect our movements in 3D and allow games to tell us that we are superb at a video game or exercising with incorrect form. We can take pictures with our handheld video game and view the result in 3D on the game's screen without 3D glasses. We now have ads for "3D" products throughout stores, eg, "3D whitening" in tooth care products, etc. With the inertia of large commercial success of 3D, "3D" is now mainstream. This means widespread, increasingly sophisticated 3D tools (if anything, to support the entertainment industry), better quality 3D imaging, and ultimately less expensive 3D tools with optimized user interfaces. No longer will 3D tools only be the domain of an engineer designing a car or fabricating a machine or part. Now homebuyers will be designing and decorating homes in 3D; families will have 3D home movies, and surgeons will employ a world of useful 3D tools for understanding the 3D intricacies of the anatomy of patients before or during surgery.

It follows that, as developments in 3D became more mainstream, there has been expansion of the application of 3D tools in medicine, and facial plastic surgery.

The public is becoming increasingly aware of this burgeoning technology. Facial plastic surgeons, who once advertized the ability to discuss surgical options using digital images on a computer screen, now advertise the ability to discuss proposed

Facial Plast Surg Clin N Am 19 (2011) xix–xxi
doi:10.1016/j.fsc.2011.07.017

surgical changes in 3D. It takes little imagination to conclude that, in the near future, it will be common place to be able to utilize 3D tools in our surgical practices. (See the Dream Machine description in the Introduction.)

As described below, this collection of articles shows a wide range of applications in which 3D tools have been shown to be advantageous over previous methods of utilizing and analyzing images for facial plastic surgery. In the table of contents, the synopses for each article provide summaries for the reader, but I will mention here the thought behind the selection and sequencing of the articles. The review starts with a broad description of the technology of the 3D tools available. The articles then discuss the use of 3D tools for planning surgery including aesthetic considerations and creation of the virtual patient. The next group of articles delineates the use of 3D tools in surgery. Last, articles describe the use of 3D to assess the changes resulting from surgery.

The descriptions of the technology include a broad overview of many of the capabilities of various 3D imaging modalities (Schendel, Duncan, Lane) and then additional useful background information about the development of 3D technology including guidelines for shopping for a 3D system (Tzou and Frey). For 3D esthetic considerations, the article by Cingi and Oghan brings a different perspective as the authors describe how their course provides facial plastic surgeons with a real and tactile 3D experience, and also cerebral practice, that very much overlaps the 3D appreciation of how a surgeon will interact with anatomy obtained from 3D image analysis. It touches also on communication with the patient.

Further surgical preparation uses the virtual patient described in Kau's article, with integration of different imaging technologies. A system of landmarks for comparison with other populations, growth, or surgical change is described. Mazza and Barbarino, in their article, show the state of the art as far as including the biomechanical behavior of the underlying tissues in the virtual 3D rendering. This is one of the facets of the 3D image analysis that will present the greatest challenges as progress continues. The further dimension in analysis using 3D is the novel method for study of facial motion in the article by Frey and coworkers.

The applications of 3D in surgery start with the description of a 3D template for complex nasal reconstruction (Sultan and Byrne). Markiewicz and Bell's article then reveals the myriad of ways that CAD/CAM technology can be used in facial plastic surgery including not just stents, but implants, templates, jigs, and models, to assess surgical progress toward a planned result. The article by

Patel and colleagues recounts case examples in different facial surgery subdisciplines, integrating the 3D tools described in the preceding articles for planning and executing surgery.

Last, measuring the 3D results of surgery includes assessment of changes with different rhinoplasty techniques (Toriumi and Dixon); volume change from autologous fat or filler injections in the midface (Meier, Glasgold, Glasgold); and changes to photo-damaged skin from IPL or laser (Clementoni et al). The latter objectively quantitates changes in vascularity, melanin distribution, and degree of individual deep wrinkles. These are exciting applications of 3D. The article by McCarn and Hilger shows the value and potential of 3D quantification in tissue expansion and the final article, by Amin and colleagues, looks at changes in midface soft tissue of the upper lip after LeFort I osteotomy.

Many of the articles include information about the technology available for 3D imaging, so it is possible for the reader to review the material without strict adherence to sequence, but either of the first two articles would be a good place to start.

Often the authors, while giving examples of the advantages of these various applications of 3D tools, also mention the numerous, not yet attained, applications to be realized in the future. An example is the 3D analysis of the results of different rhinoplasty techniques—Drs Dixon and Toriumi note that they do 3D imaging on all their patients. The article gives an excellent description of the 3D assessments that can be done, using two patients. One can imagine the wealth of information yet to come from applying these analyses to their large patient data base, eg, what are the 3D changes that occur from three different methods of tip refinement done for patients having similar presurgical tip anatomy? Clearly 3D tools are enhancing the excitement of future horizons in facial plastic surgery.

I want to thank all of the authors, the pioneers in 3D applications in facial plastic surgery, who contributed to this information source on the current use of 3D in our specialty. They have done a superb job describing the many ways that 3D tools and various methods of imaging can help us, with novel and ingenious ways to provide optimal care for our patients. These teams and individuals have spent many hours discovering which applications can shorten procedure and anesthetic time, increase the chances of success, and expand the possibilities in precise reconstruction. They are collecting data that is already helping to increase the predictability of our surgical results.

Although I used a wide network, my research may not have led to contact with some of the active pioneers in this field, and for that I am sorry and wish they were included. There are also some imaging modalities not included that have relevance in facial plastic surgery and that may soon enhance 3D information for our patients. Two examples are determination of potential flap viability and localization of surface blood vessels.

I also would like to acknowledge and thank Dr Richard Robb—ultimate guru and pioneer in 3D Biomedical Imaging—and his talented team at the Mayo Biomedical Imaging Resource, including Jon Camp and Phil Edwards, who patiently taught me various applications of 3D image analysis tools over the past 6 years. Starting 30 years ago, they developed software from scratch that could do 3D analysis of CT data from multiple cone beam scanners. (See the Introduction in this issue.)

Dr Regan Thomas had the idea for this subject but deserves the greatest credit for inspired timing on when to suggest that I take this on. Many thanks to Joanne Husovski, superwoman editor, who produces dozens of different books on different subjects each year. Clearly, this volume would not be possible without her experience and expert guidance. Finally, I want to thank Kitty Pallanch for her understanding and support of so many projects including the time and effort needed for this volume.

John Pallanch, MD, MS
ENT Department
Mayo Clinic, 200 First Street SW
Rochester, MN 55905, USA

E-mail address:
Pallanch.John@mayo.edu

REFERENCES

1. Robb RA. Biomedical imaging, visualization, and analysis. Somerset (NJ): Wiley & Sons, Inc; 2000. p. v.
2. Einstein A. Einstein Archive. Princeton: Princeton University Press; 1996. p. 33–257.

This page intentionally left blank

Image Fusion in Preoperative Planning

Stephen A. Schendel, MD, DDS[a],*, Kelly S. Duncan, BA[b],
Christopher Lane[b]

KEYWORDS

- Three dimensional • 3D • Image fusion
- Preoperative planning • Facial surface Imaging

A PATIENT-CENTRIC SURGICAL PLANNING PARADIGM

To achieve the best possible outcomes in facial cosmetic and reconstructive surgery, many clinicians are starting to embrace the use of powerful software tools that enable them to plan surgeries in a digital three-dimensional (3D) environment. The foundation of these tools is based on the patient's unique anatomic model that fuses the patient's 3D soft tissue surface with the underlying 3D skeletal structure (**Fig. 1**). Although morphing a 3D surface to generate a desired result is generally accepted in the animation and character modeling world, true surgical planning requires that the software tool incorporate a firm understanding of the various anatomic components, their relative positions to one another, and the biomechanical relationships within the craniofacial complex.

Significant technological advances in the areas of computing, 3D imaging, and the Internet in the last 10 years, in combination with the adoption of 3D patient imaging protocols, are starting to push a next-generation, truly patient-centric care paradigm. With a patient-specific anatomic model that fuses the patient's computed tomography (CT)/cone beam CT (CBCT), magnetic resonance imaging (MRI), and surface images from a single point in time, treatment planning for both the physician and patient becomes clear and understandable. Moreover, the proliferation of Web-based applications increases availability and decreases costs, enabling the virtual patient to be studied and improved treatment protocols to be developed.

Although the use of virtual anatomic reality in surgical planning can improve precision and reduce complications, it also promotes a larger health community goal of improving overall surgical results. Correctly planning and accurately simulating surgical outcome is paramount in facial surgery and the tools used should:

1. Provide a patient treatment plan to achieve the desired result
2. Give the patient a reasonable preview and understanding of the outcome
3. Serve as a communication tool among multiple specialists (eg, orthodontists, surgeons) on the treatment team.

At the center of this approach is the true digital patient or "patient-specific anatomic reconstruction" (PSAR). The PSAR is not just a series of 3D images or traditional photographs/radiographs available in a file to view separately, it is an anatomically accurate record in which all of the patient's 3D images (ie, CT/CBCT, MRI, facial surface images, teeth and so forth) are superimposed into 1 valid 3D structure and combined with the relevant biomechanical properties. This process, resulting in a single dataset from the combination of relevant information from 2 or more independent datasets, is called image fusion.

STRATEGIES FOR 3D FACIAL IMAGE FUSION

When treating the face from a maxillofacial perspective, multiple imaging modalities are required to produce an accurate PSAR model of the patient. Depending on treatment, there is typically a protocol defined that requires a series of 3D images (in 1 or several different modalities) to be

a Stanford University Medical Center, Pasteur Drive, Stanford, CA, USA
b 3dMD, 100 Galleria Parkway, #1070, Atlanta, GA 30339, USA
* Corresponding author.
E-mail address: etienne@stanford.edu

Facial Plast Surg Clin N Am 19 (2011) 577–590
doi:10.1016/j.fsc.2011.07.002
1064-7406/11/$ – see front matter © 2011 Elsevier Inc. All rights reserved.

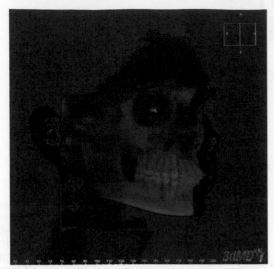

Fig. 1. 3D photogrammetric facial scan and cone beam computed tomography (CBCT) 3D radiology scan. The realistic 3D soft tissue scan has been made semitransparent to view the underlying bony anatomy.

taken at specific points in time throughout the treatment cycle. The imaging modalities currently relevant to the maxillofacial region include:

1. Traditional CT or the less invasive CBCT
2. 3D facial surface imaging (extraoral)
3. 3D dental study model surface scanning (intraoral).

Most commonly, the primary modality is CT/CBCT, to which other datasets are fused. Imaging technologies are emerging that may become important secondary modalities to which CBCT datasets may be fused, including[1,2]:

1. Ultrasound to document airway function
2. MRI to isolate muscle and generate a basic facial surface image (Takács and colleagues, 2004)[3]
3. 3D optical intraoral scanners to replace the dental impression technique and/or scanning physical study models
4. Dynamic facial (four-dimensional [4D]) surface imaging to record facial movement and expression
5. Positron emission tomography (PET).

THE IMPORTANCE OF THE 3D SURFACE IMAGE IN SURGICAL PLANNING

The face is the foundation for communications and interaction with the world, and thus patients are concerned with the effect a treatment might have on their appearance. This awareness is placing more emphasis on the importance of accurately documenting the patient's external facial features and characteristics before treatment, and then using this as a basis to plan treatment and monitor progress throughout treatment. Although a series of photographs has been used traditionally for this function, the limitations of a 2D medium significantly reduce the ability to objectively quantify treatment results for patients. How patients sees themselves in photographs may be totally different than how a clinician sees the patient in the same photograph irrespective of the lack of 3D reality (**Fig. 2**).

With a highly accurate 3D surface image of the patient's face, this debate becomes objective because the treating physician can measure the geometric shape changes that resulted from treatment and/or growth (ie, the effects of a mandibular advancement, a palate expander, cleft repair, and so forth). The need for quantification of this effect and the minimizing of subjectivity is fueling the adoption of enabling technologies. Because of the exposure risks associated with the production of 3D images using ionizing radiation, noninvasive modalities and techniques are being investigated for incorporating 3D data into a patient's PSAR. Optics-based 3D surface imaging systems are available to noninvasively capture anatomically precise 3D facial images of the patient. Not only can a patient's surface image be taken before and after treatment in conjunction with the CT/CBCT images, the clinician has the option to image the patient as often as required depending on the treatment protocol. Soft tissue only procedures can be planned and monitored only using the 3D surface imaging modality. Dental impressions can be taken producing physical

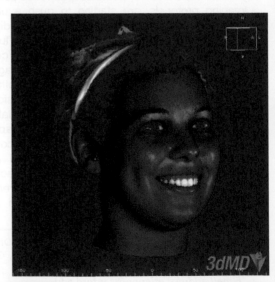

Fig. 2. 3D photogrammetric facial scan with patient smiling.

study casts that can be digitized into an in-vivo 3D dental model for incorporation into the PSAR.

3D SURFACE IMAGING TECHNIQUES

For surface 3D construction, a 3D surface image has 2 components, the geometry of the face and the color information, or texture map that is mathematically applied to the shape information. The construction of 3D surface images involves 3 steps:

1. 3D surface capture. There are 2 basic 3D surface imaging approaches. One is laser based and the other is optics based. For human form imaging, the optics-based approach has been implemented as structured light, moiré fringe projection, and stereo photogrammetric techniques.
2. Modeling. This stage incorporates sophisticated algorithms to mathematically describe the physical properties of an object. The modeled object is typically visualized as wireframe (or polygonal mesh), made up of triangles or polygons. The continuity of area between the polygons is filled in by the recruitment of surface pixels from the associated surface plane to generate a surface image or a texture map.
3. Rendering. If the 3D surface imaging system captures surface color information, at this stage the pixels are provided with values reflecting color texture and depth to generate into a lifelike 3D object viewed on the computer screen.

There are several potential advantages of registering anatomically accurate 3D facial surface images to CT/CBCT datasets (**Fig. 3**A–C).

- Surface images may correct for CBCT surface artifacts caused by patient movement (ie, swallowing, breathing, head movement, and so forth) because CBCT scans can take from 5 to 70 seconds depending on the manufacture of the CBCT unit and the imaging protocol;
- Independently acquired surface images compensate for soft tissue compression from upright CBCT device stabilization aids (ie, chin rest, forehead restraint, and so forth);
- Surface images may also the eliminate soft tissue draping from supine CBCT devices;
- Surface images may supplement missing anatomic data (ie, nose, chin, and so forth);
- Surface images may provide a more accurate representation of the draping soft tissue that reflects the patient's natural head position for condition assessment and treatment planning.

In relation to surface 3D construction, a surface image has 2 components: the geometry of the face and the color information, or texture map that is mathematically applied to the shape information. Both are required for a realistic result that is also accurate.

There are 2 basic 3D surface imaging approaches. One is laser based and the other is optics based.

Laser-based Surface Imaging

In its basic form, a laser scanner calculates the coordinate of each point on the surface of the target by measuring the time it takes for

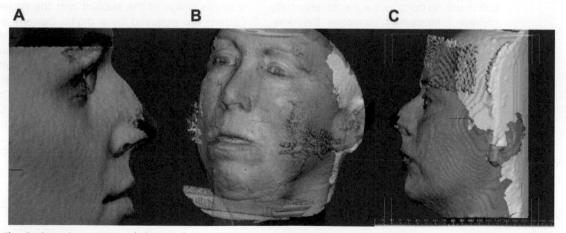

Fig. 3. Superimposition of the 3D facial photogrammetric scans and the segmented soft tissue boundary (*in white*) from CBCT scans. (*A*) Profile view in which the nasal defect from the CBCT scan is compensated for by the 3D facial photogrammetric scan. (*B*) Oblique view in which the noise defect and chin restraint device from the CBCT scan are compensated for by the 3D facial photogrammetric scan. (*C*) Left lateral view in which the nasal defect and head restraint device from the CBCT scan are compensated for by the 3D facial photogrammetric scan.

a projected light ray to return to a sensor. To improve efficiency, more complex patterns are projected, such as a light stripe. This technology of scanning the face with a laser is based on projecting a known pattern of light to infer an object's topography. This light can be in the form of a single bright light source; however, a light stripe is more commonly used. As an object is illuminated it is viewed by an offset camera. Changes in the image of the light stripe correspond with the topography of the object, and these distortions are recorded to produce 3D data for the object. Practically, the light may remain fixed and the object move or vice versa. Geometry triangulation algorithms allow depth information to be calculated, coordinates of the facial surface can be derived, and computer software can be used to create a 3D model of the object. Changes in dimensions between repeated scans or changes as a result of treatment are often shown by color differentiation or color maps. Several devices are currently commercially available (**Table 1**).

There are some disadvantages to this approach:

- The digitization process requires the subject to remain still for a period of up to 30 seconds[4] or more while the laser vertically scans the subject's face. Although the 3D model generated might be accurate on a band-by-band basis, a single human face comprises thousands of bands from top to bottom and each band is taken sequentially. Although this amount of time works adequately for inanimate objects in industrial applications, such as reverse engineering, quality inspection, and prototyping, laser technologies have proved difficult to use on conscious subjects, especially children.[5] Movement increases the likelihood of distortion, noise, and voids of the scanned image.
- Because the process involves the use of a laser, there are safety considerations related to the exposure of the eyes.
- The output can be noisy thus requiring additional processing to treat noise, outliers, and deficiencies in the generated geometry.
- The lack of soft tissue surface color texture information has also been highlighted as a possible drawback,[6] because this results in potential difficulties in the identification of landmarks that are dependent on surface color.

Several investigators have applied this approach, particularly for the assessment of facial asymmetry, treatment outcome, and relapse,[4,7–12] and reported precision of the laser scanning device to be approximately 0.5 mm on inanimate objects such as O'Grady and Antonyshyn's[10] plaster head model; however, others have reported that many measurements were unreliable (errors higher than 1.5 mm).[13] In addition, patients are scanned with their eyes closed, which may interfere with the natural facial expression and any landmarks placed around the eyes. With scan durations of 10 seconds or more, such geometry inaccuracies are likely attributed to software attempts to compensate for movement during the scanning process.

Optics-based Imaging

For human form imaging, the optics-based approach has been implemented as structured light, moiré fringe projection, and stereo photogrammetric techniques. Several systems have been commercially produced (**Table 2**).

Structured light

This is an optical technique that projects structured light patterns (usually white light), such as grids, dots, or stripes, onto the subject. Next, a single image of the subject and the projected pattern are acquired by a digital camera within the system. The reconstruction software is initially calibrated with the spatial position of the camera and the specifics of the projected light pattern. The distortion of the light pattern is then analyzed by the system's software and the 3D shape is inferred from the scale of the visible distortion. Color texture information is inherently registered with the

Table 1
Selection of commercially available laser scanning technologies

Name	Model	Manufacturer	Web Address
FastSCAN	Cobra/Scorpion	Polhemus, Colchester, VT	http://www.polhemus.com
Head & Face Color 3D Scanner	PX	Cyberware, Inc., Monterey, CA	http://www.cyberware.com
Minolta Vivid	910	Konica Minolta Sensing Americas, Inc., Ramsey, NJ	http://www.konicaminolta.com

Table 2
Selection of commercially available optics-based technologies

Name	Type	Manufacturer	Web Address
Rainbow 3D	SL	Genex Technologies, Inc., Bethesda, MD	http://www.genextech.com
3dMDface/ 3dMDcranial Systems	SP	3dMD, Atlanta, GA	http://www.3dmd.com/3dmdface.html http://www.3dmd.com/3dmdcranial.html
FaceSCAN3D	MFP	3D-shape GmbH, Erlangen, Germany	http://www.3d-shape.com
FaceSnatcher	SL	Eyetronics NV Leuven, Belgium	http://www.eyetronics.com

Abbreviations: MFP, moiré fringe protection; SL, structured light; SP, stereo photogrammetry.

xyz coordinate information. Although technically straightforward, this approach suffers from several problems including:

- Limitations in accurately capturing occluded areas and steep contours inherent in a single view point of the human face.
- Inability to generate an accurate 3D model of a human subject's face from ear to ear (180°). To image the complete craniofacial complex comprising both left and right profiles, a system with at least 2 imaging viewpoints must be used to eliminate the challenges associated with occlusions in the structure of the face, particularly the nasal region. Because of the nature of the pattern projected, these images have to be taken in sequence to avoid pattern interference (ie, a grid pattern from one viewpoint overlapping with a grid pattern from another angle). Sequential image capture extends the acquisition duration because of the time lag, which, for living human subjects, can be detrimental to the resulting data accuracy. This deficiency has reduced the application of this technique in health care.

Because of the inherent challenges for achieving accuracy, there are limited studies on the application of this technique to facial imaging in quantification of facial soft tissue changes after surgery,[14] craniofacial assessment,[15] and facial swelling.[16] Mean accuracy has been reported to be approximately 1.25%, with reproducibility being 3.27%.[16]

Moiré fringe projection

This optics-based technique projects a moiré fringe pattern onto the subject and the surface shape is calculated by analyzing the interference between projected patterns from a known point of observation. Moiré fringing is an improvement compared with simple structured light because the pattern used for reconstruction is inherently more granular or dense. In addition, more of the facial profile, especially the topology of the nose, is captured. To capture all of the facial features, up to 5 separate observations are required. Moiré 3D reconstruction suffers the same limitations as structured light because the data acquisition is interspersed with processing and has several other shortcomings including:

- It significantly increases the time taken to acquire the image. Even with the use of mirrors, each angle has to be acquired separately to avoid unwanted interference across images. In addition, the type of projectors used to project an accurate fringe requires a significant warm-up time and have a residual latency when powering down in comparison with photographic flash.
- Motion artifacts are inherent and require the use of special compensation algorithms.
- Careful control of lighting is required to avoid any stray spectral interference with the moiré patterns.

Although industrial engineering tends to uses moiré fringe projection for scanning inanimate objects, application of this methodology to facial imaging has been mainly limited to laboratory conditions for the assessment of age-related skin changes,[17,18] facial asymmetry,[19] postoperative facial changes,[20] and normal morphology.[21–23] To date, there has been little published on accuracy validation from a live patient perspective. The general issue with moiré fringe approach for live human subjects is common with other techniques requiring the projection of precalibrated structured light techniques: speed of capture. Although it has been possible to produce limited research in strictly supervised laboratory conditions, this can often entail the taking of several images of the subject until a workable model is captured. Such a workflow tends to inhibit larger data collection exercises in normal clinical environments because the workflow entailed obstructs the regular business of the clinic (**Fig. 4**).

Stereo photogrammetry

Stereo photogrammetry is a method of obtaining an extraoral image by means of 1 or more stereo pairs of photographs taken simultaneously. The concept was first applied to the face as early as 1967.[24] This technique differs from the other optics-based methods in that it requires no special pattern projection. The subject can be illuminated with regular photographic flash (**Fig. 5**). With some commercially available photogrammetric systems, the images needed to reconstruct a model are taken in a short period of time (in less than 1/500th of a second or 2 milliseconds) and then processed using highly sophisticated image analysis software. The use of industrial-grade, machine vision (MV) cameras, as opposed to single lens reflex (SLR) cameras, ensures that all of the data can be captured within 2 milliseconds no matter how many camera angles are involved because of the highly precise triggering mechanism associated with MV cameras. Stereo photogrammetry works the way a pair of human eyes measure distance (binocular vision) by taking 2 pictures of the same object, at a known distance apart, to create a stereo pair and record depth (also called stereopsis). Stereo photogrammetry uses sophisticated image analysis matching to identify and match unique external surface

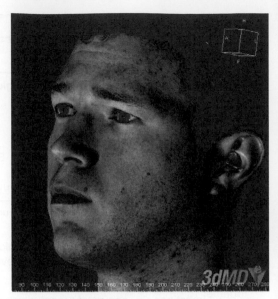

Fig. 5. 3DMD facial scan.

features between the 2 photographs and generate a composite 3D model by triangulating the points. If the system extracts a point cloud, then underlying software must know the exact position of each camera sensor relative to the others, which is calculated against a known target during the initial calibration exercise. The pattern on the surface provides the stereo algorithms with the base information required to build an accurate geometry. Once the 3D geometry model has been produced, the software maps the color texture information onto the model. Although the theory is straightforward, developing a reliable, repeatable stereo photogrammetry system is expensive because it depends on the reliability of image analysis. Several researchers have reported accurate identification of facial landmarks from 0.5 mm[25,26] to 0.2 mm.[27,28] For imaging the surface of human subjects, stereo photogrammetry seems to be superior to structured light and moiré fringe techniques in terms of:

1. Capture speed, which is mandatory for human subjects
2. Ability for more than 1 viewpoint to trigger simultaneously with other viewpoints, which is necessary for the structure of the face
3. Ability to compute the accuracy of any derived point.

Most recently, Lane and Harrell[29] reported that increased accuracy can be achieved using a hybrid of active and passive photogrammetry whereby a flat, random pattern based on white light is briefly projected onto the subject. They found that the

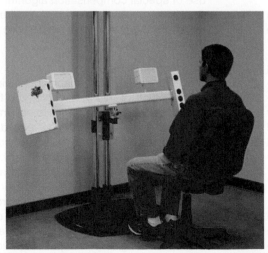

Fig. 4. 3dMD facial photogrammetric scanning system.

pattern combines with the natural skin texture to give the image analysis software more detail to perform the triangulation and helps to avoid errors and inconsistencies in establishing triangulation points caused by unpredictable reflected light in less-than-optimal lighting conditions.

Because of the limitations of all other methods of facial imaging, stereo photogrammetry systems are currently the most often clinically applied 3D surface imaging modality. Surface information of the subject's face is converted into a series of coordinates that have an xyz definition. The model is built from a series of stereo pairs, which need to be combined.

Historically, long-range photogrammetry was developed generating a separate range map 3D surface for each stereo viewpoint (each containing its own coordinate system). These range maps, or surface areas, are then subsequently stitched together to produce a new overall 3D coordinate system. Stitching multiple surface areas together has historically worked well for data input of inanimate objects and topology because subject motion is not a factor. This technique does not work well when the subjects are animate, because stitching separate 3D surfaces together to generate a single 3D model of the patient can compromise accuracy because of the discontinuity of surface information. There is no guarantee that 2 separate images taken at different points of time with the movement factor will still match, and this can result in a fracture of information along the midline, which compromises accuracy.

The preferable way to generate a 3D surface image derived from multiple stereo viewpoints is to generate a single unified and continuous coordinate system by selecting the best quality data for any given xyz coordinate from each of the stereo viewpoints. For this to work, the reconstructive algorithms must be able to place a value on the quality of each point generated. The great advantage of using hybrid photogrammetry and very fast (better than 2 millisecond) capture times incorporated in systems such as the 3dMD system is that the characteristics of the images used to generate the 3D surface are readily understood by the analysis algorithms and there is no risk of stray light causing spectral variation.

3D IMAGE FUSION FOR PREOPERATIVE PLANNING

Once the 3D images from a patient imaging session have been acquired, it is necessary to prepare the virtual patient for condition assessment, treatment planning, and outcome simulation. The imaging software environment needs to easily handle DICOM (Digital Imaging and Communications in Medicine) files, surface files such as STL or OBJ, as well as color information such as JPG or BMP. To generate an accurate PSAR, there are several steps.

Patient Workups

3D imaging adds a layer of complexity to the patient record by significantly increasing the volume of information available about a patient throughout the treatment cycle. These added components place greater demands on existing patient management software (PMS) systems, most of which were developed for textural and 2D data input to the patient record. Although multiuser Picture Archiving Communication Systems (PACS) are available, these systems are used for enterprise activities such as a hospital radiology department and are generally overly complex for a typical practice environment. Although most computerized dental practices or imaging facilities operate as limited local area networks (LANs), there are several database criteria required to facilitate image fusion from multiple devices including archiving the raw 3D images as originally generated by the imaging device; storing and easily accessing image modifications; linking relevant image sequences; and retaining virtual simulation files. To successfully implement these functions, any 3D image fusion management (3D IFM) software should apply the concepts commonly used in PC editing software to basic database management. The manner in which multimedia images are cross-referenced and presented to the user can be referred to as a patient workup. Initiation of the patient workup requires collecting, cataloging, and archiving of all relevant 3D image datasets related to 1 point in time, referred to as an episode of care. An episode of care relates to a specific point in time during the treatment cycle, such as pretreatment, 3 months into treatment, after treatment, 3 to 6 months after treatment, and so forth. Because original datasets, most likely, will need to be altered for treatment planning, the 3D IFM should be able to save these modifications without changing the raw 3D images or saving an updated DICOM. This ability is achieved through a control record, or metadata, which applies the xyz transformations to the original 3D images whenever it is loaded. The metainformation can extend to all aspects of image fusion such as reorientation, superimposition, segmentation, and simulation (discussed later). Because each patient workup is a series of episodes of care, different treatments can be planned. Ideally, a 3D IFM should be a Web-enabled, patient-centric software platform because this type of application provides many advantages, especially when treatment is provided by multiple clinicians, such as:

- Facilitating better communication between members on the treatment team;
- Providing therapeutic device suppliers with size and fit information to manufacture standard devices or design custom devices;
- Improving the patient referral process to streamline diagnosis, treatment planning, and outcome evaluation; and
- Enabling patient outcomes to be easily submitted to professional certification boards.

PSAR Registration

Because shape-based registration between the CBCT DICOM, 3D facial, or dental surface image datasets is preferable, this discussion is limited to this consideration. Although registration could be performed using fiducial markers to correlate between the skin as imaged by the DICOM dataset and the 3D surface image, there are considerable workflow and quality drawbacks to this method, including the additional time needed to place the markers themselves and the image distortion caused by the markers. The first step in shape-based registration entails segmentation of the outer surface of the CBCT data to generate a separate object that represents the outer geometry and keeps the original spatial relationship (DICOM skin). The quality of the segmented image depends on the quality of the data output from the CT/CBCT device, the lack of deformity of the facial features by structures such as the chin rest, and the quality of the segmentation routines. Next, the geometry of the 3D surface image is registered to the DICOM skin, which acts as the reference object to ensure that the 3D surface adopts the coordinate system of the DICOM on completion. The basic technique involves assessing the statistical variation between the 2 surfaces, whether the user selects the whole surface or specific areas of interest. With the surface errors that are typical with CBCT (eg, chin restraint, motion artifacts, soft tissue draping), a visual inspection of the image is recommended so the clinician can select the best regions on the face for registration. For example, the clinician would not select the region around the chin if there is a restraint. Depending on the individual DICOM skin, users typically do not select regions of the face that are subject to positional change from one modality to another, such as the mandible or the eyes. Because each 3D data set is accurate on its own, it is important to establish a consistent facial expression protocol. Registration areas that are typically

selected include regions with contour, such as the cheek and glabella areas. The nasal bridge has also been used because this region does not markedly change from childhood to adulthood.[30] These areas tend to provide a good multiaxis orientation on both images, which effectively prevents the registration algorithms from attempting to fit areas where known differences exist between the surfaces, thus improving the value of the root mean square (RMS) error. A simple color histogram can indicate the areas of displacement to determine, for example, whether the RMS variance is caused by a slightly different expression or a more fundamental issue. If the software is well designed and user friendly, area of interest superimposition should take less than 30 seconds to complete.

PSAR Assessment

After registration, numerous options allow interaction with the datasets by either rendering the volumes independently or separately, including scrolling through the volume in 3D or in the coronal, sagittal, and axial planes (Fig. 6). Although cephalometric landmark identification and analysis tracings have been the most common methods to interact with 2D radiographic and photographic data, there are well-known limitations related to the interpretation of 3D geometry on a 2D plane.[31,32] With the increasing availability of 3D imaging devices and easy-to-use software applications, there will be a transition to 3D cephalometric analysis and anthropometric surveys. When conducting landmarking exercises on nonsedated human subjects without fiducial markers or physical markings on the patient, many have noted that different facial landmarks have wide variation in their degree of reproducibility,[6,31,33–35] ranging from 2 mm to less than 0.5 mm.

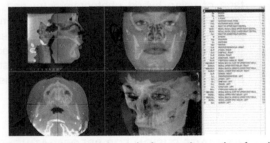

Fig. 6. Typical viewing platform where the fused image of the CBCT and photogrammetric scans are shown together with the skin semitransparent. Profile, frontal, and submentovertex views are arranged for simultaneous viewing. The lower right box shows the 3D scan, which can be rotated and manipulated.

Landmarks with well-defined borders or edges showed higher degrees of reproducibility than those placed on gently curving slopes.

Landmarks with the least reproducibility include soft tissue nasion, alar crest, gonion, and menton.[35] Currently, there are numerous leaders in this field providing various approaches to the definition of clinically relevant integrated landmark definitions[36–38] in 3D analysis[39,40] (Mayes JH, Harrell W, personal communication, 2008); (Mayes JH, Farkas LG, personal communication, 2008) and investigating transitions from point-based landmarking and measurement to shape classification and comparison.[41] The concept of using a computer-aided maxillofacial planning system to simulate a patient's facial appearance outcome was originally proposed by Vannier and colleagues[42] in 1983. There are a various computational strategies to provide this outcome simulation modeling including a nonlinear finite element model analysis (NFEMA),[43] the finite element model analysis (FEMA),[44] tetrahedral volumetric finite element model,[45] a mass spring model (MSM),[46] and, more recently, a novel mass tensor model (MTM).[47] Mean prediction error is in the order of 1 mm to 1.5 mm.[48,49]

Virtual Surgery

There are several software tools currently available for diagnosis and pretreatment assessments, but software tools are becoming available that will enable the surgeon to perform virtual surgeries/treatments in a powerful electronic 3D environment. In general terms, there are 3 expressions associated with virtual surgery/treatment: morphing, prediction, and simulation.

1. Morphing. Popularized as a marketing tool in the 2D world, this term is generally associated with creating an artist's impression of how a patient might look after treatment. As a software approach, 3D morphing is designed to show the patient surface-only changes and does not have an understanding of the various anatomic components or the biomechanical relationships within the craniofacial complex. This technique is similar to how a graphic artist would morph a character's face for a computer game (eg, chin advancement or reduction or rhinoplasty).

2. Prediction. Predictive algorithms are used to extrapolate the influence of growth, surgery, or interceptive treatment on an existing osseous platform based on normative estimates. They provide an end-point estimate of the final result but have no foundation for

accuracy. The use of this term in 3D imaging is inaccurate because it implies an assurance on the expected outcome (almost a guarantee on the virtual outcome), a result that a patient might believe is always achievable.

3. Simulation. Refers to an imitation of a real-world process in a computer program using mathematical models to study the effects of the changing parameters and conditions to make a decision.[50–55] Computer-based simulation gives the clinician the opportunity to perform virtual surgery or treatment, increasing the possibility of a successful outcome with no risk to the patient.

This allows an alternative approach; the mass spring model technique involves implementing a biomechanical model that defines the relationship between the hard and soft tissue with hundreds of thousands of nonlinear connector points (**Fig. 7**). This technique generates 3D deformable tissue models that include spring-based force computations to model the physical characteristics of real tissue reactions. This mechanism simulates deformable tissues constructed from 3D nodes, faces, tetrahedral, and edges, which include stiffness parameters to determine the ease of tissue deformation. An example is laparoscopic tools including probes, graspers, forceps, scissors, ablators, and suture needles, which provide realistic interaction with tissue models, and the numerical methods are optimized to provide real-time interaction in the 3D world. The models use force computations from physical laws and apply these forces to the 3D model components. The computations modeled include tissue deformation and relaxation; external forces

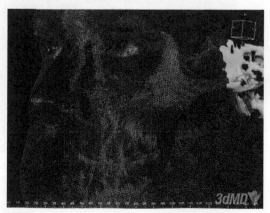

Fig. 7. Image fusion visually represented with mass spring model defining the biomechanical relationship between 3D photogrammetric facial scan and skeletal structure.

such as gravity; and 3D collision detection with force feedback. This type of simulation includes force computations that give users force feedback using a handheld haptic device. The advantage of this approach is that computations are within the power of available PCs. This type of interaction moves the world of simulation to a practical basis from the computing laboratory to the clinic's desktop computer.

The value of image fusion and virtual surgical simulation software in maxillofacial and orthognathic surgery (**Fig. 8**) is fivefold:

1. The surgeon may plan the most appropriate osteotomy sites, angulations, and depths of the cuts and then perform the surgical simulation. Based on the results from the surgical simulation, the overall management of the patient may be adjusted to include other elements that were not originally anticipated (eg, head gear or functional appliance treatment, extraction vs nonextraction treatments).

2. Unlike the physical procedure, there is opportunity to practice the procedure digitally and, if necessary, adjust the surgical or orthodontic therapy and replan the surgical treatment such as osteotomies or orthodontic appliance design. In this way, alternative dental, orthodontic, and surgical treatments can be attempted and compared.

3. The interactive process can be undertaken by the clinical team at their convenience on their own computers with each team member making changes to a centrally stored PSAR. Treatment planning can be done conjointly by treating clinicians in different physical locations, which facilitates input from other contributors to the treatment process including ear, nose, and throat specialists, pediatricians, nurses, speech pathologists, practice and counseling professionals, as well as the original referring clinician.

4. Where appropriate, the simulated patient model may also be used to discuss the treatment with the patient and/or relatives, allowing them to get a better understanding of the procedure(s). In this interaction, it must be stressed that the outcome is a simulation of a possible result and not a prediction of the final result; no guarantees are implied.

5. From a supply chain efficiency standpoint, the simulated patient model opens the possibility of interfacing directly with suppliers and custom manufacturers of therapeutic devices to order standard inventory items or patient-specific prefabricated computer-designed orthodontic and surgical apparatus and implants directly online.

To move from computer simulation to a true virtual rehearsal in which the digital environment replicates the real-world treatment/operating room environment, simulation changes from using a mouse and keyboard to a haptics-driven experience along with stereoscopic imaging. Haptics is the application of touch or force feedback sensation to the user interaction with a computer

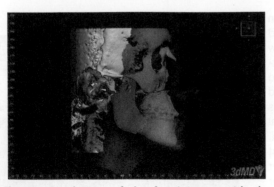

Fig. 8. Lateral view of the fused image with the maxilla cut for a Le Fort I osteotomy and the mandible cut for a sagittal split ramus osteotomy. The jaw segments can be manipulated virtually into the desired position and the soft tissue automatically reconstructs in 3D for visualization. Objective measurements of the movements are automatically recorded.

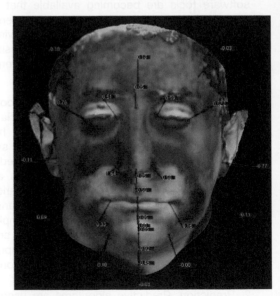

Fig. 9. Image colored to show areas of change, increase equals pink to red and decrease lighter blue with the darker blue unchanged. Objective measurements of the change from surgery can be obtained as shown by simply placing the mouse over an area and clicking.

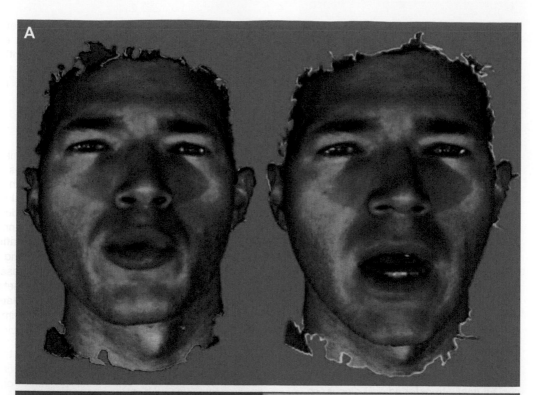

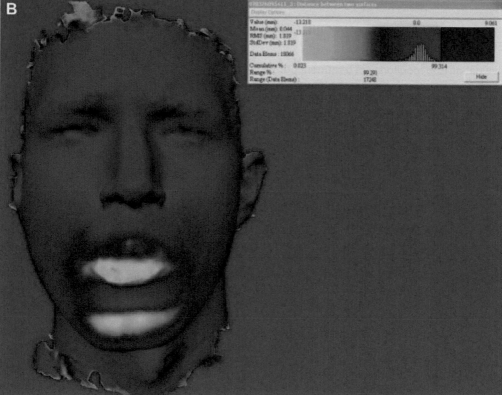

Fig. 10. 3dMD surface images captured while speaking at 60 frames per second. (*A*) Two 3dMD surface images taken a half second apart. (*B*) After the two 3dMD images from (*A*) are registered together, the 3dMDvultus software measures the change in facial expression for the half second and generates color histogram to visually inspect the differences.

application such as active forces within a surgical context or correct placement of orthodontic appliances for optimal force delivery, implant or temporary anchorage device (TAD) placement, and so forth. For example, the sensation experienced when the scalpel touches the bone, or the biomechanical force of the archwires or other types of appliances and their effect on tooth movement. In combination with visual training, haptic devices can assist with training in areas that require precise hand-eye coordination and provide for greater dexterity.[56]

Stereoscopic and autostereoscopic displays can also be used during the virtual rehearsal to further assist the treatment team's visual perception of the patient's real-world anatomy. Software can create the 2 slightly different images from the PSAR (1 for each eye), producing binocular visual depth perception. This stereopsis can be created from static and dynamic PSARs.

A computer-driven simulation is valuable when undertaking a new procedure or practicing a difficult procedure because the virtual rehearsal might conclude that the practitioner needs assistance from a specialist, in which case the patient workup can be easily transferred and discussed.

SURGICAL OUTCOME MONITORING AND EVALUATION

Evaluation and monitoring of treatment progress is an integral part of the treatment cycle. Most current postoperative assessment is limited to lateral cephalometric or photographic superimposition. However, 3D image fusion provides the ability to compare pretreatment patient data with both the virtual and actual posttreatment outcomes (**Fig. 9**).

3D IMAGE FUSION & THE 4TH DIMENSION OF TIME

An important extension of imaging fusion protocols in the near future is to expand into the fourth dimension, which includes the application of time to express motion. The addition of temporal information should enable a better understanding of the dynamics of the interaction and interrelationship of soft tissue, craniofacial complex, and dental components with mastication, speech, and deglutition. Some clinicians have extended their imaging records to include a series of static images to record relevant facial expressions and poses (**Fig. 10**A). This interim approach is referred to as 3 1/2 D. Research in this area is currently directed toward conditions including cleft lip and palate (see **Fig. 10**B)[57–59] and facial palsy.[60]

Efforts in this direction will assist in developing a powerful database of facial variations, enabling simulation software providers to continuously modify and update simulation models to separately address outcomes as they relate to facial expression.

SUMMARY

The creation of a patient-specific anatomic model by fusion of different imaging modalities creates a patient avatar that permits a specific and objective basis for making decisions. In facial surgery, this is especially important because any deviations or mistakes in surgery or treatment planning are not readily hidden and can negatively affect the quality of life. Processing and modeling of the PSAR can be accomplished now because of the recent advances in computing and Internet power. Treatment rationales can then be simulated and the best approach selected, resulting in improved patient outcomes and increased efficiency of health care delivery.

REFERENCES

1. Wolf G, Nicoletti R, Schultes G, et al. Preoperative image fusion of fluoro-2-deoxy-ᴅ-glucose-positron emission tomography and computed tomography data sets in oral maxillofacial carcinoma: potential clinical value. J Comput Assist Tomogr 2003;27:889–95.
2. Feichtinger M, Aigner RM, Santler G, et al. Case report: fusion of positron emission tomography (PET) and computed tomography (CT) images for image-guided endoscopic navigation in maxillofacial surgery: clinical application of a new technique. J Craniomaxillofac Surg 2007;35:322–8.
3. Takács B, Pieper S, Cebral J, et al, editors. Facial Modeling for Plastic Surgery Using Magnetic Resonance Imagery, SPIE Electronic Imaging, The Engineering Reality of Virtual Reality 2004 (EI06). San Jose (CA): SPIE; 2004.
4. Moss JP, Ismail SFH, Hennessy RJ. Three-dimensional assessment of treatment outcomes on the face. Orthod Craniofac Res 2003;6(Suppl 1):1–6.
5. Krimmel M, Kluba S, Bacher M, et al. Digital surface photogrammetry for anthropometric analysis of the cleft infant face. Cleft Palate Craniofac J 2006; 43(3):350–5.
6. Hajeer MY, Ayoub AF, Millett DT, et al. Three dimensional imaging in orthognathic surgery: the clinical application of a new method. Int J Adult Orthodon Orthognath Surg 2002;17:318–30.
7. Coombes A, Moss JP, Linney AD, et al. A mathematical method for the comparison of three dimensional changes in the facial surface. Eur J Orthod 1991;13: 95–110.

8. Moss JP, Linney AD, Grindrod SR, et al. A laser scanning system for the measurement of facial surface morphology. Optic Lasers Eng 1989;10: 179–90.

9. Moss JP, Coombes A, Linney AD, et al. Methods of three dimensional analysis of patients with asymmetry of the face. Proc Finn Dent Soc 1991;87:139–49.

10. O'Grady KF, Antonyshyn OM. Facial asymmetry: three dimensional analysis using laser surface scanning. Plast Reconstr Surg 1999;104:928–37.

11. Coward TJ, Scott BJ, Watson RM, et al. Laser scanning of the ear identifying the shape and position in subjects with normal facial symmetry. Int J Oral Maxillofac Surg 2000;29:18–23.

12. Ismail SF, Moss JP. The three-dimensional effects of orthodontic treatment on the facial soft tissues — a preliminary study. Br Dent J 2002;192:104–8.

13. Aung S, Ngim R, Lee S. Evaluation of the laser scanner as a surface measuring tool and its accuracy compared with direct facial anthropometric measurements. Br J Plast Surg 1995;48:551–8.

14. Techalertpaisarn P, Kuroda T. Three-dimensional computer-graphic demonstration of facial soft tissue changes in mandibular prognathic patients after mandibular sagittal ramus osteotomy. Int J Adult Orthodon Orthognath Surg 1998;13:217–25.

15. Curry S, Baumrind S, Carlson S, et al. Integrated three-dimensional craniofacial mapping at the Craniofacial Research Instrumentation Laboratory/University of the Pacific. Semin Orthod 2001;7: 258–65.

16. Yip E, Smith A, Yoshino M. Volumetric evaluation of facial swelling utilizing a 3-D range camera. Int J Oral Maxillofac Surg 2004;33:179–82.

17. Tsukahara K, Fujimura T, Yoshida Y, et al. Comparison of age-related changes in wrinkling and sagging of the skin in Caucasian females and in Japanese females. J Cosmet Sci 2004;55:351–71.

18. Ahn S, Kim S, Lee H, et al. Correlation between a cutometer and quantitative evaluation using moire topography in age-related skin elasticity. Skin Res Technol 2007;13:280–4.

19. Yuen K, Inokuchi I, Maeta M, et al. Evaluation of facial palsy by moiré topography index. Otolaryngol Head Neck Surg 1997;117:567–72.

20. Chen LH, Iizuka T. Evaluation and prediction of the facial appearance after surgical correction of mandibular hyperplasia. Int J Oral Maxillofac Surg 1995;24:322–6.

21. Kawai T, Natsume N, Shibata H, et al. Three-dimensional analysis of facial morphology using moiré stripes. Part I. Method. Int J Oral Maxillofac Surg 1990;19:356–8.

22. Kawai T, Natsume N, Shibata H, et al. Three-dimensional analysis of facial morphology using moiré stripes. Part II. Analysis of normal adults. Int J Oral Maxillofac Surg 1990;19:359–62.

23. Motoyoshi M, Namura S, Arai HY. A three-dimensional measuring system for the human face using three-directional photography. Am J Orthod Dentofacial Orthop 1992;101:431–40.

24. Burke PH, Beard FH. Stereophotogrammetry of the face. A preliminary investigation into the accuracy of a simplified system evolved for contour mapping by photography. Am J Orthod 1967;53:769–82.

25. Ayoub AF, Wray D, Moos KF, et al. Three-dimensional modeling for modern diagnosis and planning in maxillofacial surgery. Int J Adult Orthodon Orthognath Surg 1996;11:225–33.

26. Ayoub A, Garrahy A, Hood C, et al. Validation of a vision-based, three-dimensional facial imaging system. Cleft Palate Craniofac J 2003;40:523–9.

27. Littlefield TR, Cherney JC, Luisi JN, et al. Comparison of plaster casting with three-dimensional cranial imaging. Cleft Palate Craniofac J 2005; 42(2):157–64.

28. Khambay B, Nairn N, Bell A, et al. Validation and reproducibility of a high-resolution three-dimensional facial imaging system. Br J Oral Maxillofac Surg 2009;46:27–32.

29. Lane C, Harrell W. Completing the 3D Picture. Am J Orthod Dentofacial Orthop 2008;133(4):612–20.

30. Enlow DH, Hans MS. Essentials of facial growth. Philadelphia (PA): WB Saunders; 1996.

31. Ferrario VF, Sforza C, Schmitz JH, et al. A three-dimensional computerized mesh diagram analysis and its application in soft tissue facial morphometry. Am J Orthod Dentofacial Orthop 1998;114:404–13.

32. Swennen GRJ, Schutyser F, Hausamen JE. Three-dimensional cephalometry. A color atlas and manual. Heidelberg: Springer; 2005.

33. Ferrario VF, Sforza C, Dalloca LL, et al. Assessment of facial form modifications in orthodontics: proposal of a modified computerized mesh diagram analysis. Am J Orthod Dentofacial Orthop 1996; 109:263–70.

34. Ferrario VF, Sforza C, Puleo A, et al. Three-dimensional facial morphometry and conventional cephalometrics: a correlation study. Int J Adult Orthodon Orthognath Surg 1996;11:329–38.

35. Gwilliam JR, Cunningham SJ, Hutton T. Reproducibility of soft tissue landmarks on three-dimensional facial scans. Eur J Orthod 2006;28:408–15.

36. Jacobson A, Jacobson RL. Radiographic cephalometry: from basics to 3D imaging. 2nd edition. New Malden (UK): Quintessence Publishing; 2006. ISBN: 0-86715-461-6.

37. Swennen GRJ, Schutyser F, Barth E-L, et al. A new method of 3-D cephalometry. Part I: the anatomic cartesian 3-D reference system. J Craniofac Surg 2006;17:314–25.

38. Swennen GR, Barth EL, Eulzer C, et al. The use of a new 3D splint and double CT scan procedure to obtain an accurate anatomic virtual augmented

model of the skull. Int J Oral Maxillofac Surg 2007; 36:146–52.

39. Olszewski R, Zech F, Cosnard G, et al. Three-dimensional computed tomography cephalometric craniofacial analysis: experimental validation in vitro. Int J Oral Maxillofac Surg 2007;36(9):828–33.

40. Schendel S, Jacobson R. Three-dimensional imaging and computer simulation for office-based surgery. J Oral Maxillofac Surg 2009;67(10):2107–14.

41. Kau CH, Richmond S. A three-dimensional analysis of surface changes to the facial morphology in a longitudinal study of 12 year normal untreated children. Am J Orthod Dentofacial Orthop 2008;134(6): 751–60.

42. Vannier MW, Gado MH, Marsh JL. Three-dimensional display of intracranial soft-tissue structures. AJNR Am J Neuroradiol 1983;4:520–1.

43. Koch RM, Gross MH, Carls FR, et al, Simulating facial surgery using finite element models, Proceedings of SIGGRAPH. New Orleans (LA): ACM Press 1996. p. 421–8.

44. Sarti A, Gori R, Lamberti C. A physically based model to simulate maxillo-facial surgery from 3D CT images. Future Generat Comput Syst 1999;15: 217–21.

45. Zachow S, Gladiline E, Hege HC, et al. Finite-element simulation of soft tissue deformation. In: Proceedings of Computer Assisted Radiology and Surgery (CARS), Elsevier Science BV; 2000. p. 23–8.

46. Keeve E, Girod S, Kikinis R, et al. Deformable modelling of facial tissue for craniofacial surgery simulation. Comput Aided Surg 1998;3:228–38.

47. Mollemans W, Schutyser F, Van Cleynenbreugel J, et al. Tetrahedral mass spring model for fast soft tissue deformation. Lect Notes Comput Sci (IS4TM) 2003;2673:145–54.

48. Westermark A, Zachow S, Eppley B. Three-dimensional osteotomy planning in maxillofacial surgery including soft tissue prediction. J Craniofac Surg 2005;16:100–4.

49. Mollemans W, Schutyser F, Nadjmi N, et al. Predicting soft tissue deformations for a maxillofacial surgery planning system: from computational strategies to a complete clinical validation. Med Image Anal 2007;11:282–301.

50. Pieper S, Laub D Jr, Rosen J. A finite element facial model for simulating plastic surgery. Plastic Reconstr Surg 1995;96:1100–5.

51. Delingette H. Towards realistic soft tissue modeling in medical simulation. Proceedings of the IEEE Journal: Special Issue on Surgery Simulation, April 1998. p. 512–23.

52. Haasfeld S, Zöller J, Albert FK, et al. Preoperative planning and intraoperative navigation in skull base surgery. J Craniomaxillofac Surg 1998;26: 220–5.

53. Cotin S, Delingette H, Ayache N. A hybrid elastic model allowing real-time cutting, deformations and force-feedback for surgery training and simulation. Vis Comput 2000;16:437–52.

54. Montgomery K, Heinrichs L, Bruyns C, et al. Surgical simulator for operative hysteroscopy and endometrial ablation. Proceeding of the 15th International Congress and Exhibition: Computer-Aided Radiology and Surgery (CARS 2001). Berlin, June 27–30, 2001.

55. Cutting C. A deformer-based surgical simulation program for cleft lip and palate surgery. Presented at: Medicine Meets Virtual Reality (MMVR05), Long Beach (CA), January 26–29, 2005.

56. Morris D, Tan H, Barbagli F, et al. Haptic feedback enhances force skill learning. Published in Proceedings of the 2007 World Haptics Conference (WHC07): The Second Joint EuroHaptics Conference and Symposium on Haptic Interfaces for Virtual Environment and Teleoperator Systems. Tsukuba (Japan). March 22–24, 2007. p. 21–6.

57. Trotman CA, Faraway JJ, Losken HW, et al. Functional outcomes of cleft lip surgery. Part II: quantification of nasolabial movement. Cleft Palate Craniofac J 2007;44:607–16.

58. Trotman CA, Barlow SM, Faraway JJ. Functional outcomes of cleft lip surgery. Part III: measurement of lip forces. Cleft Palate Craniofac J 2007;44:617–23.

59. Trotman CA, Faraway JJ, Phillips C. Visual and statistical modeling of facial movement in patients with cleft lip and palate. Cleft Palate Craniofac J 2005;42:245–54.

60. Mishima K, Yamada T, Fujiwara K, et al. Development and clinical usage of a motion analysis system for the face: preliminary report. Cleft Palate Craniofac J 2004;41:559–64.

Evolution of 3D Surface Imaging Systems in Facial Plastic Surgery

Chieh-Han John Tzou, MD*, Manfred Frey, MD

KEYWORDS

- 3D Surface imaging • Three-dimensional • Facial analysis
- Stereo photogrammetry • Structured light • 3dMD
- Axis Three • Canfield • Di3d • 3D photography

HISTORY OF THREE-DIMENSIONAL SURFACE IMAGING SYSTEMS
Introduction of Systems

The three-dimensional (3D) quantitative analysis of facial morphology is vitally important in plastic and reconstructive surgery. Past attempts to measure the complexities of the human face include stereophotogrammetry,[1–8] image subtraction technique,[9] moiré topography,[10–12] liquid crystal scanning,[13–15] light luminance scanning,[16,17] laser scanning,[18–20] stereolithography,[21] and video systems.[22–32] A few of these have used instruments that provided 3D measurements with promising results,[13,26–33] but only more recently have these instruments found a greater place in routine clinical use.

Stereophotogrammetry

Thalmaan[1] made one of the first attempts to capture the 3D surface of the face in 1944. It was also the first attempt to use stereophotogrammetry in clinics. This technique was based on measurements from photographs. Thalmaan examined an adult with facial asymmetry and a baby with Pierre Robin syndrome. Images of the subject from two different views were taken and inserted into a plotting machine to draw 3D contour maps. In 1967, Burke and Beard[2] improved on Thalmaan's method by using simpler and less-expensive cameras. They improved and shortened the time-consuming method through applying a multiplex plotting system. Their method was applied to assess facial deformities (eg, cleft palate, cleft lip palate) in children[3] and the growth spurt of soft tissue in the face,[6,34] and to measure faces preoperatively and postoperatively.[5] They expected that the modified method would allow a wider application of this technique to document facial deformations.

In 1995, Ras and colleagues[7] concluded that stereophotogrammetry was an appropriate 3D registration method for quantifying and detecting development and changes in facial morphology. Deacon and colleagues[35] greatly improved the stereophotogrammetric technique in 1999. They replaced the precalibrated metric cameras and film emulsion with low-cost charge coupled device (CCD) cameras, which offered the advantage of digitized image capture for 3D automatic analysis, drastically shortening the manual analysis of stereophotogrammetry.

Liquid Crystal Range Finder

In 1984, Inokuchi and colleagues[13] developed the liquid-crystal rangefinder for recognizing facial deformities in three dimensions. This device was an

Financial Disclosure: No financial arrangements with the investigators have been made whereby the study outcome could affect compensation; moreover, the investigators have no proprietary interest in the tested products and do not have a significant equity interest in them. The investigators have not received payments of other sorts.

Division of Plastic and Reconstructive Surgery, Department of Surgery, Medical University of Vienna, Waehringer Guertel 18-20, A-1090 Vienna, Austria

* Corresponding author.

E-mail address: chieh-han.tzou@meduniwien.ac.at

imaging system that used gray-coded pattern projection to generate 3D images. The exposure time, approximately 1 second for a recording session, was considered advantageous over the 8 to 30 seconds of scanning time in laser systems; therefore, time-motion artifacts could be eliminated.[15,36]

Laser Systems

Laser scanning systems have high resolution and are accurate. They have been widely used in anthropometric studies,[37–40] and some have been applied in clinics.[19,33,41] The first 3D laser system to be routinely used in a clinic was devised by Moss and colleagues[19] in 1991 at the Department of Orthodontics at University College in London. They monitored the growth of children with facial deformities for more than a decade. Data acquisition took approximately 10 seconds, and its accuracy was ± 0.5 mm.

In 1993, Vannier and colleagues[33] reported examination of the human head with an optical laser system consisting of six scanners. The acquisition process took less than a second for a 360° image, which was the shortest time among laser scanning systems. The system proved sensitive enough to detect subtle dimensional changes resulting from surgery, including postoperative edema and surface changes from facelift procedures, and it provided accurate and complete 3D coverage of the complex facial surface. In 1995, Cacou and colleagues[41] were the first to combine electromyography and laser scanner technology to study facial muscle functions. Their system showed highly accurate measurements and was said to be suitable for monitoring changes during facial treatments. Accuracy and highly repeatable imagery improved over the years and was proven to produce accurate 3D images. Kohn and colleagues[42] reported that most errors in the scanning process were in the location procedure of landmarks; therefore, Bush and Antonyshyn[20] recommended setting up a standardized head position to attain an optimal laser image.

Subtraction Technique

In 1992, Neely and colleagues[9] developed an image subtraction technique, wherein a black-and-white video camera captured the subject's maximal facial movements, which were then analyzed by computer software. This technique was rapid and region-specific, and quantified the images objectively along a dimensional data scale. This method produced promising results, which were correlated with the House-Brackmann[43] facial nerve grading system, illustrating facial functional deficit at measured distances.

Moiré Topography

Takasaki[10] devised Moiré topography in 1970. Moiré is a French word for "watered," describing the geometric design that results when a set of straight or curved lines is superposed onto another.[44] This technique is based on the light interference theory, in which illumination through a grid creates contour lines on an object. Takasaki used moiré photographs to assess facial asymmetry and surface deformation during facial expression. Using this system in 1992, Inokuchi[45] applied Moiré topography to probe the "Moiré Index," a method to quantitatively assess facial movements and the severity of facial palsy. Yuen and colleagues[46] reported in 1997 that this system was extremely time-consuming in the evaluation procedure.

Light Luminance

OSCAR (objective scaling of facial nerve function based on area analysis), developed in 1998 by Meier-Gallati and colleagues,[16] was an objective scaling system of facial nerve function. It used a black-and-white camera to capture the variations of luminance produced by changes of facial expression and thereby assess dynamic facial asymmetry.[17] This method proved to be objective, reproducible, fast, and simple to use; however, it allowed no absolute measurement of distances in the face.

Video Systems

In 1989, Caruso and colleagues[26] attempted to assess 3D facial movements. Three video cameras (50 Hz), based on a 3D kinematic system (VICON, Oxford Metrics, Inc., Tampa, Florida), were used to collect the data. They showed the feasibility of obtaining 3D trajectories of lip and jaw landmarks during chewing movements.

In 1994, Ferrario and colleagues[27] developed a videotaping system to quantify facial asymmetry. Standardized facial landmarks were collected by two 50-Hz cameras (ELITE system, BTS, Milan, Italy). These landmarks were automatically recognized. The x, y, and z coordinates were reconstructed and calculated with software (Laboratorio di Anatomia Funzionale dell'Apparato Stomatognatico, Milan, Italy). This study reported the feasibility of 3D quantification and the assessment of facial asymmetry.

In 1994, Paletz and colleagues[22] devised one of the first video systems to access facial morphology and movements. This two-dimensional (2D) video assessment of facial movements studied trajectories of lip landmarks during a natural smile. They quantified the amplitude and direction of the landmarks in motion by using a 16-mm cine camera.

Trotman and colleagues[28–30] showed a video analysis system in 1996, which provided data of facial movements in three dimensions. Facial motions were captured by three 60-Hz video cameras (Motion Analysis, Motion Analysis Corporation, Santa Rosa, California), whereupon 3D maximum motion amplitudes were calculated by a computer workstation (Sun Sparc, Sun Corporation, Palo Alto, California). This video-based tracking system showed impairment and habilitation of facial movements, determining which regions of the face show the greatest excursion during specific facial animation.

In 1997, Bajaj-Luthra and colleagues[23,24] devised the maximal static response assay, a study using a 2D video system to focus on the quality and quantity of synkinetic movements in healthy faces. Here, facial movements with defined landmarks were recorded and analyzed through subtracting their position-in-repose image from images depicting their maximal motion. This system contributed to the fundamental knowledge of synkinesis in faces; however, it was capable only of 2D measurements.[25]

However, assessing absolute measurements of facial movements was impossible. Frey and colleagues[31] concentrated their efforts on quantitatively and qualitatively assessing facial movements in 1994 on a computer-assisted video system with four cameras (VICON, Video Systems, Inc., West Palm Beach, Florida). Three-dimensional facial landmark movements were calculated as a percent of reference distances. In 1999, Frey and colleagues[32] improved the principle of the VICON video system through replacing three of four cameras with a simple mirror system. This innovation needed only one camera to capture 3D movements in the face and has been reported to be in clinical routine use ever since.[47–52]

RECENT DEVELOPMENTS IN 3D SURFACE IMAGING SYSTEMS

Technological advances in the past 2 decades have made 3D surface imaging accessible to patient protocols; moreover, imaging management and 3D analysis and treatment planning software applications are being reengineered to handle and analyze these highly precise 3D data formats efficiently. Laser and optical-based surface imaging technologies have evolved and are widely used in the medical fields. Optical-based surface imaging technologies include structured light imaging and stereophotogrammetry imaging systems. The basic principles of structured light imaging and stereophotogrammetry imaging systems are described; particulars can vary depending on business focus from one manufacturer to another.

Laser Imaging Technology

Laser imaging acquires 3D data through scanning a laser beam (spot or stripe) across a target object. It normally uses a straightforward geometric calculation to determine the surface coordinates of the object. The object scatters the light, which is collected at a known triangulation distance from the laser. Through using trigonometry, the x, y, and z coordinates of a surface point are calculated.[53]

Structured Light Technology

Structured light technology projects organized patterns of white light (grids, dots, or stripes) onto the surface of a target object while photographing the subject with a camera calibrated with the specifics of the projected light pattern. The distortion of the light pattern is captured and processed to generate the shape data and inherently register pertinent color and texture information. To generate an accurate 3D model, a two-viewpoint capture must be taken in sequence to avoid pattern interference.[54]

Stereophotogrammetric Technologies

Stereophotogrammetric techniques take a sophisticated software approach based on the fundamental principle of taking two pictures of the same object to create a stereo pair, recording depth to generate a composite 3D model. The recorded pattern on the surface provides the stereo algorithms with the base information required to build accurate 3D geometry. Once the 3D geometry model has been produced, software maps the color and texture information onto the model. Two basic triangulation strategies exist for stereo photogrammetry: active and passive.

Active Stereophotogrammetric Technology

Active stereophotogrammetry deploys the projection of a focused random unstructured light pattern on the actual surface of the target object. It combines this pattern with the visible natural pattern of the object's surface (if any) to give the stereo algorithms as much information as possible to generate a quality 3D geometry. No special external lighting conditions are needed for this technique, and it is resilient to the effects of ambient lighting.

Passive Stereophotogrammetric Technology

In contrast, passive stereophotogrammetry generates 3D geometry solely based on the natural patterns of the target object's surface. High-resolution cameras are needed to ensure that enough surface detail is available to generate the

3D geometry. Care must be taken to avoid the effects of strong directional ambient light to avoid glare on the surface.

Current Status

Currently, the promising methods of 3D surface imaging are stereophotogrammetry (passive and active) and structured light. Five companies currently provide the most notable commercialized 3D imaging software and hardware that is sold and supported worldwide, and each offers different approaches toward 3D surface imaging techniques:

- 3dMD (www.3dmd.com), based in London, United Kingdom, and Atlanta, Georgia
- Axis Three (www.axisthree.com), based in Belfast, Ireland
- Canfield (www.canfield.com), based in Fairfield, New Jersey
- Di3D (www.di3d.com), based in Glasgow, Scotland, United Kingdom
- Genex (www.genextech.com), based in Bethesda, Maryland

The following sections give an overview of these systems.

3DMD
3dMD History

The 3dMD company started in 1999 with the first delivery of a 3dMD system. 3dMD had already launched into the United States health care market and started to develop breast reconstruction imaging and cosmetic imaging technologies. Subsequently, it delivered 3dMD products to MD Anderson Cancer Center, Procter & Gamble, and the National Institutes of Health (NIH/NIDCR). Because of significant positive feedback from clinical users worldwide, which specified and validated its systems, it was able to launch the first four-dimensional (4D) motion capture version of the 3dMDface System in 2005. In 2007, it introduced the 3dMDvultus software application for 3D surface image fusion with CT and CBCT (cone beam CT), which is a lower radiation dose CT, compared with the conventional CT. Its hardware is smaller, and therefore easily fits into almost any clinical routine. At this moment, 3dMD is focusing on extending its 3dMDvultus software and refining its 4D motion technique. 3dMD reports that their 60-frame-per-second 4D face system with a two-viewpoint perspective is now in approximately 20 universities around the world that are focused on research in this field. Some

published research is referenced on 3dMD's Web site.[55–58]

3dMD Technology

The 3dMDface System (http://www.3dmd.com/3dmdface.html) uses a hybrid of active and passive stereophotogrammetry for 3D surface imaging (Fig. 1), wherein the software algorithms use a combination of the projected random pattern and the natural surface patterns, such as pores and freckles on the skin. This modular system consists of two pods, each of which contains one full color and two black-and-white machine vision cameras. Pictures are captured by light photography with industrial-grade cameras. The capture time is approximately 1.5 ms (1/650th of a second), limiting the risk of motion artifacts. The six simultaneous photographs of the face are rendered with professional personal computer equipment for approximately 30 seconds to reconstruct the 3D stereophotogrammetric picture (in the form of a .TSB file and any industry-standard 3D file format), to be viewed in the 3dMDvultus software program and other commercially available 3D software programs. The typical data file size of a 3dMD capture is approximately 20 MB. Advantages of the 3dMD system are ultra high speed capture (1.5 ms), eliminating errors caused by patient movement (ideal for children), ease of use, short calibration (<2 minutes), and a software platform that supports CT/CBCT initiatives, radiation-free planning, outcome simulation, and treatment follow-up. Most of the technique ensures high-quality geometry capturing, regardless of lighting conditions. Geometry accuracy is less than 0.2 mm root mean square or better. The 3dMDface

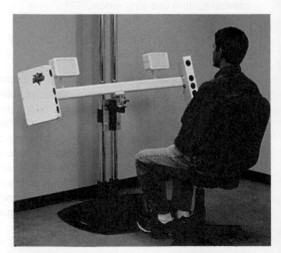

Fig. 1. 3dMD hybrid (active & passive) stereophoto-grammetry face system. (*Courtesy of* 3dMD, Atlanta, GA; with permission.)

System is designed to be compact and extremely robust. Many of these systems are regularly transported as standard airline luggage to remote locations and treatment facilities around the world. This robustness easily enables use at home in the practice or clinic.

According to the company, more than 1000 3D surface imaging units have been supplied around the world, and the 3dMDface System is exceptionally reliable. In the rare event of an operational issue, the company's technicians can diagnose the problem remotely and rectify the situation within hours. The 3dMDvultus software simulates real-time soft tissue changes from the mass spring biomechanical model, based on long-term published scientific research.[59]

3dMD Scientific Validation

At least four medical groups have validated the face and breast system so far.

In 2005, Aldridge and colleagues[60] investigated the precision, error, and repeatability associated with anthropometric landmark coordinate data collected from the 3dMD system. Data collected from images with the 3dMDface System were highly repeatable and precise: the average error associated with the placement of landmarks was submillimeter. The investigators concluded that anthropometric data collected using the 3dMDface System are highly reliable.

In 2005 by Losken and colleagues[61,62] validated the ability to qualitatively determine differences in shape, size, and contour of the breast. The relative difference between the measured volume and the calculated volume was approximately −2%, with a standard deviation of ± 13% to 16%. The coefficient of reproducibility for each reader was excellent, between 0.80 and 0.92. Surface measurement of nipple to notch showed the mean relative difference between the measured and calculated distances for raters was approximately −6%, with a standard deviation of ± 6% to 7%. They concluded that the ability to determine breast volume and surface measurements objectively with 3D imaging technology is now available with consistent and reproducible accuracy. Three-dimensional technology provides invaluable information, particularly in the longitudinal evaluation of results.

Maal and colleagues[63] objectively evaluated treatment outcomes in oral and maxillofacial surgery via pretreatment and posttreatment 3D photographs of the patient's face. Three-dimensional images and facial expressions were captured with Maxilim (Medicim NV, Mechelen, Belgium) and 3dMD (3dMD LLC, Atlanta, Georgia). They found a strong correlation between the results of hardware and

software packages. The intraobserver and interobserver error for the reference-based registration method was found to be 1.2 and 1.0 mm, respectively, in the Maxilim software. No significant difference was found between the software packages that were used to perform surface-based registration.

In 2010, Lubbers and colleagues[64] evaluated the handling of the 3dMD system in matters of data acquisition and analysis. They found the system to be very reliable, with a mean global error of 0.2 mm (range, 0.1–0.5 mm) for mannequin head measurements; neither the position of the head nor that of the camera influenced these parameters. They recommended the system for evaluation and documentation of the facial surface and suggested it could offer new opportunities in reconstructive surgery.

AXIS THREE
Axis Three History

Axis Three, "a pioneer in 3D solutions for cosmetic and plastic surgery"[59] since 2002 has been developing high-precision 3D imaging equipment for engineering, design sector, and medical applications. Its current 3D imaging technology platform results from partnership with Siemens in 2006, a technology that was pursued for biometrical identification. This partnership supports Axis Three's continuous refining of a 3D capturing and imaging solution. Axis Three's technical vision is to open up its technology to third-party development, facilitating and leveraging its reach to various medical 3D imaging applications.

Axis Three Technology

Axis Three's face system (http://www.axisthree. com/products/face-surgery-simulation) applies structured light technology to create 3D data (Fig. 2). It has created a 3D capture engine applying CCT (color coded triangulation), a patented capture technology developed in conjunction with Siemens. CCT is a structured light technology that requires sequential firing from different camera viewpoints. It has three pods. Each pod has a single camera, which requires approximately 300 ms (one-third of a second) to capture the image. Total time for the image-capturing process is approximately 1 second. The typical data file size of an Axis Three capture is 3 MB. CCT technology can capture millions of measurement points to create a 3D cast of the patient. Axis Three claims a high level of anatomic accuracy, at .05 mm with the patient 1 m from the focal plane. According to Axis Three, capturing and processing an image takes 2 to 3 minutes. Axis Three claims to supply the only 3D simulation science-based software on

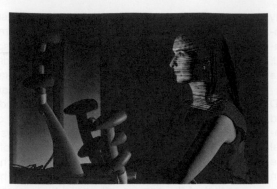

Fig. 2. Axis Three face simulation system with structured-light technology, applying CCT (color-coded triangulation by Siemens. (*Courtesy of* Axis Three, Belfast, Ireland; with permission.)

physics-driven tissue typing for use in aesthetic surgery. The company ensures that TBS (tissue behavior simulation), its soft tissue modeling software, generates highly accurate simulations to the specific implant's placement shape and composition. Axis Three claims that this is the only system on the market that creates a virtual volume of the inner breast tissue and allows the user to assign a tissue-elasticity type for each patient, on-site and in real time.

Axis Three Scientific Validation

No peer-reviewed scientific papers about validation of the system were found.

CANFIELD
Canfield History

Canfield is a global imaging system company for scientific research and health care applications, including the pharmaceutical, biotechnology, cosmetics, medical, and skin care industries. Canfield was founded in 1988 to develop and supply specialized photographic systems to the medical and skin care industries worldwide. It focuses on developing off-the-shelf solutions, primarily for plastic surgeons and dermatologists. Its best-known application is the Mirror medical imaging software for simulating surgical procedures on 2D images. In 2005, Canfield introduced its first 3D imaging system.

Canfield Technology

The Canfield VECTRA M3 face system (http://www.canfieldsci.com/imaging_systems/facial_systems/VECTRA_M3_Imaging_System.html) uses passive stereophotogrammetry (**Fig. 3**). It is a modular 3D image capturing system that consists of three

pods, including two color SLR cameras in each pod. According to Canfield, synchronized 2D images of the subjects are captured within 3.5 ms (one three-hundredth of a second). High-resolution color capture of 36 MB assures photorealistic rendering of the finest details.

Canfield Scientific Validation

To test the accuracy and reproducibility of an earlier-generation version of the Canfield VECTRA system previously based on active stereophotogrammetry, in 2010 de Menezes and colleagues[65] calculated the systematic and random errors between operators, calibration steps, and acquisitions. No systematic errors were found for all tests performed (P>.05, paired t-test). The investigators stated that the method was repeatable, and random errors were always lower than 1 mm.

In 2010, Rosati and colleagues,[66] performed a technical evaluation of the Canfield system, digitally integrating dental virtual model and soft-tissue facial morphologies from adults using a 3D stereophotogrammetric imaging system. The greatest mean relative error of measurements was smaller than 1.2%, and no significant differences in repeatable reproductions were found.

Also in 2010, Quan and colleagues[67] used the VECTRA system to measure ptotic breast tissue advancement. They documented pseudoptosis in the first postoperative year, which showed migration of breast tissue from the upper pole to the lower pole of the breast by 6% (P<.05), and concluded that 3D photography is a useful tool, enabling plastic surgeons to monitor postoperative changes in breast morphology objectively.

A scientific validation of the current passive stereophotogrammetry system was not yet present in the literature.

DI3D
Di3D History

Founded in 2002 and based in Glasgow, Scotland, Dimensional Imaging Ltd. is a world-leading supplier of human body 3D and 4D surface image capture and analysis solutions. Dimensional Imaging supplied systems are already in use in 13 countries on four continents, for a range of applications such as oral and maxillofacial surgery, orthodontics, burn treatment, facial recognition, and entertainment. Dimensional Imaging recently launched a groundbreaking 4D surface image capture system, which can capture 3D video sequences of dynamically changing surfaces. This system is proving to be a particularly attractive solution for high-resolution facial performance capture.

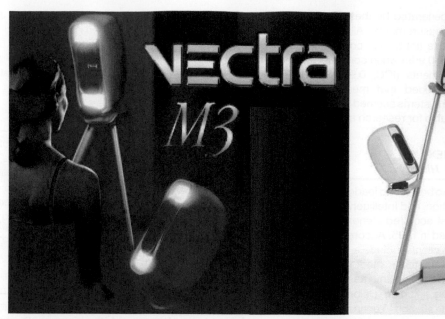

Fig. 3. VECTRA M3 face imaging system, applying passive stereophotogrammetry technology. (*Courtesy of* Canfield, Fairfield, NJ; with permission.)

Di3D Technology

The Di3D 3D surface capture system (http://www.di3d.com/products/3d_systems/) uses 3D passive stereophotogrammetry to produce a fully textured 3D surface image with ultra-high resolution (**Fig. 4**). The Di3D system uses four high-resolution 8 megapixel Canon EOS350D color digital cameras with 50-mm lenses. All 3D surfaces were captured and reconstructed using the standard system settings as prescribed by the manufacturer for imaging the

face (flash brightness, ¼; camera shutter speed, 1/200s). A personal computer requires less than 5 minutes to produce a 3D model of the captured facial casts.

Di3D Scientific Validation

In 2008, Winder and colleagues[68] assessed the technical performance of a 3D surface imaging system for geometric accuracy and maximum field of view on a mannequin head with black ink dots serving as facial landmarks. They found that the Di3D system had a mean error in the 3D surfaces of 0.057 mm, a repeatability error (variance) of 0.0016 mm, and a mean error of 0.6 mm in linear measurements, compared with manual measurements.

Also in 2008, Khambay and colleagues[69] assessed the accuracy and reproducibility of a high-resolution 3D imaging system (Di3D) using 12 adult facial plaster casts with landmarks marked. They reported that the reproducibility of the Di3D capture was 0.13 mm, with a range of 0.11 to 0.14 mm, and the system error averaged 0.21 mm, with a range of 0.14 to 0.32 mm. They concluded that the Di3D system error was within 0.2 mm, which is clinically acceptable.

In 2010, Fourie and colleagues[70] published the results of an evaluation of accuracy and reliability of standard anthropometric linear measurements on seven cadaver heads made with three different 3D scanning systems: laser-surface scanning (Minolta Vivid 900), CBCT, and 3D stereophotogrammetry (Di3D system). They compared the

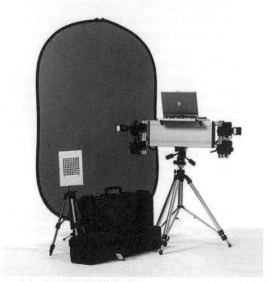

Fig. 4. Di3D 3D capture systems, applying passive stereophotogrammetry technology. (*Courtesy of* Dimensional Imaging Ltd., Glasgow, Scotland, UK; with permission.)

measure-ments generated by these systems with physical linear measurements. All three systems proved very reliable (intraclass correlation coefficient [ICC] >0.923–0.999) when compared with the physical measurements (ICC, 0.964–0.999). The investigators concluded that measurements recorded with these systems seemed to be sufficiently accurate and reliable for research and clinical use.

TECHNEST/GENEX
Technest/Genex History

Technest claims to be a world leader in 3D imaging, 3D facial recognition, and intelligence surveillance. In 2005, Technest acquired Genex Technologies, which was founded in 1995. According to the company's profile, its clients include a diverse array of government, commercial, medical, and dental organizations. The company has won national recognition, being listed in Deloitte & Touche's Technology Fast 50 and Technology Fast 500 program for 2 years consecutively, and having received the prestigious National Tibbetts Award. The company is further developing and commercializing the unique Rainbow method of capturing 3D data. Technest has become a market leader in advanced imaging, including 3D and 360° technologies. Its first commercial product was the Rainbow 3D camera, which generated significant presence in the medical research market. Clients include Harvard Medical School, Johns Hopkins University School of Medicine, and Walter Reed Army Medical Center. The most recent version of Technest's 3D technology is the 3D FaceCam, which offers a wide range of interesting applications for commercial and governmental uses.

Technest/Genex Technology

The Rainbow 3D camera model 250 (http://www.genextech.com/pages/601/Rainbow_3D_Camera.htm) is designed for capturing large objects, such as the full face (**Fig. 5**). According to Genex, it is an instantaneous full-frame 3D imaging system.[71] It uses three coordinated sensors to capture a high level of detail around key feature areas, such as nose and eyes, with coverage of the shoulders and ears. The camera has a field of view of 250 by 200 mm and an accuracy rating of 250 μm. It uses structured light technology. According to the company's brochure, image acquisition takes 400 to 500 ms (0.4 s) and requires only 30 seconds to generate the 3D model. However, Weinberg and colleagues[72] claimed that large horizontal measurements (eg, bizygomatic width) could not be obtained from the 3D captures because these regions were outside the camera's field of view.

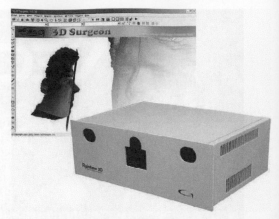

Fig. 5. Genex Rainbow 3D camera system, applying structured light technology. (*Courtesy of* Technest Holdings, Inc., Bethesda, MD; with permission.)

Technest/Genex Scientific Validation

In 1996, Geng[71] reported that the repeatability, or internal consistency, of the Genex 3D system shows differences of only a fraction of a millimeter among captures. Therefore, the repeatability of the Genex 3D system was determined to be sufficiently high to proceed with data collection.

In 2004, Lee and colleagues[73] studied the accuracy of the Rainbow 250. They found that substantial image distortion occurred when images were captured at sharp angles (90°, side views). Images captured from the frontal perspective, ± 15°, were the most accurate. They stated that the lenses were located somewhat close to each other, resulting in a limited field of view and difficulty in getting an accurate z-coordinate measurement.

In 2005 and 2006, Weinberg and colleagues[72,74] studied the precision and accuracy of the Genex 3D facial measuring system. They found that the 3D photos were clearly better than direct anthropometry. Good congruence was observed between means derived from the 3D photos and direct anthropometry, and the magnitude of these differences was often clinically insignificant (<2 mm). They concluded that this camera system is sufficiently precise and accurate for anthropometric research designs.

No validation studies were found for Genex's more recent 3D FaceCam.

RECOMMENDATIONS FOR EVALUATION OF WHICH SYSTEM WOULD BE OPTIMAL FOR A SURGEON'S PRACTICE

Searching for a proper 3D imaging system is like purchasing the most suitable personal computer for one's field of application. After having defined the requirement and assignment of 3D imaging, the following aspects should be taken into consideration for the final decision.

Technical Aspects

The entire process of the system is important to understand, from calibrating the system, capturing the patient data, and processing the 3D surface image to the final display and use in 3D surgical planning software tools. The system should be checked while in use at a busy office; one should talk to its users—patients and medical staff—and pay attention to the following points: (1) calibration routine (is it simple, and can it be handled by one person); (2) actual data capture time and surface coverage (must the patient stay still for a certain amount of time, how many images are taken to obtain ear-to-ear coverage, and does the system generate a quality surface image every time or does the operator have to take a series of captures to get one usable image); (3) image processing procedure (does the 3D data process automatically or is there a batch mode option, and how long does it take before the 3D image is ready for display); (4) integration with a practice management system[53] and 3D analysis and treatment planning software; and (5) use of space in the office. Moreover, one should consider the system's user-friendliness, durability, and manpower to operate; the manufacturer's reputation for responsive and effective customer service; and the cost for purchasing and maintenance.

Space Requirements

Because space is limited in offices, this aspect should be evaluated thoroughly. From a patient workflow perspective and a use standpoint, a few considerations must be evaluated when locating the system in the practice. The entire space requirement is important to understand; not just the system's footprint, but also the space required for the patient, the calibration, and any additional features to operate, because some systems require a backdrop behind the patient. Because these systems typically rely on calibration, placing them in high-traffic areas, such as a hallway, greatly increases the chance that the system will get bumped and go out of calibration. Wall-mounted systems are recommended, because they maintain consistency of patient positioning across visits. Moreover, standardizing a consistent patient imaging protocol will assure an accurate registration of the 3D surface image to a CBCT or traditional CT image for surgical planning and an accurate registration of the pretreatment and posttreatment 3D surface image for clinical audit and outcome evaluation.

Accuracy and Validity

Accuracy and validity are fundamental factors for reliable analysis. Accuracy has two principal components: absolute accuracy with respect to the physical reference of an object, and repeatable accuracy (consistency between discrete scans). One should ask for an accuracy validation study conducted by an independent third-party organization, and make sure that the validation tests are run, using live unsedated subjects.[75] Moreover, one should confirm that the validation test was conducted on a similar technology platform to the system being evaluated for purchase. For the 3D surface image to have any validity, the geometry generated must reflect the true contours of the actual anatomic surface, down to a small fraction of a millimeter.

Supplier Company

When evaluating 3D surface imaging system suppliers, surgeons should take a close look at the customer base, such as: (1) the number of 3D systems sold to date and the geographic location of the customers in relation to the surgeon's practice; (2) the percentage of these customers working with the system in a busy practice or hospital; (3) whether the company is committed to supporting open access to software from other software suppliers; (4) the number of customers in the surgeon's particular field (plastic reconstructive surgeon, orthodontists, radiologist, and so on); and (5) the organization's track record to date. This last question is extremely important because a customer base dictates future functionality and technology advancements.[53]

SUMMARY

The articles in this issue show that 3D surface imaging is taking surgeons to a new level of communication with patients, surgical planning, and outcome evaluation. It allows patients to see 3D images in multiple views. Moreover, 3D surface imaging provides quick and standardized image documentation, compared with well-known limitations in recording 3D geometry on a 2D plane.[76] This article provides surgeons with the background information for evaluating the type of systems used in current studies applying 3D imaging technology, and information about the systems they might incorporate into their practice. The surgeon contemplating purchasing a 3D acquisitions system could benefit from considering the recommendations given when evaluating the different systems.

REFERENCES

1. Thalmaan D. Die Stereogrammetrie: ein diagnos-tisches Hilfsmittel in der Kieferorthopaedie [Stereopho-togrammetry: a diagnostic device in orthodontology]. Zurich (Switzerland): University Zurich, Switzerland; 1944 [German].

2. Burke PH, Beard FH. Stereophotogrammetry of the face. A preliminary investigation into the accuracy of a simplified system evolved for contour mapping by photography. Am J Orthod 1967;53(10):769–82.

3. Burke PH. Stereophotogrammetric measurement of normal facial asymmetry in children. Hum Biol 1971;43(4):536–48.

4. Leonard MS, Johnson GW, Starfield AM, et al. Computer graphics in facial morphology analysis. Int J Oral Surg 1981;10(Suppl 1):273–5.

5. Burke PH, Banks P, Beard LF, et al. Stereophoto-graphic measurement of change in facial soft tissue morphology following surgery. Br J Oral Surg 1983; 21(4):237–45.

6. Burke PH, Hughes-Lawson CA. The adolescent growth spurt in the soft tissues of the face. Ann Hum Biol 1988;15(4):253–62.

7. Ras F, Habets LL, van Ginkel FC, et al. Method for quantifying facial asymmetry in three dimensions using stereophotogrammetry. Angle Orthod 1995; 65(3):233–9.

8. Ras F, Habets LL, van Ginkel FC, et al. Quantification of facial morphology using stereophotogrammetry–demonstration of a new concept. J Dent 1996;24(5): 369–74.

9. Neely JG, Cheung JY, Wood M, et al. Computerized quantitative dynamic analysis of facial motion in the paralyzed and synkinetic face. Am J Otol 1992; 13(2):97–107.

10. Takasaki H. Moire topography. Appl Opt 1970;9: 1467–72.

11. Kawano Y. Three dimensional analysis of the face in respect of zygomatic fractures and evaluation of the surgery with the aid of Moire topography. J Craniomaxillofac Surg 1987;15(2):68–74.

12. Yuen K, Kawakami S, Ogawara T, et al. Evaluation of facial palsy by Moire topography. Eur Arch Otorhino-laryngol 1994;(Suppl):S541–4.

13. Inokuchi I, Sato K, Ozaki Y. Range-imaging system for 3-D range imaging. Paper presented at: 7th ICPR Proceeding; Montreal, Canada, 1984. p. 806.

14. Sato K, Inokuchi I. A range-imaging system utilizing a nematic liquid crystal mask. Presented at the First International Conference on Computer Vision. Lon-don, 1987. p. 657.

15. Yamada T, Sugahara T, Mori Y, et al. Rapid three-dimensional measuring system for facial surface structure. Plast Reconstr Surg 1998;102(6):2108–13.

16. Meier-Gallati V, Scriba H, Fisch U. Objective scaling of facial nerve function based on area analysis

17. (OSCAR). Otolaryngol Head Neck Surg 1998; 118(4):545–50.

17. Scriba H, Stoeckli SJ, Veraguth D, et al. Objective evaluation of normal facial function. Ann Otol Rhinol Laryngol 1999;108(7 Pt 1):641–4.

18. Vanezis P, Blowes RW, Linney AD, et al. Application of 3-D computer graphics for facial reconstruction and comparison with sculpting techniques. Forensic Sci Int 1989;42(1–2):69–84.

19. Moss JP, Coombes AM, Linney AD, et al. Methods of three dimensional analysis of patients with asymmetry of the face. Proc Finn Dent Soc 1991;87(1):139–49.

20. Bush K, Antonyshyn O. Three-dimensional facial anthropometry using a laser surface scanner: vali-dation of the technique. Plast Reconstr Surg 1996; 98(2):226–35.

21. Moss JP, Grindrod SR, Linney AD, et al. A computer system for the interactive planning and prediction of maxillofacial surgery. Am J Orthod Dentofacial Or-thop 1988;94(6):469–75.

22. Paletz JL, Manktelow RT, Chaban R. The shape of a normal smile: implications for facial paralysis recon-struction. Plast Reconstr Surg 1994;93(4):784–9.

23. Bajaj-Luthra A, Mueller T, Johnson P. Quantitative analysis of facial motion components: anatomic and nonanatomic motion in normal persons and in patients with complete facial paralysis. Plast Reconstr Surg 1997;99(7):1894–902 [discussion: 1903–4].

24. Bajaj-Luthra A, VanSwearingen J, Thornton R, et al. Quantitation of patterns of facial movement in patients with ocular to oral synkinesis. Plast Re-constr Surg 1998;101(6):1473–80.

25. Johnson P, Bajaj-Luthra A, Llull R, et al. Quantitative facial motion analysis after functional free muscle re-animation procedures. Plast Reconstr Surg 1997; 100(7):1710–9 [discussion: 1720–2].

26. Caruso AJ, Stanhope SJ, McGuire DA. A new technique for acquiring three-dimensional orofa-cial nonspeech movements. Dysphagia 1989;4: 127–32.

27. Ferrario VF, Sforza C, Poggio CE, et al. Distance from symmetry: a three-dimensional evaluation of facial asymmetry. J Oral Maxillofac Surg 1994; 52(11):1126–32.

28. Trotman C, Gross M, Moffatt K. Reliability of a three-dimensional method for measuring facial animation: a case report. Angle Orthod 1996;66(3):195–8.

29. Trotman CA, Faraway JJ, Silvester KT, et al. Sensi-tivity of a method for the analysis of facial mobility. I. Vector of displacement. Cleft Palate Craniofac J 1998;35(2):132–41.

30. Trotman CA, Faraway JJ. Sensitivity of a method for the analysis of facial mobility. II. Interlandmark sepa-ration. Cleft Palate Craniofac J 1998;35(2):142–53.

31. Frey M, Jenny A, Giovanoli P, et al. Development of a new documentation system for facial movements as a basis for the international registry for

neuromuscular reconstruction in the face. Plast Reconstr Surg 1994;93(7):1334–49.

32. Frey M, Giovanoli P, Gerber H, et al. Three-dimensional video analysis of facial movements: a new method to assess the quantity and quality of the smile. Plast Reconstr Surg 1999;104(7):2032–9.

33. Vannier MW, Pilgram TK, Bhatia G, et al. Quantitative three-dimensional assessment of face-lift with an optical facial surface scanner. Ann Plast Surg 1993;30(3):204–11.

34. Burke PH, Beard LF. Growth of soft tissues of the face in adolescence. Br Dent J 1979;146(8):239–46.

35. Deacon AT, Anthony AG, Bhatia SN, et al. Evaluation of a CCD-based facial measurement system. Med Inform (Lond) 1991;16(2):213–28.

36. Yamada T, Sugahara T, Mori Y, et al. Development of a 3-D measurement and evaluation system for facial forms with a liquid crystal range finder. Comput Methods Programs Biomed 1999;58(2):159–73.

37. Farkas LG, Ross RB, James JS. Anthropometry of the face in lateral facial dysplasia: the bilateral form. Cleft Palate J 1977;14(1):41–51.

38. Farkas LG, Hreczko TA, Kolar JC, et al. Vertical and horizontal proportions of the face in young adult North American Caucasians: revision of neoclassical canons. Plast Reconstr Surg 1985;75(3):328–38.

39. Farkas LG, Kolar JC. Anthropometrics and art in the aesthetics of women's faces. Clin Plast Surg 1987;14(4):599–616.

40. Farkas LG, Ross RB, Posnick JC, et al. Orbital measurements in 63 hyperteloric patients. Differences between the anthropometric and cephalometric findings. J Craniomaxillofac Surg 1989;17(6):249–54.

41. Cacou C, Greenfield BE, Richards R, et al. Studies of co-ordinated lower facial muscle function by electromyography and surface laser scanning techniques. Paper presented at: 4th International Muscle Symposium, Zurich, Switzerland, 1995. p. 183.

42. Kohn LA, Cheverud JM, Bhatia G, et al. Anthropometric optical surface imaging system repeatability, precision, and validation. Ann Plast Surg 1995;34(4):362–71.

43. House JW, Brackmann DE. Facial nerve grading system. Otolaryngol Head Neck Surg 1985;93:146–7.

44. Britannica E. Moiré pattern. Encyclopædia Britannica 2011. Available at: http://www.britannica.com/EBchecked/topic/387754/moire-pattern. Accessed February 6, 2011.

45. Inokuchi I. Quantitative assessment of facial palsy by Moire topography. Nippon Jibiinkoka Gakkai Kaiho 1992;95(5):715–25 [in Japanese].

46. Yuen K, Inokuchi I, Maeta M, et al. Evaluation of facial palsy by Moire topography index. Otolaryngol Head Neck Surg 1997;117(5):567–72.

47. Frey M, Giovanoli P. The three-stage concept to optimize the results of microsurgical reanimation of the paralyzed face. Clin Plast Surg 2002;29(4):461–82.

48. Giovanoli P, Tzou CH, Ploner M, et al. Three-dimensional video-analysis of facial movements in healthy volunteers. Br J Plast Surg 2003;56(7):644–52.

49. Tzou C, Giovanoli P, Ploner M, et al. Are there ethnic differences of facial movements between Europeans and Asians? Br J Plast Surg 2005;58(2):183–95.

50. Frey M, Giovanoli P, Michaelidou M. Functional upgrading of partially recovered facial palsy by cross-face nerve grafting with distal end-to-side neurorrhaphy. Plast Reconstr Surg 2006;117(2):597–608.

51. Frey M, Michaelidou M, Tzou C, et al. Three-dimensional video analysis of the paralyzed face reanimated by cross-face nerve grafting and free gracilis muscle transplantation: quantification of the functional outcome. Plast Reconstr Surg 2008;122(6):1709–22.

52. Michaelidou M, Tzou C, Gerber H, et al. The combination of muscle transpositions and static procedures for reconstruction in the paralyzed face of the patient with limited life expectancy or who is not a candidate for free muscle transfer. Plast Reconstr Surg 2009;123(1):121–9.

53. Lane C, Harrell W Jr. Completing the 3-dimensional picture. Am J Orthod Dentofacial Orthop 2008;133(4):612–20.

54. Olesen OV, Paulsen RR, Hojgaar L, et al. Motion tracking in narrow spaces: a structured light approach. Med Image Comput Comput Assist Interv 2010;13(Pt 3):253–60.

55. Edge JD, Hilton A, Jackson P. Model-based synthesis of visual speech movements from 3D video. EURASIP Journal on Audio, Speech, and Music Processing 2009;2009(2009):12.

56. Popat H, Henley E, Richmond S, et al. A comparison of the reproducibility of verbal and nonverbal facial gestures using three-dimensional motion analysis. Otolaryngol Head Neck Surg 2010;142(6):867–72.

57. Popat H, Richmond S, Playle R, et al. Three-dimensional motion analysis—an exploratory study. Part 2: reproducibility of facial movement. Orthod Craniofac Res 2008;11(4):224–8.

58. Popat H, Richmond S, Playle R, et al. Three-dimensional motion analysis—an exploratory study. Part 1: assessment of facial movement. Orthod Craniofac Res 2008;11(4):216–23.

59. Schendel SA, Montgomery K. A Web-based, integrated simulation system for craniofacial surgical planning. Plast Reconstr Surg 2009;123(3):1099–106.

60. Aldridge K, Boyadjiev SA, Capone GT, et al. Precision and error of three-dimensional phenotypic measures acquired from 3dMD photogrammetric images. Am J Med Genet A 2005;138(3):247–53.

61. Losken A, Seify H, Denson DD, et al. Validating three-dimensional imaging of the breast. Ann Plast Surg 2005;54(5):471–6 [discussion: 477–8].

62. Losken A, Fishman I, Denson DD, et al. An objective evaluation of breast symmetry and shape differences

using 3-dimensional images. Ann Plast Surg 2005;
55(6):571–5.

63. Maal TJ, van Loon B, Plooij JM, et al. Registration of
3-dimensional facial photographs for clinical use.
J Oral Maxillofac Surg 2010;68(10):2391–401.

64. Lubbers HT, Medinger L, Kruse A, et al. Precision
and accuracy of the 3dMD photogrammetric system
in craniomaxillofacial application. J Craniofac Surg
2010;21(3):763–7.

65. de Menezes M, Rosati R, Ferrario VF, et al. Accuracy
and reproducibility of a 3-dimensional stereophotogrammetric imaging system. J Oral Maxillofac Surg
2010;68(9):2129–35.

66. Rosati R, De Menezes M, Rossetti A, et al. Digital
dental cast placement in 3-dimensional, full-face
reconstruction: a technical evaluation. Am J Orthod
Dentofacial Orthop 2010;138(1):84–8.

67. Quan M, Fadl A, Small K, et al. Defining pseudoptosis (bottoming out) 3 years after short-scar medial
pedicle breast reduction. Aesthetic Plast Surg
2011;35(3):357–64.

68. Winder RJ, Darvann TA, McKnight W, et al. Technical
validation of the Di3D stereophotogrammetry surface
imaging system. Br J Oral Maxillofac Surg 2008;46(1):
33–7.

69. Khambay B, Nairn N, Bell A, et al. Validation and
reproducibility of a high-resolution three-dimensional facial imaging system. Br J Oral Maxillofac
Surg 2008;46(1):27–32.

70. Fourie Z, Damstra J, Gerrits PO, et al. Evaluation of
anthropometric accuracy and reliability using different
three-dimensional scanning systems. Forensic Sci Int
2011;207(1–3):127–34.

71. Geng ZJ. Rainbow three-dimensional camera: new
concept of high-speed three-dimensional vision
systems. Opt Eng 1996;35(2):376–83.

72. Weinberg SM, Naidoo S, Govier DP, et al. Anthropometric precision and accuracy of digital three-
dimensional photogrammetry: comparing the Genex
and 3dMD imaging systems with one another and
with direct anthropometry. J Craniofac Surg 2006;
17(3):477–83.

73. Lee JY, Han Q, Trotman CA. Three-dimensional
facial imaging: accuracy and considerations for clinical applications in orthodontics. Angle Orthod 2004;
74(5):587–93.

74. Weinberg SM, Scott NM, Neiswanger K, et al. Digital
three-dimensional photogrammetry: evaluation of
anthropometric precision and accuracy using a Genex 3D camera system. Cleft Palate Craniofac J 2004;
41(5):507–18.

75. Rockwell K. The importance of flash sync speed.
2009. Available at: http://www.kenrockwell.com/tech/
syncspeed.htm. Accessed February 6, 2011.

76. Honrado CP, Lee S, Bloomquist DS, et al. Quantitative
assessment of nasal changes after maxillomandibular surgery using a 3-dimensional digital imaging
system. Arch Facial Plast Surg 2006;8(1):26–35.

Teaching 3D Sculpting to Facial Plastic Surgeons

C. Cingi, MD[a],*, F. Oghan, MD[b]

KEYWORDS

- 3D • Three dimensional • 3D sculpting • Facial sculpting
- Image analysis • Preoperative planning
- Patient consultation

The human body is a 3-dimensional (3D) object; and any changes, whether from movement during facial expression or from surgery, occur in 3 dimensions. The importance of thinking in 3D when doing facial plastic surgery extends to[1] preoperative planning,[2] consideration of esthetics,[3] discussion with patients,[4] surgical simulation, and[5] manual dexterity in execution of the steps to attain the desired 3D goal.

Although ethnic differences exist in Turkey, we can describe the general structure of the Mediterranean nose as large and arched. The most common nasal surgery in this country currently is reduction rhinoplasty. Most patients requesting this surgery have a large nose associated with a nasolabial angle less than 90°, thick skin, and a deviated nose.

The interest in plastic surgery interventions has rapidly increased during the last 15 years and continues to rise. The interest in facial plastic surgery interventions is consistent with the general socioeconomic levels of society. The increased interest in rhinoplasty surgery began 25 years ago in the United States and was subsequently observed in European countries, including Turkey. Because of the increased interest in rhinoplasty, many otolaryngologists are keen to be taught rhinoplasty procedures and several courses and symposia continue to be organized to meet this need. These meetings are typically designed to improve theoretical knowledge in an engaging and educational manner. In accordance with the increased interest in rhinoplasty, the incidence of overcorrected noses has increased. This report is about 3D sculpting courses that the authors developed after realizing the need for education regarding planning the way to attain a suitable nose as an important element of plastic surgical interventions.

The authors have found clay to be an inexpensive, readily available medium that allows facial plastic surgeons to further explore the relationship between their 3D handwork and the 3D esthetic result. This article describes the authors' course and study, taking facial plastic surgeons through specific exercises to demonstrate the esthetic impact of 3D manipulations of the nose and face. The authors describe the course components, which include 3D assessment, exercises in manual dexterity, and improving imagination in sculpting facial and nasal features for the optimal esthetic result and match to a given facial shape. In addition, the authors discuss the overlap and relationship between a course in 3D sculpting in facial plastic surgery and current 3D tools for design and image analysis that are used now for facial plastic surgery. This has implications for the 5 previously mentioned areas incorporating 3D thinking in facial plastic surgery: planning, esthetics, discussion, simulation, and performance.

[a] Department of Otorhinolaryngology, Faculty of Medicine, Osmangazi University, Hasan Polatkan Street, Meselik 26020, Eskisehir, Turkey
[b] Department of Otorhinolaryngology, Faculty of Medicine, Dumlupinar University, Tavsanli 10 km Street, Central Campus, Kutahya 43270, Turkey
* Corresponding author.
E-mail address: ccingi@gmail.com

Facial Plast Surg Clin N Am 19 (2011) 603–614
doi:10.1016/j.fsc.2011.07.004

TEACHING 3D SCULPTING TO FACIAL PLASTIC SURGEONS

Using clay, the authors produced and duplicated sample masks for these education courses (**Figs. 1** and **2**). The objectives of the course are

- Internalization of nose ratios
- Development of eye measurements
- 3D thinking
- 3D planning
- Improving manual dexterity and eye-hand coordination
- Improving imagination.

Internalization of Nose Ratios

The face is divided into 3 equal parts. These parts include 3 horizontal planes and a vertical division of the face with 5 vertical lines. To know these ratios in theory is not enough. Thus, the course starts with practice in measuring these ratios with a compass on a mud mask (**Fig. 3**), learning to equalize these portions by making appropriate changes, and observing the results. Such practice is beneficial in the internalization of nose ratios and giving an appreciation of the relationship between measurements and the 3D facial esthetic.

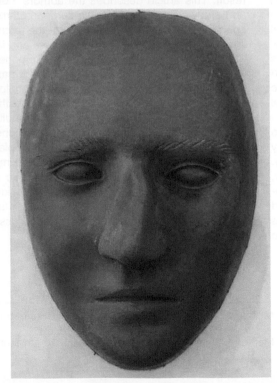

Fig. 1. Clay masks are made for the course participants.

3D measurements for anthropometric and esthetic purposes have raised great interest among artists and researchers who have designed useful methods to define and measure human facial features. The assessment of facial dimensions is of prime importance in medical fields for both diagnosis and treatment planning. Given that otorhinolaryngological, maxillofacial, and plastic reconstructive surgeons often require quantitative information regarding the relationships of hard and soft tissue, image processing algorithms using 3D image acquisition tools described at the end of this article may be applied to facial images to develop and improve anthropometric applications that reduce the time required for examination and improve measurement reliability. Additionally, the detection of clinically important distances and angles and the analysis and comparison of different forms can be enabled by such applications.

Three-Dimensional Thinking and Planning

Thinking and seeing in 3D is rarely included in classical medical training. Realizing the effects of the minor modifications of the tip of the nose on the profile appearance or on a three-quarter view may be described by some as 3D planning. However, to truly be 3D planning, it should take into consideration the view of patients during daily social interactions, not only from the front or side but also from all angles by evaluating the view from all perspectives. Many people describe their profiles (side views) as improving when they lift the tip of their nose with their fingertip, a process termed unidirectional evaluation. If a surgical process to achieve this lifting effect is performed, the profile lines may be improved; but this exact profile view is rarely achieved in daily life, which highlights the necessity of 3D planning. The surgeon, and others, will view patients in 3D after surgery not from a single direction.

In the case of facial plastic surgery, it is important to perform detailed surgical planning before surgery to ensure that the optimal and appropriate surgical methods are applied. Historically, esthetic surgical practice did not include 3D planning, but current advances in 3D technology are changing that.

Development of Eye Measurements

Eye measurement is a skill that can be developed through practice. Precise eye measurements are important to ensure equalization of the 3 horizontal facial areas. During the clay study, the participants first assess sizes, shapes, and angles with their eyes, followed by measurements with a compass.

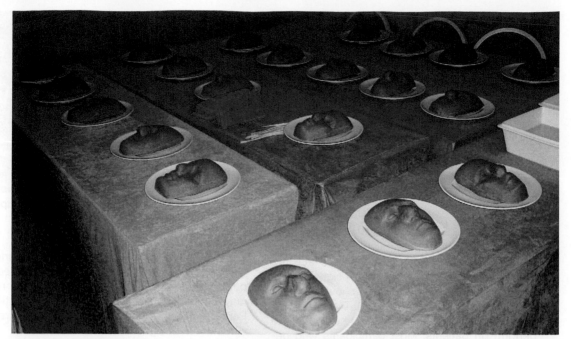

Fig. 2. Each participant has his or her own mask to work on for each phase of the course.

The aim of this evaluation is to allow the participants to become accustomed to eye measurements, which will foster improvement in their accuracy.

As an example, we might describe the basic technique of placing a suture as beginning 2 mm outside the upper edge of the lip of the wound and exiting inside the wound 2 mm from the surface. This procedure is followed by entering 2 mm below the surface of the incision at the opposite lip of the wound and exiting 2 mm outside the upper edge of the lip of the wound. The suture is tightened by tying a knot. Good eye measurements, as well as excellent manual dexterity and hand-eye coordination, are all required to ensure that this procedure is performed correctly.

Improving Manual Dexterity

Fine-motor movements of the hands improve during the kindergarten period, and exercises are performed during preschool for this purpose. Some individuals increase their manual dexterity during their youth, whereas others do not have the opportunity to do so. Thus, if individuals who have graduated from medical school continue their otorhinolaryngology education and perform exercises that improve their manual dexterity, one can predict an improvement in the success of their operations. Exercises to both assess and improve manual dexterity include

- Cutting pictures from a newspaper without missing the borders: This exercise serves to identify those participants who are neater and faster. This practice can persuade participants who are unsuccessful to spend extra time practicing these exercises.
- A competition attempting to align 100 beads in the shortest time possible: At the end of this exercise, a bell curve is generated. Most of the group can complete this in an average or very short period of time. Some take longer to complete the exercise, and this group might be offered further exercises to improve manual dexterity.

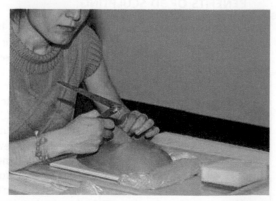

Fig. 3. The participants start with practice in measuring the ratios with a compass on a mud mask.

- Suturing 4 sides of a 2 × 2-mm section of cartilage on gauze with 4 sutures: This exercise simulates difficulties encountered during suturing of a graft, including when cartilage graft placement is necessary during rhinoplasty. These difficulties include disruption of the graft when crossing the suture and tearing of the graft caused by excessive tightening of the suture. Those who are unsuccessful at the end of this exercise are frequently motivated to pursue additional training and to do exercises to improve their manual dexterity.

Improving the Imagination

When the clay masks are provided to participants, they are initially required to distribute the face into the appropriate proportions and design an ideal nose for these proportions. **Box 1** shows the tools that are used in the course (**Fig. 4**). The aim is then to perform changes that would not be possible to perform on patients. Most participants who become accustomed to training with clay frequently request clay masks to perform the exercise outside of the training period.

STEPS OF THE COURSE
Study Phases on Large-Nosed Clay Masks

1. First, facial proportions are assimilated using sample clay masks derived from patients. An assessment of the horizontal and vertical components of the face is performed by measuring the face with a compass.
2. The deformed nose on the mask is then optimized to the known desirable proportions of the face (**Fig. 5**).
3. Interventions that will esthetically improve the face (apart from the nose) are performed, including chin advancement and raising the eyebrows.
4. The final goal is to design the ideal nose for this face (**Figs. 6** and **7**).

Box 1
Nasal study materials and instruments for surgeon training with clay

- Clay and water
- Ceramic hand tools
- Sponge
- Brush
- Compass

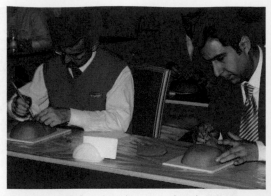

Fig. 4. Ceramic hand tools are used as the participants design the ideal nose.

Once this stage is complete, the aim is to perform changes to the mask that cannot be performed on patients and to create an ideal nose. This nose may be incongruous with the facial proportions. Participants in the training can observe directly whether the designed nose fits the face.

Studies on Sculptures Without a Nose

This study is more difficult to perform and is regarded as the second phase. In phase 1, the participants begin with a nose on the clay mask that is typically deformed. In this instance, it is easy to observe and correct the defect. Adding a nose to a noseless sculpture (**Fig. 8**) during the second phase is more difficult, but it is an important skill to master for 3D planning and training.

At this stage, the determination of the nasofrontal angle is ensured by directing the participants. The next goal is to create the dorsum and to decide the level of nasal projection. Once this is completed, the nostrils and columella are created. The basal view of the nose is frequently the most difficult section for the participants.

BENEFITS OF 3D SCULPTING

For a long time, automobile designers have created automobile prototypes, sometimes in full size, in clay to appreciate the true esthetic effect of a given design. Furthermore, designers have made smaller clay models and scanned this model using a 3D optical or laser scanning system to put the model into a computer-aided design (CAD) program for further design work (reverse engineering). Designers have used special 3D viewing devices to appraise their designs, but nothing as truly simulates the esthetic impact to a viewer as seeing it as an actual 3D object. Just as multiple photographic views would give patients more information than a single view, the ability to move

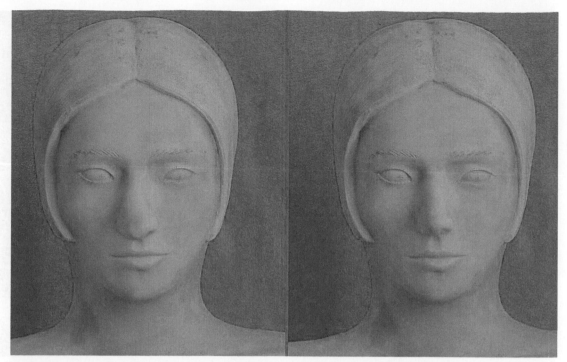

Fig. 5. The deformed clay nose is optimized to the known desirable dimensions of the face.

an image in 3D looking at the esthetic effect of any changes from different angles gives an even greater appreciation of changes that can occur with surgery. Stereophotogrammetry (see the section at the end of this article) now allows facial plastic surgeons to capture the 3D image of their patients and to analyze the esthetics of the nose and face while viewing it in 3D from an infinite number of perspectives. Further enhancement of

3D appreciation is gained by viewing an actual 3D object. Studying facial relationships and esthetics with clay sculpting is like the automobile designers creating a full-size prototype in clay.

The exercises in sculpting for Facial Plastic Surgeon's Course have implications that carry over directly to facial plastic surgery. Besides the obvious value of exercises in 3D assessments of dimension and esthetics, there is the less-obvious

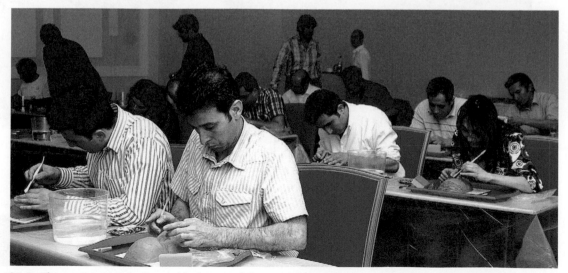

Fig. 6. The participants design an ideal nose of the appropriate proportions for their mask.

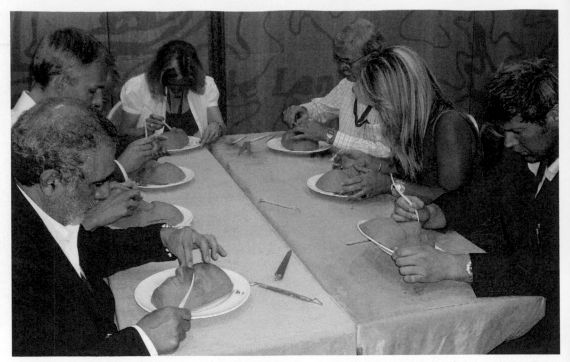

Fig. 7. The participants in phase 1 are designing the ideal nose for the face on their mask.

role of insight regarding preoperative planning and communication with patients.

Planning for facial plastic surgery includes

- Deciding the surgical procedure to be performed and determining the most appropriate method whereby the surgeon can achieve this outcome

- Explaining the result-oriented planning to patients
- Discussing the expected or desired outcome of the operation with patients
- Reaching a clear conclusion about the objective of the surgery
- Achieving an understanding of the surgeon's and the patients' points of view using 1 or

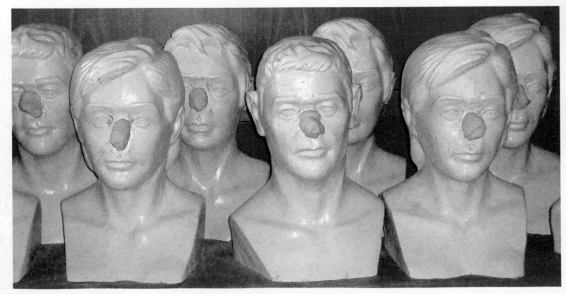

Fig. 8. In phase 2, a nose is added to a noseless sculpture. This exercise is more difficult.

more tools for communication: These tools include verbal description while pointing to certain features on patients, drawings, photographs, or digital images in 2-dimensional (2D) or 3D renderings to demonstrate elements of the process that would be difficult to describe without such media.

Preoperative Planning and Communication With Patients

Surgical procedures done in the setting of tumor or trauma to cure disease and repair damaged anatomic structures differs from elective facial plastic surgical procedures in that there may not be as detailed a discussion about the details of the surgical approach before surgery because of the imperative nature of the surgery, particularly when medical treatment proves insufficient. The primary objective in a surgery for a malignant parotid tumor is total resection with ample surgical margins, and the secondary aim is to repair the skin defect or fill the empty cavity of the tumor. Three-dimensional tools can aid appreciably in reconstruction after tumor removal (eg, contour defects attributable to parotidectomy[1] or in mandibuloplasty). However, in these cases, the hope of patients is to have some return toward their previous appearance, whereas in elective facial plastic procedures, patients hope for a change to something better than what they had. In this case, the surgery targets the same region, but the primary objective of the surgery is for an improved new appearance. In elective plastic surgical procedures, the patients have planned carefully and considered their choice to proceed. For this reason, expectations may be higher, and the results obtained may not fit with the patients' intended outcome, which emphasizes the importance of communication regarding planning and possible outcomes of surgery.

The next step beyond using 3D tools at a console to communicate preoperatively with patients and to do 3D preoperative planning is to work with a true 3D model of the patients' face or nose.

Clay studies for surgery planning before the operation

1. It is not always possible for patients to describe the changes they require without visual aids. Conducting a clay study with patients allows the translation of a 3D idea into a tangible objective. This process can be considered as the next stage of 3D image processing.
2. A clay study conducted before the operation is useful for patients to recognize, in a tangible

way, any visible nasal pathologies that should be addressed, in addition to esthetic issues. This study is particularly important when patients with prominently asymmetric faces realize this asymmetry following surgery and are unhappy on careful examination, having not realized that the asymmetry existed previously.
3. A clay study makes it possible to show the patients any severe nasal pathologic condition and demonstrate that the nose shape requested by patients may not be possible.
4. The preoperative clay study should be conducted 24 hours in advance of surgery, and changes in the procedure, once confirmed by patients, should be minimized during this period.

Although manipulating clay during a discussion with patients may not be practical for many surgeons, one can imagine an extension of the 3D software user interface to accomplish an actual tactile 3D model–based discussion. Facial plastic surgeons can already discuss changes on preoperative digital images using touch screens or light pens. Some surgeons are now doing this using 3D images and a 3D display. The next step is to have a facial model with a surface that can be manipulated and that will be given the 3D shape of a given patient from the 3D images acquired by stereophotogrammetry or similar capture techniques. Then the surgeon, using his or her hands or instruments similar to the ones used in the authors' course, could demonstrate to themselves away from patients, or even in mutual discussion with patients, the effect of various subtle manipulations of the 3D model.

The technology for such a user interface for a simulator/patient communication device is already tangible. One only needs a modifiable 3D surface that could serve as both a 3D printout but also allow a 3D input device sending the computer the surface spatial alterations occurring on the 3D object. It is already possible to use stereophotogrammetry to capture the external 3D dimensions of any face and print a matching 3D object. From this a mold can be made to create clay models for the authors' course. This practice would allow various kinds of noses to be modified by surgeons to immediately appreciate what each type of manipulation can accomplish. It would also allow 3D printing of a model of patients that the surgeon could use to communicate about their mutual desired surgical goals.

The most important thing, however, is the appreciation of the consequence of 3D changes on the esthetic of the patients' nose and face. The 3D manipulations done by the surgeons in the authors' course bring together the surgeon's 3D vision, sense of touch, feel for what is attractive, appreciation of what is possible, and immediate awareness of the result rendered by any 3D manipulation. This appreciation is accomplished with a depth that is one step beyond even 3D design changes done with 3D glasses or in a 3D design hood because of the additional feedback element of touch, a sense so integral to a surgeon's work.

RELATING 3D SCULPTING TO COMPUTER-BASED 3D IMAGING AND COMPUTER-BASED 3D MODELING

Facial model reconstruction and surgical simulation are increasingly important to today's facial plastic surgeons. Precise presurgical planning can help surgeons reduce the potential risks in facial plastic surgery. Koch and colleagues[2] proposed algorithms for both presurgical planning and postsurgical evaluation using surgery realistically simulated with finite element methods. Lee and colleagues[3] developed a physically based model to generate facial expression. At the time, this approach was computationally expensive and, therefore, not readily available for real-time surgical simulation.

The authors have found clay to be an inexpensive, readily available medium that allows facial plastic surgeons to further explore the relationship between their 3D handwork and the 3D esthetic result. This article describes the authors' course and study taking facial plastic surgeons through specific exercises to demonstrate the esthetic impact of 3D manipulations of the nose and face.

The authors noted the possibility of using the patients' 3D images to print or render a 3D moldable model of the patients' face, thus, enhancing the ability to conceptualize and visualize planned surgical modifications for any given patient. New technologies of CAD and computer-aided manufacturing that can be used in facial plastic surgery and to premanufacture facial reconstructive elements or prostheses have increased rapidly in the last decade.[4]

COMPUTER-BASED 3D IMAGING AND COMPUTER-BASED 3D MODELING

Current advances in 3D imaging technology now offer powerful options for planning and simulation that can be used by the facial plastic surgeon. Using data from a normal side, modeling (more reverse engineering) can be done in mirror image in 3D to fashion sizing templates or reconstructive plates or implants for patients with head and neck tumors that will be resected.

These 3D tools are essential for the practical implementation of 3D anthropometrics. In particular, it is possible to obtain information on the 3D facial features of a person. Not only does this allow 3D rendering as the authors have discussed previously but it allows study in 3D of the anthropometrics that are appreciated as attractive.

For many years, Farkas[5] applied the direct anthropometry technique for studying facial morphology.[5] This approach has been applied to study facial growth and to compare patients' phenotype with the norms of the population. Anthropometrics is an objective tool for assessing the facial form and detecting changes over time, diagnosing genetic or acquired deformities, planning and evaluating interventions for surgery, studying normal and pathologic growth, and verifying the outcome of treatments. Anthropometry has the advantages of being inexpensive, simple to be applied, and noninvasive. Limitations of this approach include the need for patient cooperation and longer time for data acquisition and capturing.[6]

Cephalometric radiographs have been widely applied in the study of hard-tissue morphology, prediction of changes related to the growth, and quantitative assessment of references data.[7,8] It is also an important tool for the diagnosis of craniofacial abnormalities and planning of treatment modalities.[9] Errors in analysis caused by magnification, superimposition of structures, limited experience, and difficulty in landmark determination are common in this method.[10]

Photogrammetric digital imaging is a noninvasive, inexpensive, and commonly used method to investigate preoperative and postoperative changes and provides a permanent record of patients.[11] The recent spread and development of digital 2D imaging has made it an essential and routine part of medical practice.[12] Digital imaging has many advantages, such as the immediate display of the image and simplicity in manipulation. Furthermore, data can be stored or managed in a digital format that makes measurements applicable.[11] This approach has been used to acquire facial norms of populations, detect interethnic variations, and in the diagnosis of dysmorphic children.[13]

Three-dimensional imaging methods include 3D cephalometry, morphoanalysis, moire topography, computed tomography (CT)-assisted 3D imaging, 3D ultrasonography, 3D laser scanning, and stereophotogrammetry. Advances in technology have now allowed 3D imaging, such as CT.[14,15] Some of these technologies require expensive equipment and the ability to determine soft-tissue features is limited.[16,17] Moreover, concerns have been raised about the use of radiation for facial studies.[18] For these reasons, 3D surface imaging techniques, such as laser scanning and stereophotogrammetry, have been developed to capture the soft-tissue facial structures.[19–21] Three-dimensional surface imaging has become more common in computer animation and movies, but its application in medicine is more recent. Among the earliest systems of measuring the spatial relationships, Ras and colleagues[22] presented 3D imaging as a new method for quantifying facial morphology and detecting changes in facial growth. The rapid development in computer technology opens new perspectives to improve 3D imaging.

After data acquisition, several steps are needed to create 3D surface images.[23,24] The first step includes the production of geometric mode of visualization or wireframe, which is made up of a series of x, y, and z landmark coordinates. Mathematical algorithms are used to connect the points with each other and express the 3D model in triangles or polygons. In the second step, color information is added to the wireframe, which consists of a layer of pixels called texture mapping. A further step is to add shading and lighting, which brings more reality to the 3D object obtained. The final step is called rendering, in which the computer converts the anatomic data into a lifelike 3D object viewed on the computer screen. Improvement in computer-vision tools makes it possible to perform all measurements in 3D, and subsequently, statistical shape analysis can be applied.[25,26]

Laser Scanning

This technology depends on projecting a known pattern of laser light onto the object of interest and then using geometric principles to create a 3D model of the object.[27] Many studies test the accuracy and precision of laser scanner measurements versus those obtained using digital calipers.[28,29] The results showed that the accuracy of laser scanner was less than 2 mm in the plaster model with a precision of 0.8 to 1.0 mm on the human face. Laser scanning gives a noninvasive, accurate, and reproducible tool for medical applications.[14] However, this technology does have its shortcoming, such as a long scan time (making it difficult to apply for children)[30] and the inability of the laser scanner to capture soft-tissue texture, which results in difficulties in the identification of landmarks. Moreover, patients' eyes must also be closed for protection and the head must be kept in a fixed position.[16]

Stereophotogrammetry

Stereo photography has been in existence for many years. As with laser scanning, it also relies on the method of triangulation. The basic principle of stereophotogrammetry is the use of 2 or more cameras configured as a stereo pair to capture simultaneous images of the subject.[31] The cameras are placed apart from each other and the patients' face is enclosed by a calibration frame or placed in a space in which a calibration object was previously imaged.[32] The cameras focal lengths, their exact position to each other and to the object, are calculated during the calibration procedures.[32] After that, a 3D facial image can be captured and displayed on the monitors so that landmarks can be selected either manually or by using image-processing algorithms.[15] The acquired 3D coordinates are used to calculate distances between points allowing subsequent 3D reconstruction of the entire face.[33] Many 3D stereophotogrammetric commercial systems are available in the markets. One system that was developed at Glasgow University Dental School[34] consists of 2 camera stations, each with a pair of monochrome cameras to capture the stereo image and a color digital camera to capture the skin texture. The face illumination depends on random projected light or on natural lighting.[31] Picture capture takes 50 ms and a computer program constructs a 3D image from the data transferred from each camera station. The system has been validated and its accuracy was reported to be within 0.5 mm.[19] This system has been tested in the facial morphology of patients who are orthognathic to detect the magnitude of surgical change, along with the possible postsurgical relapse.[15] Another stereophotogrammetric system is called 3dMD FACE (3dMD; Atlanta, GA, USA). It uses multiple cameras to capture facial images (1 color and 2 infrared) with random light projected on the object's surface.[31] The capture time is 1.5 to 2.0 ms, which creates less distortion and is more useful for data capture for children.[26,35] The 3dMD system can also accommodate additional cameras with no reduction in capture speed.[26] The 3dMD systems can overlap the random light pattern to allow a full 360° view of patients to be digitally captured in a single acquisition. The picture accuracy is within 1 mm, with a resolution of up to 40,000 polygons per square inch, and the texture image is in 24-bit color. Distances, angles, and volumetric data can subsequently be calculated using the computer software, in addition to facial shape, texture, and skin tone in 3 dimensions. The 3dMD FACE system is also capable of capturing more than 22 frames per second, making the technology's real-time mode an option for speech or motion analysis requirements.

This system has been applied in studies of facial morphology[36] and assessment of facial anomalies.[37,38] In comparison with laser scanning, stereophotogrammetry eliminated the need for direct contact and reduced the need for patients' cooperation because of the high speed of data acquisition.[19] Moreover, the patients' image can be repeated without any harmful effects on the participant.[35] When using a laser scanning system, to achieve good acquisition, the person has to cooperate by staying motionless throughout the scanning (15 s) because even small movements could produce errors in the resultant point cloud. A special device (cephalostat) must be used to hold the head still during 3D acquisition. The equipment developed for the photogrammetric acquisition is simple: 3 or 4 digital cameras and photogrammetric software are enough to obtain the 3D information. With the photogrammetric technique, data processing is slower but the information acquisition (the time spent to take photographs) is very fast (1/5000 s, the flashing time). Stereophotogrammetry has been reported to be accurate and reliable for landmark digitization[39,40] and distance acquisition.[26,35] Moreover, although less information about facial shape is obtained using photogrammetry (less points), the points where 3D information is acquired are equally spaced and, after estimation of their spatial localization, need no further processing. Previous studies have shown that the photogrammetric method is very promising for the digital reconstruction of 3D shapes of human faces. Indeed, photogrammetry seems to offer the best compromise regarding all parameters used to evaluate systems of digitization of human faces: a realistic reproduction of the shape, short processing times of the model, simplicity and low cost, noninvasive equipment, and accuracy.

Facial variations among ethnic groups and populations have been studied using direct anthropometry or by 2D imaging.[41] With the development of the 3D technologies, additional methods in facial evaluation can be applied, such as statistical shape analysis.[38] Another application for 3D imaging is the assessment of differences between genders. Three-dimensional surface imaging can evaluate growth changes by studying the variation in sequential captures of faces superimposed on one another.[31] This method of facial assessment offers an excellent opportunity for the possibility of greater accuracy than 2D cephalometric studies.[10,12]

Facial morphology plays an important role in the diagnosis and treatment planning for many dysmorphic syndromes.[42,43] Classical anthropometry and 2D approaches have been applied in the study of craniofacial anomalies[5,13]; but technical approaches, including 3D surface imaging, are now available for further differentiation of facial distortions.[44] Stereophotogrammetry was used to compare craniofacial morphology of unaffected relatives of individuals with nonsyndromic clefts and matched controls.[38] Three-dimensional imaging technologies were also used to compare postsurgical nasal changes after orthognathic surgery.[37] Other studies were conducted to evaluate the treatment outcome of facial augmentation in upper-lip reconstructive surgery,[45] assess the 3D facial soft-tissue response to transverse palatal expansion,[46] or to localize and quantify differences in facial soft-tissue morphology in patients with obstructive sleep apnea.[47] Samson Lee and Wayne F. Larrabee (unpublished data, 2006) were able to demonstrate quantitative changes by generating a histogram of color-based differences taken from 3D images of preoperative and postoperative patients undergoing a facelift procedure. Decreases in jowl volume, neck volume, and neck surface area were calculated, as well as relative changes to the nasolabial fold. Current research focuses on changes as a result of nasal surgery and looks at possible new cephalometric measurements that may not be easily calculated from regular 2D photographs. In the literature, 3D analysis of facial esthetics has involved cadaveric study, such as that of Nemoto and colleagues,[48] who studied cadaveric forehead skin attachments to the underlying galea to determine planes of dissection for facial rejuvenation. Smith and colleagues[49] used histologic sections from a cadaver to recreate a 3D image using computer-modeling software.

Three-dimensional technology has improved in the last decade and is rapidly becoming mainstream. Recently, surgeons have been using 3D image viewing to aid in presurgical planning and discussion. The surgeon has the possibility of making modifications virtually using the presurgical anatomy of the nose. This practice allows the option of correcting the anatomy by taking into account the potential pursuit of facial symmetry. Three-dimensional tools may also be used for an immediate provisional adhesive prosthesis that can be delivered to patients in a few days after surgical resection to restore an acceptable esthetic appearance.

Stereophotogrammetric systems can now provide 3D surface imaging. This capability allows comparing the pretreatment and posttreatment facial status of the patient, ensures monitoring of postsurgery results of various postures and various facial expressions during the treatment process, and allows follow-up of the effectiveness of the treatment. These systems are used in facial plastic surgery and orthognathic surgery cases for selecting and planning possible therapies and operations, evaluating and simulating the treatment visually, and for following up with comparison of presurgical and postsurgical changes. In many studies, such as cleft lip and palate, airway studies, orthodontic treatment, and speech therapy, diagnostic and treatment planning can be made by combining the anatomic and biomechanical characteristics of patients with the surface tone characteristics captured by stereophotogrammetry.

Available software (compatible with Mimics, SimPlant OMS, SimPlant Ortho) allows combining (registering) the surface data with CT/cone beam CT images and digital medical model studies and even the corresponding tissue biomechanical characteristics (see the article in this publication by Mazza and Barbarino), which allows enhanced 3D diagnostic and treatment planning technology.

Technical capabilities of stereophotogrammetric systems are detailed in other articles. These capabilities include surface data corrections when combined with cone beam CT surface data, documentation of natural head movements and facial expressions of the patient, and enabling the surgeon to perform digital surface angle and distance as well as volume measurements.

SUMMARY

The 3D manipulations done by the surgeons in the authors' course allow the appreciation of the consequence of 3D changes on the esthetic of the patients' nose and face. This appreciation incorporates the surgeon's sense of touch, which is an integral element in surgery.

Presurgical planning with 3D tools, like any preoperative planning, can help surgeons reduce risk and improve the course and outcome of surgery. These tools also offer new means of optimizing preoperative communication with patients.

The authors' course includes facial measurements. Various current 3D techniques for measuring surface facial morphology are reported. The 3D imaging system that will be most widely adapted will be one that is accurate and reliable in capturing, archiving, and storing data and will do so in a cost-effective way.

REFERENCES

1. Lin SJ, Patel N, O'Shaughnessy K, et al. A new three-dimensional imaging device in facial aesthetic and reconstructive surgery. Otolaryngol Head Neck Surg 2008;139:313–5.

2. Koch RM, Gross MH, Carls FR, et al. Simulating facial surgery using finite element models. In ACM SIGGRAPH'96. Annu Conf Proc 1996;421–8.

3. Lee Y, Terzopoulos D, Waters K. Realistic face modeling for animation. In ACM SIGGRAPH'95. Annu Conf Proc 1995;55–62.

4. Ciocca L, Bacci G, Mingucci R, et al. CAD-CAM construction of a provisional nasal prosthesis after ablative tumour surgery of the nose: a pilot case report. Eur J Cancer Care 2009;19:97–101.

5. Farkas LG. Examination, photogrammetry of the face, craniofacial anthropometry in clinical genetics. In: Farkas LG, editor. Anthropometry of the head and face. New York: Raven Press Ltd; 1994. p. 22, 80, 104, 192.

6. Guyot L, Dubuc M, Richard O, et al. Comparison between direct clinical and digital photogrammetric measurements in patients with 22q11 microdeletion. Int J Oral Maxillofac Surg 2003;32(3):246–52.

7. Thilander B, Persson M, Adolfsson U. Roentgen-cephalometric standards for a Swedish population. A longitudinal study between the ages of 5 and 31 years. Eur J Orthod 2005;27(4):370–89.

8. Inada E, Saitoh I, Hayasaki H, et al. Cross-sectional growth changes in skeletal and soft tissue cephalometric landmarks of children. Cranio 2008;26(3):170–81.

9. Uysal T, Yagci A, Basciftci FA, et al. Standards of soft tissue Arnett analysis for surgical planning in Turkish adults. Eur J Orthod 2009;31(4):449–56.

10. Sayinsu K, Isik F, Trakyali G, et al. An evaluation of the errors in cephalometric measurements on scanned cephalometric images and conventional tracings. Eur J Orthod 2007;29(1):105–8.

11. Ettorre G, Weber M, Schaaf H, et al. Standards for digital photography in cranio-maxillo-facial surgery - part I: basic views and guidelines. J Craniomaxillofac Surg 2006;34(2):65–73.

12. Paredes V, Gandia JL, Cibrián R. Digital diagnosis records in orthodontics. An overview. Med Oral Patol Oral Cir Bucal 2006;11(1):E88–93.

13. Boehringer S, Vollmar T, Tasse C, et al. Syndrome identification based on 2D analysis software. Eur J Hum Genet 2006;14(10):1082–9.

14. Hajeer MY, Ayoub AF, Millett DT, et al. Three-dimensional imaging in orthognathic surgery: the clinical application of a new method. Int J Adult Orthodon Orthognath Surg 2002;17(4):318–30.

15. Hajeer MY, Millett DT, Ayoub AF, et al. Applications of 3D imaging in orthodontics: part I. J Orthod 2004;31(1):62–70.

16. Honrado CP, Larrabee WF Jr. Update in three dimensional imaging in facial plastic surgery. Curr Opin Otolaryngol Head Neck Surg 2004;12(4):327–31.

17. Ayoub AF, Xiao Y, Khambay B, et al. Towards building a photo-realistic virtual human face for craniomaxillofacial diagnosis and treatment planning. Int J Oral Maxillofac Surg 2007;36(5):423–8.

18. Bourne CO, Kerr WJ, Ayoub AF. Development of a three-dimensional imaging system for analysis of facial change. Clin Orthod Res 2001;4(2):105–11.

19. Ayoub A, Garrahy A, Hood C, et al. Validation of a vision-based, three-dimensional facial imaging system. Cleft Palate Craniofac J 2003;40(5):523–9.

20. Holberg C, Schwenzer K, Mahaini L, et al. Accuracy of facial plaster casts. Angle Orthod 2006;76(4):605–11.

21. De Menezes M, Rosati R, Allievi C, et al. A photographic system for the three-dimensional study of facial morphology. Angle Orthod 2009;79(6):1070–7.

22. Ras F, Habets LL, van Ginkel FC, et al. Quantification of facial morphology using stereophotogrammetry–demonstration of a new concept. J Dent 1996;24(5):369–74.

23. Seeram E. 3-D imaging: basic concepts for radiologic technologists. Radiol Technol 1997;69(2):127–44 [quiz: 145–8].

24. Riphagen JM, van Neck JW, van Adrichem LN. 3D surface imaging in medicine: a review of working principles and implications for imaging the unsedated child. J Craniofac Surg 2008;19(2):517–24.

25. Moss JP. The use of three-dimensional imaging in orthodontics. Eur J Orthod 2006;28(5):416–25.

26. Weinberg SM, Naidoo S, Govier DP, et al. Anthropometric precision and accuracy of digital three-dimensional photogrammetry: comparing the Genex and 3dMD imaging systems with one another and with direct anthropometry. J Craniofac Surg 2006;17(3):477–83.

27. Majid Z, Chong AK, Setan H. Important considerations for craniofacial mapping using laser scanners. Photogramm Rec 2007;22(120):290–308.

28. Kau CH, Richmond S, Zhurov AI, et al. Reliability of measuring facial morphology with a 3-dimensional laser scanning system. Am J Orthod Dentofacial Orthop 2005;128(4):424–30.

29. Gwilliam JR, Cunningham SJ, Hutton T. Reproducibility of soft tissue landmarks on three dimensional facial scans. Eur J Orthod 2006;28(5):408–15.

30. Bozic M, Kau CH, Richmond S, et al. Facial morphology of Slovenian and Welsh white populations using 3-dimensional imaging. Angle Orthod 2009;79(4):640–5.

31. Kau CH, Richmond S, Incrapera A, et al. Three-dimensional surface acquisition systems for the study of facial morphology and their application to maxillofacial surgery. Int J Med Robot 2007;3(2):97–110.

32. Majid Z, Chong AK, Ahmad A, et al. Photogrammetry and 3D laser scanning as spatial data capture techniques for a national craniofacial database. Photogramm Rec 2005;20(109):48–68.

33. Littlefield TR, Kelly KM, Cherney JC, et al. Development of a new three dimensional cranial imaging system. J Craniofac Surg 2004;15(1):175–81.

34. Siebert JP, Marshall SJ. Human body 3D imaging by speckle texture projection photogrammetry. Sensor Rev 2000;20(3):218–26.

35. Wong JY, Oh AK, Ohta E, et al. Validity and reliability of craniofacial anthropometric measurement of 3D digital photogrammetric images. Cleft Palate Craniofac J 2008;45(3):232–9.

36. Seager DC, Kau CH, English JD, et al. Facial morphologies of an adult Egyptian population and an adult Houstonian white population compared using 3d imaging. Angle Orthod 2009;79(5):991–9.

37. Singh GD, Levy-Bercowski D, Yanez MA, et al. Three-dimensional facial morphology following surgical repair of unilateral cleft lip and palate in patients after nasoalveolar molding. Orthod Craniofac Res 2007;10(3):161–6.

38. Weinberg SM, Neiswanger K, Richtsmeier JT, et al. Three-dimensional morphometric analysis of craniofacial shape in the unaffected relatives of individuals with nonsyndromic orofacial clefts: a possible marker for genetic susceptibility. Am J Med Genet A 2008;146(4):409–20.

39. Lee JY, Han Q, Trotman CA. Three-dimensional facial imaging: accuracy and considerations for clinical applications in orthodontics. Angle Orthod 2004;74(5):587–93.

40. Khambay B, Nairn N, Bell A, et al. Validation and reproducibility of a high-resolution three-dimensional facial imaging system. Br J Oral Maxillofac Surg 2008;46(1):27–32.

41. Ngeow WC, Aljunid ST. Craniofacial anthropometric norms of Malays. Singapore Med J 2009;50(5):525–8.

42. Grobbelaar R, Douglas TS. Stereo image matching for facial feature measurement to aid in fetal alcohol syndrome screening. Med Eng Phys 2007;29(4):459–64.

43. Hammond P. The use of 3D face shape modeling in dysmorphology. Arch Dis Child 2007;92(12):1120–6.

44. Hammond P, Hutton TJ, Allanson JE, et al. Discriminating power of localized three-dimensional facial morphology. Am J Hum Genet 2005;77(6):999–1010.

45. Downie J, Mao Z, Rachel Lo TW, et al. A double-blind, clinical evaluation of facial augmentation treatments: a comparison of PRI 1, PRI 2, Zyplast and Perlane. J Plast Reconstr Aesthet Surg 2009;62(12):1636–43.

46. Ramieri GA, Nasi A, Dell'acqua A, et al. Facial soft tissue changes after transverse palatal distraction in adult patients. Int J Oral Maxillofac Surg 2008;37(9):810–8.

47. Banabilh SM, Suzina AH, Dinsuhaimi S, et al. Craniofacial obesity in patients with obstructive sleep apnea. Sleep Breath 2009;13(1):19–24.

48. Nemoto M, Uchinuma E, Yamashina S. Three-dimensional analysis of forehead wrinkles. Aesthetic Plast Surg 2002;26:10–6.

49. Smith D, Aston S, Cutting C, et al. Designing a virtual reality model for aesthetic surgery. Plast Reconstr Surg 2005;116:893–7.

Creation of the Virtual Patient for the Study of Facial Morphology

Chung How Kau, BDS, MScD, MBA, PhD, MOrth, FDS, FFD, FAMS

KEYWORDS

- 3 dimensional • Virtual patient • Facial morphology
- Preoperative planning • Craniofacial structure

For clinicians, the head and neck region is a complex area to work in. Multiple craniofacial anomalies and dentofacial deformities are treated on a daily basis. With better techniques and less-invasive procedures, the face is also an area where cosmetic procedures are performed routinely.

Unlike other areas of the body, the face is unique and gives an individual identity; it relays who we are, where we come from, and what we think or feel. The heavy emphasis on facial beauty and aesthetics has recently shifted the way orthodontists, cosmetic dentists, oral and maxillofacial surgeons, and plastic and reconstructive surgeons look at the human face. For any given face, diagnosis and treatment start from the outside in, meaning from the soft tissue surface to the hard tissue structures. Some in the profession have termed this procedure the soft tissue paradigm.[1,2]

Many craniofacial teams still rely on the traditional methods for diagnosis and treatment planning. However, this should not be the case. With modern techniques and technologies, a realistic 3-dimensional capture of the face to which texture and color are added is achievable and should be of prime importance to all craniofacial researchers and clinicians.

The advances in technology allow us to reconstruct the human face layer by layer, integrating bone, teeth, and skin together to generate a volumetric model of the actual patient. This article describes how the virtual patient is created and manipulated to reach the best treatment outcome. In addition, it also proposes a method of analysis of the human form.

3-DIMENSIONAL DIAGNOSTIC RECORDS

In the image capture of the facial form, 3 primary areas are easily reproduced with current techniques. These are

1. The surface texture of the face
2. The skeletal structure of the head and neck
3. The teeth and its corresponding occlusion.

SURFACE ACQUISITION TECHNOLOGY

Traditionally, extraoral photographs are taken to represent the face before treatment. This photograph serves as a baseline record and also as a planning material. Careful orientation of the head and control of the lens magnification are important for the clinician; however, these photographs are only 2 dimensional, and, even though many views are usually taken, they do not reflect a 3-dimensional reality of the result.

There are a multitude of 3-dimensional surface acquisition systems[3] that are described by Kau and colleagues in other articles in the literature. The most popular technique is stereophotogrammetry. This system is a technology that allows the capture of volumetric surfaces. Usually, 2 or more cameras on each side work as stereo pairs, and a method of triangulation using complex algorithms are used to merge the obtained pictures and create a volume.

The 3dMD system (3dMDface, Atlanta, GA, USA) was used in this article. This machine is equipped with 6 cameras, 3 on each side, that acquire volume, texture, and color.[4] Its capture

Department of Orthodontics, University of Alabama at Birmingham, School of Dentistry, 1919 7th Avenue South, Birmingham, AL 35294, USA
E-mail address: ckau@uab.edu

Facial Plast Surg Clin N Am 19 (2011) 615–622
doi:10.1016/j.fsc.2011.07.005
1064-7406/11/$ – see front matter

time is 1.5 milliseconds. The system produces 1 continuous point cloud from the 2 camera viewpoints and generates a 3-dimensional composite model.[3] Texture and colors are layered over the model. The cameras can only read the well-illuminated anatomic parts of the face; therefore, the submental area, the inside of the nostrils and ears, and the hairline sometimes show as voids.[5] Well-groomed facial hair, on the other hand, does not seem to affect the scanning procedure.[6] Images are stored as proprietary software versions as *.tsb files from the 3dMD files. The 3dMD system presents multiple advantages. Other than the speed of data acquisition and the reported geometric accuracy (<0.2 mm root mean square or better) (depending on exact configuration), it allows the capture of the face in natural head position (NHP).

NHP is considered to be the most natural physiologic and anatomic orientation of the head.[7] This position is internally regulated by each individual and results from a combination of visual, sensory, and postural reflexes.[8] This position is usually achieved by asking patients to look at a distant point in the horizon or at their own reflection in a mirror. NHP has been proven to be clinically reproducible[9] and has been used in all studies of the author.[10]

Another important component of surface texture capture is the facial pose. It is important that a technique be used to capture a reproducible pose. A previously published study has shown that facial pose is reproducible up to 0.85 mm over a 3-day period.[10] This possibility is remarkable considering the variation of facial form that can exist between 2 periods.

The techniques used require the patient to be seated on an adjustable stool preventing strain to the muscles of the neck. The patients are asked to level their eyes to the horizontal line and to align the midline of their faces with the vertical line drawn on a mirror facing them. The subjects are told to swallow hard and to keep their jaws in

a relaxed position just before the images are taken.[11,12] The 3-dimensional image is captured almost instantaneously with a click of a button.

CONE BEAM COMPUTERIZED TOMOGRAPHY

To create the virtual patient, the 3dMD image is combined with an imaging source that captures the skeletal tissues. There are 2 main methods for skeletal hard tissue capture, one being the traditional spiral computerized tomography and the other the cone beam computerized tomography (CBCT). Because of irradiation concerns for routine patient care, a lower-dosimetry emitting machine is recommended. Like the surface acquisition system, the subjects are placed in NHP when the CBCT images are taken . CBCT allows the acquisition of 3-dimensional images of the skull and teeth. It can also capture soft tissue surfaces, but the rendered quality of soft tissue is not ideal. Furthermore, the extent of the field of view does not include the cranium or go past the cephalometric point glabella. Hence, CBCT images need to be combined with stereophotogrammetry.[13]

The cone beam produces a more-focused beam and much less radiation scatter compared with the conventional fan-shaped computed tomographic (CT) devices.[14] The estimated radiation dose is between about 60 and 1000 μSv.[15] Capture time is less than 20 seconds during which the machine revolves once or twice around the patients' head. The machine is equipped with a conventional low-radiation x-ray tube that focuses the beam on a flat-panel detector or charge-coupled device. It is estimated that the total radiation involved in a CBCT is equivalent to 20% of that of conventional CT and corresponds to the dose generated by full-mouth periapical radiographs.[16] Raw data are stored in Digital Imaging and Communications in Medicine (DICOM) file formats. Further reading on the device may be found in the literature.[17]

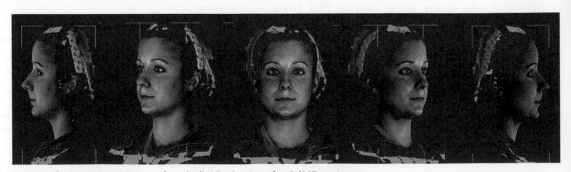

Fig. 1. Soft tissue acquisition of an individual using the 3dMD system.

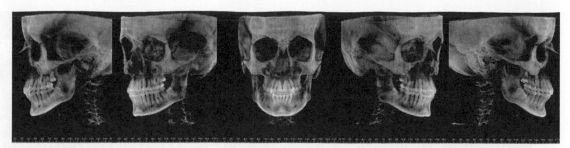

Fig. 2. CBCT acquired with the Kodak 9500 machine. The views correspond to the soft tissue views in **Fig. 1**.

DENTAL MODEL INTEGRATION

Traditionally, dental stone casts have been used by clinicians to visualize the occlusion, perform analysis, and fabricate appliances. The introduction of 3-dimensional digital casts has tremendously decreased chairside time and reduced storage space in orthodontic offices. Digital dental casts have been reported to provide an accurate and reliable representation of the dentition.[18] These virtual models can be produced in 2 ways. In the first method, dental impressions are scanned and the generated models can be viewed with the adequate software. Some investigators have tried to integrate these dental images in the CBCTs, stating that raw dental arches derived from CBCT itself can be inaccurate because of metallic scatters.[19]

The new challenge is then to integrate these 3-dimensional dental models in the virtual patient reconstruction. The technique used by Gateno and colleagues[19,20] allows an accurate incorporation of the teeth in the skull but causes soft tissue distortion because of the jig they use. Swennen and colleagues[21] report an interesting approach to merge the models with the hard tissue but use 3-stage scans to achieve their goal, which increased the radiation dose in the patient. The second method is to use appropriate software to create study models directly from the CBCT. A good example is InVivo Anatomage (Anatomage, San Jose, CA, USA) that can create study models from CBCT scans taken by a Galileos cone beam scanner with a field of view of 15 × 15 × 15 cm[22] and a voxel resolution of 0.125 mm. The CBCT images are then electronically sent via a secure Web site to the company Anatomage in a DICOM format. This approach significantly cuts down the record acquisition steps because no impressions are required and the teeth are already integrated in the skull.

Some preliminary works on the direct rendering of dental casts directly from CBCT DICOMs have shown some promise. However, these representations are not enough for appliance fabrication.

A study using the Little's index compared CBCT study models with OrthoCAD models (CADENT, Fairview, NJ, USA) and found them to be as accurate as the digital models for measuring overjet, overbite, and crowding. Moreover, CBCT models offer diagnostic information on bone level, root orientations, and temporomandibular situation.[23] The advantages of digital models are numerous. Recovery of the right dental occlusal relations allows a more-accurate treatment diagnosis, planning, and adequate appliance design.[24] Canine impactions or multidisciplinary treatments, especially those involving surgery, can benefit from this technology.[25]

CREATING THE VIRTUAL PATIENT
3dMDvultus Software

Some software platforms permit the fusion of the surface texture (acquired by the 3dMD system) with the hard tissue (CT/CBCT/digitized dental study models). One such platform is the 3dMDvultus system. Because both soft and hard tissue images are taken in NHP, fusing the CBCT-generated soft tissue surface with the stereophotogrammetric image allows total visualization and manipulation of the created virtual head.

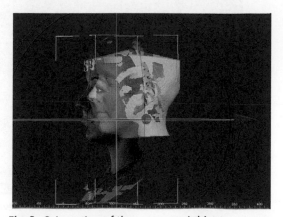

Fig. 3. Orientation of the segmented skin structure to the 3dMD surface skin structure.

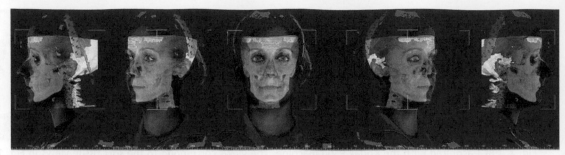

Fig. 4. Surface-to-surface merging of the soft and hard tissue 3-dimensional images (*frontal to lateral view*).

The steps needed to merge soft tissue to hard tissue in this software are described by the manufacturer and consist of the following:

1. The patient-acquired surface images and CBCT results are loaded in the software, and segmentations into surfaces are created.
2. After unlocking rotation and translation functions, the operator manually fits the soft tissue generated by the CBCT on the 3dMD surface.
3. The registration is surface based. The operator selects anatomically stable surfaces, and the software refines the initial manual registration.
4. Once the surfaces are registered, it becomes possible to visualize volumes or cuts in different degrees of transparency.

The following section illustrates the sequence in which data are acquired and the virtual model created for a patient who presented at the Craniofacial Clinic at the Department of Orthodontics, University of Alabama at Birmingham.

The sequence used is as follows:

1. Soft tissue acquisition: the soft tissue surface is acquired with the 3dMD system in NHP (**Fig. 1**).
2. Hard tissue acquisition: the CBCT presented in this article was generated using a Kodak 9500 3D system. This machine captures dualjaw (9 × 15 cm) or dentomaxillofacial (18.4 × 20.6 cm) anatomy. It allows radiation dose control through variable milliampere and kilovolt settings. The voxel resolution is 0.2 mm (**Fig. 2**).
3. Merging of surfaces: surface-to-surface merginging on anatomically stable regions associates the CBCT and 3dMD surfaces (**Figs. 3** and **4**).
4. Landmarks: soft tissue and hard tissue landmarks can be identified at this stage (discussed in next paragraph) (**Figs. 5** and **6**).
5. Surgical simulation: the 3dMDvultus software allows surgical simulation. Virtual cuts similar to the real surgical cuts are possible and allow the practitioner to replicate bony movements. The software calculates and applies soft tissue changes for better visualization of the end result (**Fig. 7**).

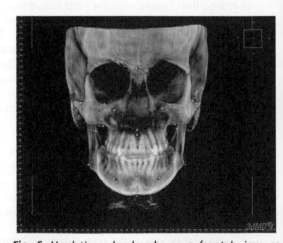

Fig. 5. Soft tissue landmarks on a frontal view, as listed in **Box 1**. Lateral landmarks are not shown in this view.

Fig. 6. Hard tissue landmarks on a frontal view, as listed in **Box 2**. Lateral and internal landmarks are not shown in this view. Foramina are used as landmarks for their ease of location and reproducibility.

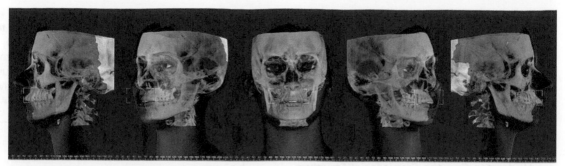

Fig. 7. Maxillary (*top*) and mandibular (*bottom*) surgical cuts performed to simulate maxillary advancement and mandibular setback, respectively.

MULTIPLE APPLICATIONS
Traditional Studies

Soft tissue surfaces can be compared to evaluate growth,[26] gender differences,[27,28] population differences,[29–31] changes after surgical interventions such as orthognathic surgery, or craniofacial corrections.[32,33] The steps needed to perform the fusion using the best-fit method have been described in previous publications. This software not only represents a great tool for communication with the patient but also puts all the craniofacial team on the same page because all surgical movements and their repercussions on the soft tissue can be simulated and viewed in 3 dimensions. Treatment evaluation is also possible by superimposing different images taken at different time points.

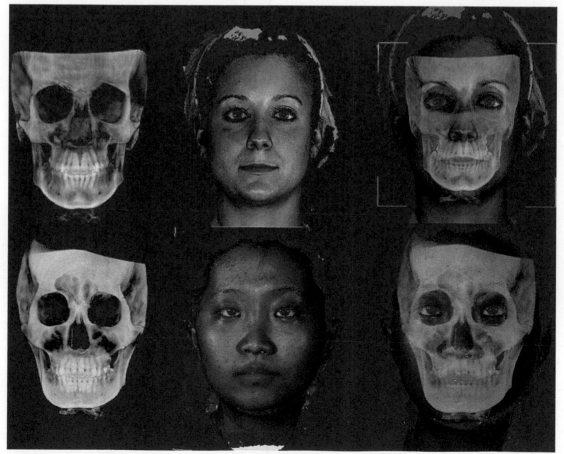

Fig. 8. Similar phenotypic expression of the skeletal hard tissue but variations of the facial or soft tissue phenotype.

Genomic Studies

Another type of study of interest is the expression of the genome in relation to the facial phenotype. A simple example (**Fig. 8**) is used to illustrate where the skeletal structures appear similar but the facial phenotype represents 2 different population types. This study certainly represents a novel area of work for the future.

Understanding the Craniofacial Structure

Another possible relevance in the virtual patient is the true quantification of the head and neck within a reference framework. Landmarks have been used in anthropometry and cephalometry to study craniofacial dimensions and establish norms for each gender and population.[34,35]

Using the 3dMDvultus software, the Kau analysis system allows each landmark position to be captured on the surface (soft tissue, bone, and teeth) of the virtual patient. **Boxes 1** and **2** present the soft and hard tissue landmarks that we use in the facility (27 and 36 landmarks, respectively).

Box 1
Soft tissue landmarks

G': glabella

N': nasion

En_R: endocanthion right

En_L: endocanthion left

Ex_R: exocanthion right

Ex_L: exocanthion left

Or'_R: orbitale right

Or'_L: orbitale left

Prn: pronasale

Sn: subnasale

Al_R: alare right

Al_L: alare left

Sbal_R: subalare right

Sbal_L: subalare left

Ls: labiale superius

Cph_R: cristi philtri right

Cph_L: cristi philtri left

Sto: stomion

Li: labiale inferius

Ch_R: cheilon right

Ch_L: cheilon left

Pog': pogonion

Gn': gnathion

Po'_R: porion right

Po'_L: porion left

Zy_R: zygion right

Zy_L: zygion left

Box 2
Hard tissue landmarks

S: sella

N: nasion

Or_R: orbitale right

Or_L: orbitale left

ZT_R: zygotemporal point right

ZT_L: zygotemporal point right

ZM_R: zygomaxillary point right

ZM_L: zygomaxillary point left

ANS: anterior nasal spine

PNS: posterior nasal spine

Point A: subspinale

Point B: supramentale

Pog: pogonion

Gn: gnathion

Me: menton

GP: genial point

Go_R: gonion right

Go_L: gonion left

Po_R: porion right

Po_L: porion left

Co_R: condylion right

Co_L: condylion left

LCo_R: lateral mandibular condyle right

LCo_L: lateral mandibular condyle left

MCo_R: medial mandibular condyle right

MCo_L: medial mandibular condyle left

RP_R: ramus point right

RP_L: ramus point left

CP_R: coronoid point right

CP_L: coronoid point left

L_R: lingula right

L_L: lingula left

InfO_R: infraorbital foramen right

InfO_L: infraorbital foramen left

Mf_R: mental foramen right

Mf_L: mental foramen left

These points are easily identifiable and were chosen to map the entire hard and soft tissues in the face. Each patient now has unique x-, y-, and z-coordinates. Moreover, these points allow the creation of a unique intrinsic system for each individual. This concept represents a major paradigm shift in treating patients, especially those in need for orthognathic/reconstructive surgery.

With a 3-dimensional coordinate system, it becomes possible to relate different parts of the same face to each other, taking into account the individual proportions. The goal is then to correct the malformation to a harmonious result within this particular system. This statement supports the need for standardized normative data but redefines the boundaries. It emphasizes the need for such norms for each ethnic group to be able to assemble individuals on the basis of common features. However, when it comes to treating one particular patient, the collective norms serve as guidelines and the intrinsic system is the ultimate guide to individually achieve optimal results.

SUMMARY

Imaging technology is constantly being refined and improved. The tools that the craniofacial team has allow the team to gather all diagnostic records from a single CBCT scan and a single surface imaging shot. These new opportunities will surely take orthodontics, dentofacial orthopedics, and craniofacial surgery to a whole new level. Volumetric imaging finally captures the patient's 3-dimensional essence and is a valuable tool to longitudinally monitor growth and treatment interventions.

REFERENCES

1. Ackerman JL, Wr P, Dm S. The emerging soft tissue paradigm in orthodontic diagnosis and treatment planning. Clin Orthod Res 1999;2:49–52.
2. Sarver DM, Ackerman JL. Orthodontics about face: the re-emergence of the esthetic paradigm. Am J Orthod Dentofacial Orthop 2000;117(5):575–6.
3. Kau CH, Richmond S, Incrapera A, et al. Three-dimensional surface acquisition systems for the study of facial morphology and their application to maxillofacial surgery. Int J Med Robot 2007;3(2): 97–110.
4. Incrapera AK, Kau CH, English JD, et al. Soft tissue images from cephalograms compared with those from a 3D surface acquisition system. Angle Orthod 2010;80(1):58–64.
5. Heike CL, Upson K, Stuhaug E, et al. 3D digital stereophotogrammetry: a practical guide to facial image acquisition. Head Face Med 2010;6:18.
6. Lane C, Harrell W Jr. Completing the 3-dimensional picture. Am J Orthod Dentofacial Orthop 2008; 133(4):612–20.
7. Ackerman JL, Proffit WR, Sarver DM, et al. Pitch, roll, and yaw: describing the spatial orientation of dentofacial traits. Am J Orthod Dentofacial Orthop 2007; 131(3):305–10.
8. Cooke MS, Wei SH. The reproducibility of natural head posture: a methodological study. Am J Orthod Dentofacial Orthop 1988;93(4):280–8.
9. Chiu CS, Clark RK. Reproducibility of natural head position. J Dent 1991;19(2):130–1.
10. Kau CH, Richmond S, Zhurov AI, et al. Reliability of measuring facial morphology with a 3-dimensional laser scanning system. Am J Orthod Dentofacial Orthop 2005;128(4):424–30.
11. Kau CH, Richmond S, Savio C, et al. Measuring adult facial morphology in three dimensions. Angle Orthod 2006;76(5):773–8.
12. Kau CH, Zhurov A, Bibb R, et al. The investigation of the changing facial appearance of identical twins employing a three-dimensional laser imaging system. Orthod Craniofac Res 2005;8(2):85–90.
13. Kau CH, Richmond S, Palomo JM, et al. Three-dimensional cone beam computerized tomography in orthodontics. J Orthod 2005;32(4):282–93.
14. Mah J, Hatcher D. Current status and future needs in craniofacial imaging. Orthod Craniofac Res 2003; 6(Suppl 1):10–6 [discussion: 179–82].
15. De Vos W, Casselman J, Swennen GR. Cone-beam computerized tomography (CBCT) imaging of the oral and maxillofacial region: a systematic review of the literature. Int J Oral Maxillofac Surg 2009; 38(6):609–25.
16. Sukovic P. Cone beam computed tomography in craniofacial imaging. Orthod Craniofac Res 2003; 6(Suppl 1):31–6 [discussion: 179–82].
17. Kau CH, Bozic M, English J, et al. Cone-beam computed tomography of the maxillofacial region—an update. Int J Med Robot 2009;5(4):366–80.
18. Quimby ML, Vig KW, Rashid RG, et al. The accuracy and reliability of measurements made on computer-based digital models. Angle Orthod 2004;74(3): 298–303.
19. Gateno J, Xia JJ, Teichgraeber JF, et al. Clinical feasibility of computer-aided surgical simulation (CASS) in the treatment of complex cranio-maxillofacial deformities. J Oral Maxillofac Surg 2007;65(4):728–34.
20. Xia JJ, Gateno J, Teichgraeber JF, et al. Accuracy of the computer-aided surgical simulation (CASS) system in the treatment of patients with complex craniomaxillofacial deformity: a pilot study. J Oral Maxillofac Surg 2007;65(2):248–54.
21. Swennen GR, Mollemans W, De Clercq C, et al. A cone-beam computed tomography triple scan procedure to obtain a three-dimensional augmented

virtual skull model appropriate for orthognathic surgery planning. J Craniofac Surg 2009;20(2): 297–307.

22. Kamel SG, Kau CH, Wong ME, et al. The role of cone beam CT in the evaluation and management of a family with Gardner's syndrome. J Craniomaxillofac Surg 2009;37(8):461–8.

23. Kau CH, Littlefield J, Rainy N, et al. Evaluation of CBCT digital models and traditional models using the Little's Index. Angle Orthod 2010;80(3):435–9.

24. Chenin DL, Chenin DA, Chenin ST, et al. Dynamic cone-beam computed tomography in orthodontic treatment. J Clin Orthod 2009;43(8):507–12.

25. Kau CH, Pan P, Gallerano RL, et al. A novel 3D classification system for canine impactions—the KPG index. Int J Med Robot 2009;5(3):291–6.

26. Kau CH, Richmond S. Three-dimensional analysis of facial morphology surface changes in untreated children from 12 to 14 years of age. Am J Orthod Dentofacial Orthop 2008;134(6):751–60.

27. Gor T, Kau CH, English JD, et al. Three-dimensional comparison of facial morphology in white populations in Budapest, Hungary, and Houston, Texas. Am J Orthod Dentofacial Orthop 2010;137(3): 424–32.

28. Kau CH, Zhurov A, Richmond S, et al. The 3-dimensional construction of the average 11-year-old child

face: a clinical evaluation and application. J Oral Maxillofac Surg 2006;64(7):1086–92.

29. Seager DC, Kau CH, English JD, et al. Facial morphologies of an adult Egyptian population and an adult Houstonian white population compared using 3D imaging. Angle Orthod 2009;79(5):991–9.

30. Kau CH, Richmond S, Zhurov A, et al. Use of 3-dimensional surface acquisition to study facial morphology in 5 populations. Am J Orthod Dentofacial Orthop 2010;137(Suppl 4):S56.e51–9 [discussion: S56–7].

31. Bozic M, Kau CH, Richmond S, et al. Novel method of 3-dimensional soft-tissue analysis for Class III patients. Am J Orthod Dentofacial Orthop 2010; 138(6):758–69.

32. McCance AM, Moss JP, Fright WR, et al. A three dimensional analysis of soft and hard tissue changes following bimaxillary orthognathic surgery in skeletal III patients. Br J Oral Maxillofac Surg 1992;30(5):305–12.

33. Hajeer MY, Ayoub AF, Millett DT. Three-dimensional assessment of facial soft-tissue asymmetry before and after orthognathic surgery. Br J Oral Maxillofac Surg 2004;42(5):396–404.

34. Farkas L. Anthropometry of the head and face. New York: Raven Press; 1994.

35. Jacobson A. The proportionate template as a diagnostic aid. Am J Orthod 1979;75(2):156–72.

3D Mechanical Modeling of Facial Soft Tissue for Surgery Simulation

Edoardo Mazza, PhD[a,b,]*,
Giuseppe Giovanni Barbarino, PhD[a]

KEYWORDS

- 3D mechanical modeling • Face • Soft tissue
- Surgery simulation

Computer-based design and simulation methods enable engineers to optimize functionality, reliability, manufacturing process, and costs of new devices and machines. To this end, computer models are developed that represent the three-dimensional (3D) geometry of the system, the interaction of its parts, the changes in shape caused by the application of loads, as expected in the different conditions of service. Recent improvements in the procedures for 3D geometric data acquisition and representation, advances in the understanding and the mathematical description of the force-displacement relationship in the case of large deformations and nonlinear time-dependent behavior of materials, and the continuous enhancement in the performance of modern computer systems have allowed application of this approach to complex design problems, such as, for example, the optimization of the crash resistance behavior of a car. Application of computer-based design and simulation procedures to medical problems is one of the main objectives of current research in biomechanics. Examples of recent developments are simulations of trauma, calculations for predicting the outcome of surgery, real-time simulations for intraoperative navigation, and surgical training using virtual reality.[1–5] This article presents the 3D numerical model of the face developed in our laboratory at ETH Zurich for simulation of soft facial tissue response to physiologic loads, and for investigation of plastic and reconstructive surgery procedures and devices.

Modeling the changes in shape of the face caused by the application of external force vectors or internal (muscle) contractions is a challenging mechanical problem. It requires an accurate representation of the anatomic elements, their interactions, the kinematic boundary conditions (ligament fixations), and the nonlinear and time-dependent force-deformation characteristics of all involved tissues and organs. Although numerical models were intended initially to realize realistic animations of facial expressions (eg, Terzopoulos and colleagues[6]), more detailed representation of face anatomy and the force-deformation characteristics were developed for simulations related to the physiology and pathology of face deformation, such as for modeling human mastication,[7] facial outlook or expressions of emotion in craniofacial[8] and maxillofacial[9,10] surgery planning, and for the prediction of the outcome of reconstructive surgery after burns injuries.[11]

The so-called finite element (FE) method is a calculation tool that provides accurate simulations of the mechanical behavior of deformable bodies. The large computational time associated

Financial support by J&J Medical and the Swiss National Science Foundation (project "Computer Aided and Image Guided Medical Intervention," NCCR CO-ME) is gratefully acknowledged.

[a] Institute of Mechanical Systems, ETH-Swiss Federal Institute of Technology, Zurich 8092, Switzerland
[b] Mechanics for Modeling and Simulation, EMPA - Materials Science and Technology, Dübendorf 8600, Switzerland
* Corresponding author. Institute of Mechanical Systems, ETH, Zurich 8092, Switzerland.
E-mail address: mazza@imes.mavt.ethz.ch

Facial Plast Surg Clin N Am 19 (2011) 623–637
doi:10.1016/j.fsc.2011.07.006
1064-7406/11/$ – see front matter © 2011 Elsevier Inc. All rights reserved.

with FE calculations has motivated the development of alternative numerical approaches allowing for fast (in certain cases, even real-time) surgery simulation, such as mass-spring or mass-tensor models.[12,13] FE models are often used as the benchmark for evaluation of the predictive capabilities of these simplified numerical algorithms (see, eg, Mollemans and colleagues[9]).

FE models of the face proposed in the literature were mostly based on the external contour of the face and the shape of the bones. In the study by Keeve and colleagues,[12] uniform mechanical properties for soft facial tissue were applied. Chabanas[14] distinguished 2 layers and modeled 4 muscles using elements running through the layers. Zhachow and colleagues[15] and Gladilin and colleagues[8] proposed a more accurate model from the anatomic point of view: magnetic resonance images were segmented to extract the shape of 18 face muscles, which were embedded into homogeneous soft tissue. The muscles were activated through the definition of a contractile force acting in the direction of predefined muscle fibers. Active muscle behavior was considered also in the work by Nazari and colleagues[16] for simulation of orofacial movements.

In most of these models, linear elastic material behavior is assumed for soft facial tissue.[17] Nonlinear mechanical model equations are required in the case of large deformations of facial tissue (see, eg, Har-Shai and colleagues[18]). Mazza and colleagues[19] used hyperelastic-viscoplastic constitutive equations with internal variables (including a so-called aging function) to simulate gravimetric descent such as that resulting from a progressive loss of stiffness of the aging facial tissue. The corresponding FE model consists of 4 layers of uniform thickness obtained from laser scan data of the external face surface.

Although still far from the realization of computer models capable of quantitative and reliable patient-specific prediction of surgical outcome, today's numerical simulations, with an increasing level of realism, are intended to provide objective criteria for comparison of alternative surgical procedures, improve visualization and prediction of soft tissue deformation for surgery planning and intraoperative navigation, and to complement trials on cadavers and clinical studies for the development of new tools for plastic and reconstructive surgery. This article reports on the development of a 3D FE model of a face designed to give a faithful representation of (1) the anatomy, (2) the mechanical interactions between different tissues, and (3) the nonlinear force-deformation characteristics of all tissues. The model presented in this paper is one of the most accurate numerical models of the

face available so far. The geometry of each anatomic part is based on reconstructions from magnetic resonance images; shape, constraints, and interactions of tissues and organs have been verified to be consistent with state-of-the-art knowledge on face anatomy; nonlinear constitutive equations are used for modeling the mechanical behavior of each tissue.

The procedure for model generation is presented, including the reconstruction based on segmented contours of the anatomic parts, the realization of the corresponding FE mesh for numerical simulations, the anatomic aspects considered for defining kinematic boundary conditions, and interactions between the anatomic parts. The mechanical model equations used for describing the mechanical behavior of facial tissues are introduced later in this article. Materials parameters were initially selected based on data from the literature. Specific information on the mechanical behavior of the face being investigated was obtained from a series of experiments. The response of facial tissues to gravity loads and to the application of a measured pressure inside the oral cavity has been quantified using magnetic resonance images and holographic techniques and compared with the results of the corresponding FE calculations. Information on the local mechanical response of the superficial soft tissue (skin, superficial musculoaponeurotic system [SMAS], and superficial fat) in different regions of the face, was obtained using suction experiments (Cutometer and aspiration device). Results of predictions of gravimetric soft tissue descent will be presented as an example of application of the face model. Aging predictions were evaluated comparing the contour of the simulated aged face with the results of contour extraction from frontal photos of volunteers at different ages. This article also includes a discussion of the capabilities and limitations of the present model and an outlook to possible applications and further development of this approach.

MODEL DEVELOPMENT
Representation of Bones, Muscles, Tissue Layers, Ligaments

High-resolution magnetic resonance imaging (MRI) data were acquired for determination of the shape of bones, soft layers, and muscles. This procedure is commonly used to generate 3D anatomic models.[15,20] Using a Philips Achieva 1.5T scanner, 150 slices at a distance of 2 mm with an in-plane resolution of 0.5 mm were obtained for the head and neck of a 27-year old man lying in the supine position. The high quality of images obtained resulted from an iterative optimization considering acquisition time and ability of the tested person to maintain a relaxed position, without muscular contractions. **Fig. 1** shows an example of a transverse MRI image.

The most challenging step for extraction of geometric data to be used in the FE model is the segmentation and reconstruction of all anatomic elements. Skull and mandibula could be obtained using a semiautomated procedure based on a simple threshold segmentation algorithm, with manual adjustments applied to separate mandibula and skull in the articulation temporomandibular (ATM) region, and upper and lower teeth. The good contrast and resolution of the MRI images allowed in this case a quick and reliable reconstruction of bones, for which computed tomography scans are usually preferred. The definition of the external contour of the face was almost fully automated, requiring only minor adjustments.

Reconstruction of the muscles was obtained through a time-consuming procedure, illustrated in **Fig. 2** for the case of the masseter muscle. The commercial software AMIRA (Konrad-Zuse-Zentrum Berlin, Mercury Computer Systems) was used for segmentation and reconstruction of each anatomic part. The software creates a polygonal surface model of each segmented feature. The triangulated surface is imported into the commercial software package Geomagic Studio (Geomagic, Inc., Triangle Park, NC) for a manual correction of incomplete parts. The FE model is then created based on this geometry (discussed later). All muscles required manual segmentation

and reconstruction; in regions where they intersect or run close to each other, a manual separation of the contours had to be made. Identification of the muscle boundaries in some cases needed the evaluation of information from literature and consultation with anatomy experts. Not all muscles and local tissue parts were modeled, to limit both the effort related to anatomy extraction and the computational power, which increases with model complexity. Barbarino and colleagues[21] describe the selection of the muscles to be included in the model along with the considerations related to their relevance to the mechanical behavior of the face. As indicated in **Fig. 3**, the following muscles were included in the model: buccinator, zygomaticus major and minor, levator anguli oris, levator labii, levator labii alaeque nasi, depressor labii, depressor anguli oris, mentalis, and masseter. Orbicularis oris, risorius, temporalis, and pterygoidei medialis and lateralis are among the muscles neglected in the present model.

Skin (epidermis and dermis) is modeled with a soft layer of constant thickness (2 mm, an average of the values observed in the MRI images) covering the whole face. Mucosa is a continuous layer, similar in structure to the skin. It was thus modeled with the same thickness as the skin. The SMAS is an important structure for plastic surgery, but there is not a consistent anatomic definition of this layer.[22,23] The MRI images did not allow the SMAS to be distinguished from deeper connective tissue. The model assumption adopted was therefore to introduce the SMAS along

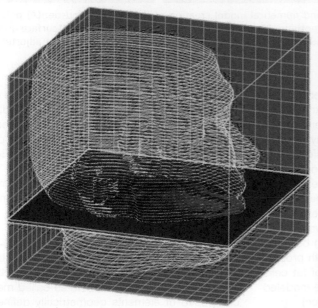

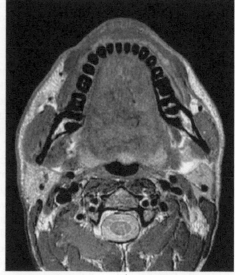

Fig. 1. High-resolution MRI scan used for segmentation and reconstruction of face muscles, bones, and superficial layers.

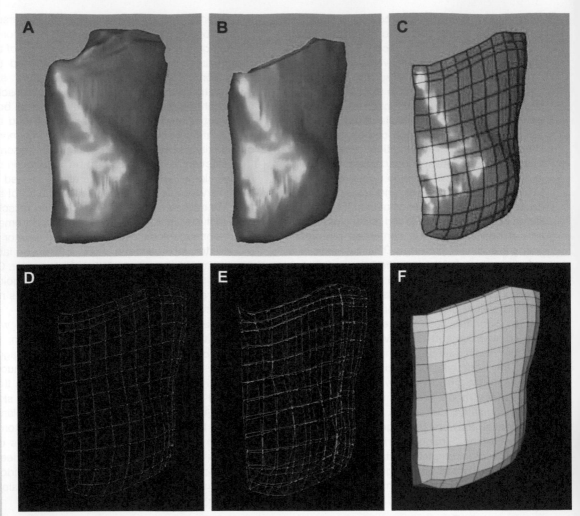

Fig. 2. The procedure for reconstruction and numerical model creation of the masseter muscle: (*A*) polygonal surface model; (*B*) shape correction and smoothing; (*C*) basis surface, subdivided in patches; (*D*) surface quadrangular mesh; (*E*) 3D mesh extruded and nodes projected on the original geometry; (*F*) manually adjusted final mesh.

with the superficial fat as a homogeneous layer parallel to the skin with a general thickness of 3 mm. The thickness of this layer has been suitably reduced in different regions to not overlay muscles or bones. This procedure led to a nonuniform layer interfacing the skin to muscle, bone, or deeper connective tissue. Further details concerning the representation of SMAS and platysma muscle are reported by Barbarino and colleagues.[21]

Soft tissue deeper to the SMAS was represented as filler of the empty spaces in between mucosa, muscles, SMAS, and skin, with properties determined by the large number of fat cells included in this tissue. All interfaces are modeled as tied contacts (no sliding, no separation).

Retaining ligaments are not explicitly represented in the FE model, but their effect is considered in terms of boundary conditions: following the nomenclature of La Trenta,[24] zygomatic, mandibular, and platysma-auricular ligaments were modeled by constraining the displacement of the corresponding regions of the FE model (see **Fig. 3**). The masseteric-cutaneous ligaments were modeled by locally increased resistance to deformation for the connective tissue between the anterior border of the masseter muscle and the skin.

Generation of the FE Mesh

The FE calculation of face deformations is based on a local definition of the relationship between forces and displacements. The so-called mesh is composed of elements geometrically defined by the nodes located at the outer boundaries of each element. Depending on the mechanical

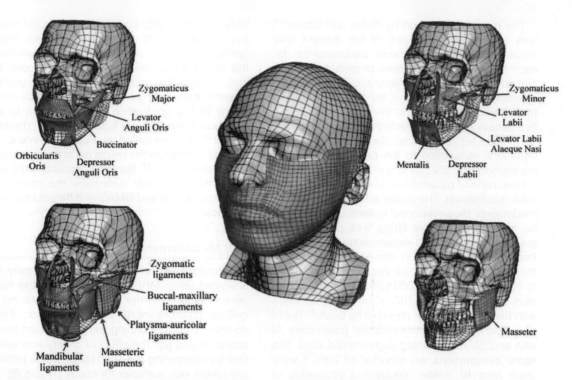

Fig. 3. Overview of FE model of the face with indication of muscles and ligaments.[21]

properties of the material, the forces applied at the nodes are transmitted through adjacent elements, and result in node displacements and element deformations. The computational time is proportional to the number of degrees of freedom, and thus to the number of elements and nodes. The FE mesh of the face was defined with the objective of creating a model with sufficient spatial discretization, providing good performance in terms of computational time and accuracy. A semiautomatic procedure has been applied that generates a mesh composed of hexahedron elements starting from an object in the form of a triangulated surface.[2]

As illustrated in **Fig. 2**, each object is divided in parts with a simple geometry (close to a parallelepiped) and a basis surface is defined for each part. The surface is subdivided in patches using a grid of splines and a quadrilateral surface mesh is generated. This two-dimensional (2D) mesh is extruded by an average thickness of the part, thus creating a 3D hexahedron mesh. Then, an algorithm is used to project the nodes of this mesh to the original triangulated surface of the object. Manual adjustments are often required to correct distorted elements or to increase the correspondence with the object geometry at some locations. The mesh of each object is then imported into the commercial software ABAQUS

(Simulia, Providence, RI), used as solver and postprocessor for the FE calculations (see **Fig. 3** for the whole numerical model).

Model Equations for the Mechanical Behavior of Soft Facial Tissue

The local relationship between forces (stresses) and deformation is defined for each material through the so-called constitutive equations. Har-Shai and colleagues[18] evaluated the nonlinear viscoelastic mechanical properties of skin and SMAS with experiments on excised tissue samples. Corresponding constitutive equations were developed by Rubin and Bodner.[25] The original model considers history-dependent variables and corresponding evolution equations to reproduce the observed mechanical response caused by the microscopic morphology of the tissues. A direct link between tissue microstructure and macroscopic mechanical behavior cannot be achieved at present. Instead, the equations and the material parameters are determined by comparing predictions of the model with macroscopic experimental data. The constitutive model was implemented as a user-defined algorithm into the commercial FE software ABAQUS (Papes O, PhD thesis, in preparation), and used for aging simulations by Mazza and colleagues.[26]

The model formulation by Rubin and Bodner[25] was applied to all tissues of the present face model, with a specific model parameter set for each tissue. Steady response of facial tissue was considered in the experiments and corresponding simulations. For this reason, the parts of the model that describes short-term, transient, and dissipative behaviors were neglected for the calculations performed so far. Further details on the model equations as applied to the present face model are reported by Barbarino and colleagues.[21]

Five material parameters have to be assigned to each facial tissue. The values selected for this face model were those reported in literature. Note that no material parameter fitting was performed to match simulations and experimental observations that are reported later in this article. Because of the high water content, all tissues were assumed to have a density of 1000 g/cm³, except for the skin, with a value of 1100 g/cm³, in accordance with the measurements reported by Duck.[27] Rubin and Bodner[25] determined model parameters of skin and SMAS by fitting experimental data. The same assumptions we reported in 2005[26] were used here to define mechanical properties of mucosa and deep fat; the material constants of the mucosa were taken to be the same as those of the skin, because they have a similar structure. For the deep fat, the stiffness was taken to be 1 order of magnitude less than the SMAS. Mechanical properties of muscles were selected to provide a factor of 10 higher value of the stiffness compared with SMAS. For simplicity, muscles were selected as passive isotropic tissue.

Local measurements of the mechanical response of the superficial layers of the specific face modeled in this work were performed, providing specific values for the corresponding model parameters (discussed later).

In all simulations, skull, mandibula, and the parotid gland have been modeled as rigid bodies, because these parts are stiffer than all other facial tissues considered in the model.

EXPERIMENTAL OBSERVATION AND SIMULATION OF FACE DEFORMATION

The FE model as described earlier can be used for simulation of face deformation for specified force applications, related to physiologic conditions of loading or to medical intervention. The uncertainties of the simulation results are related to model assumptions such as (1) constitutive model parameters, (2) spatial discretization (mesh density), (3) boundary conditions (ligaments, fixations), and (4) organ interactions. The purpose of the experiments reported here was to compare simulations

with physical reality and thus evaluate the predictive capabilities of the model, and to provide further information on the mechanical behavior of the face for improvement of the FE model. MRI and holographic measurements were used to determine the change in shape of the face consequent to the application of simple (and known) distributed mechanical loads or given displacements.[21] The so-called pull-up experiment was applied to analyze the response to the application of a force vector.[28] Suction measurements were performed to locally determine the mechanical behavior of skin and SMAS in different regions of the face.[29]

MRI Measurements

Deformation of the face caused by gravity was analyzed using MRI scans taken with the tested person lying (1) in the supine position facing the ceiling, (2) horizontally facing the floor. **Fig. 4** compares corresponding transversal sections for scans (1) and (2). The effect of gravity was quantified by computing the shortest distance between the whole skin surfaces for cases (1) and (2). The same procedure was applied to determine skin surface displacements for corresponding FE simulations of a distributed gravity field with a magnitude of 2 × g, corresponding to the difference between configurations (1) and (2). Measurements and FE calculations are compared in **Fig. 5** showing a good qualitative correspondence in the distribution of the deformation, with the calculated values lower than the measurements, indicating a too-stiff behavior of the model. Note that no adjustment of material parameters was applied for these results.

MRI measurements with 2 wooden balls with a diameter of 2.5 cm inserted between the cheeks and the tooth were conducted to analyze the model response to a known imposed internal deformation. **Fig. 6** shows a representative transversal section for this case and compares the MRI scan with the corresponding numerical results. The simulation considered the wooden balls as rigid bodies placed inside the oral cavity and displaced to the final position in contact with the mucosa. The calculated external surface displacement and the internal distribution of deformations agree to a great extent with the experiment. The redistribution of connective tissue (deep fat and SMAS) is well represented and the corresponding displacements of the buccinator and masseter muscles confirm the selection of the corresponding boundary conditions. Differences are evident toward the lips region, probably related to the muscles being modeled as passive,

A

B

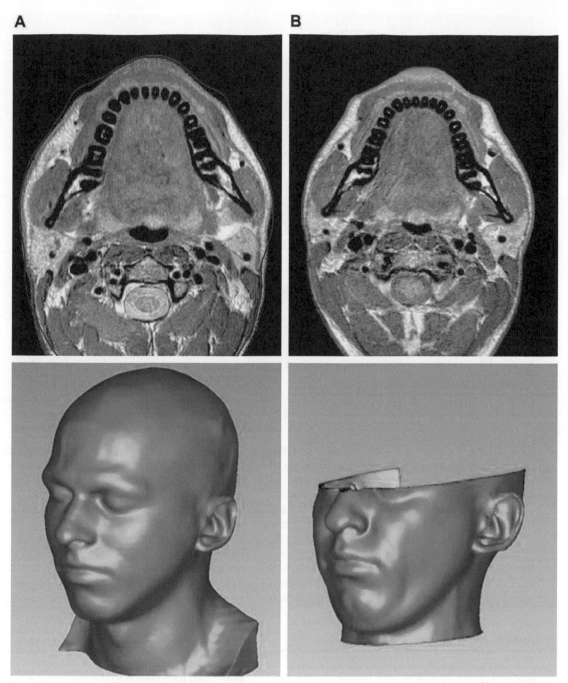

Fig. 4. Comparison of transversal sections showing the deformation caused by gravity load.[21] (*A*) reference measurement with (*red*) superimposed contour from the corresponding section with the face upside down (*B*).

whereas a contraction of the orbicularis oris muscle is necessary to keep the lips closed.

Holographic Measurements

In holographic measurements, phase and intensity information are recorded from the interference pattern of light reflected from the observed surface and reference light from the same source.[30] The analysis of these data allows determination of the 3D surface shape of the face with short acquisition time and high resolution.

Two measurements have been performed: (1) with the tested person standing vertically in front of the holographic camera system with no face muscle contractions; (2) in the same position, but

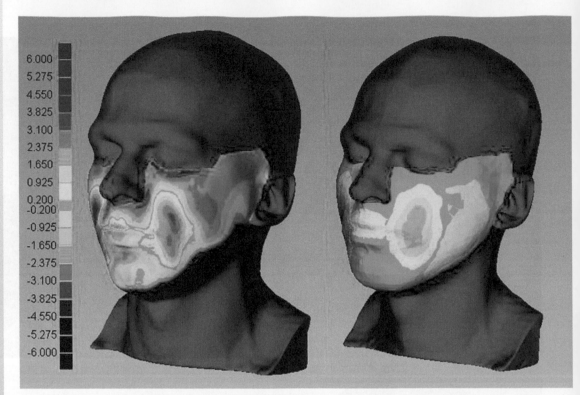

Fig. 5. Measured (*left*) and calculated (*right*) face surface displacement caused by gravity load. Colors indicate the distance of the deformed surface from the reference surface, in millimeters.

with a tube inserted between the lips and the subject blowing into it with a relative pressure of approximately 10 mbar (measured with a pressure sensor connected with the tube). The result of this experiment was the displacement field as the distance map between the face surfaces (1) and (2), **Fig. 7**B. Using the same color code, **Fig. 7**C reports the result of the corresponding FE simulation with overpressure applied inside the oral cavity. The comparison shows good qualitative correspondence, with the FE model providing lower displacement.

Pull-up Experiments

The basic principle for these experiments is to apply a given displacement vector on the skin surface, pulling the tissue in a predefined direction, and measure the corresponding time-dependent reaction force in a time interval. The setup used for this type of measurement is shown in **Fig. 8**. The system is designed to allow selection of the direction and magnitude of the pulling vector. The firm attachment to the skin was developed to minimize relative movement between pull-up device and face surface. To reduce unwanted movements, tested persons place their chins on a chin rest and their foreheads are stabilized

against the frame using a stiff elastic headband. The force transducer is connected to a computer. Measurements were performed on the jaw, midface, and parotid regions. The observed transient relaxation behavior is related to the time-dependent, dissipative response of the tissue, which is not considered in the mechanical model formation. Instead, the measured long-term reaction force is compared with the corresponding FE calculations (**Fig. 9**). The force values predicted by the model are in the right order of magnitude, but generally too high.

Cutometer and Aspiration Experiments

Two instruments based on the suction method were used for measuring the mechanical behavior of the superficial layers (ie, skin and SMAS) in 5 different regions of the face. The Cutometer MPA 580 applies negative pressure on the skin, which is drawn into the aperture of the probe (2 mm diameter). An optical system measures the elevation of the skin. Tests were performed in the jaw, nasolabial, parotid, zygomatic, and forehead regions (**Fig. 10**). A linearly increasing pressure from 0 to 500 mbar was applied at low rate. Details of the measurement protocol are reported by Barbarino and colleagues.[29] The aspiration device

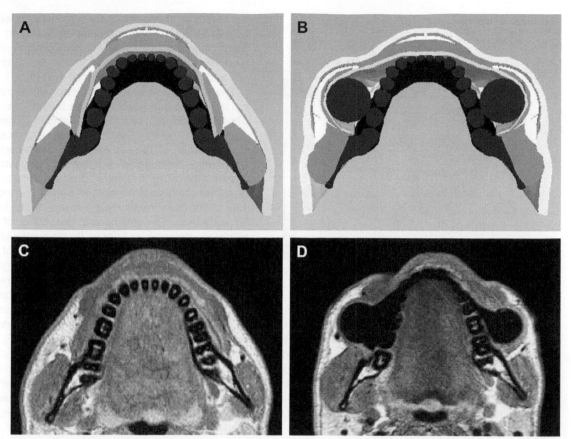

Fig. 6. Calculated (*A, B*) and measured (*C, D*) shape change caused by the insertion of wooden balls between cheeks and tooth.[21]

works with the same principle but has a larger aperture (8 mm), thus deeper tissues are involved in the suction experiment. Measurements were performed by the application of a linearly increasing pressure for 5 seconds, followed by a constant load for 30 seconds. The maximum elevation at the end of the measurement is considered as the long-term response of the tissue.

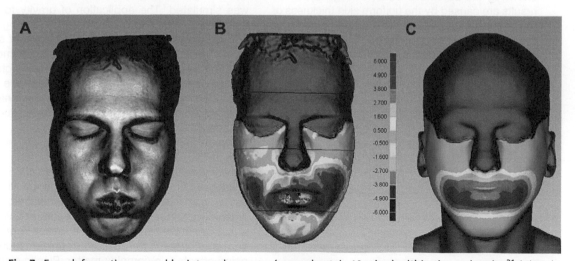

Fig. 7. Face deformation caused by internal pressure (approximately 10 mbar) within the oral cavity.[21] (*A*) Holographic measurements (*B*) and FE calculation (*C*) of outer skin displacement are displayed. Colors indicate the distance of the deformed surface from the reference surface, in millimeters.

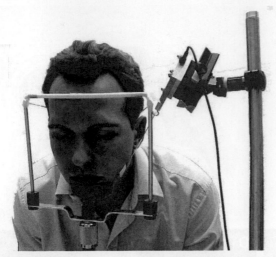

Fig. 8. Experimental setup for pull-up experiments.

The interpretation of the measured tissue deformation is based on the layered structure of the face, with the skin as the outermost layer and the SMAS plus the superficial fat as the next deeper layer. To investigate the specific layer morphology of the measurement locations in the parotid, forehead, and jaw regions, a set of high-resolution MRI images were acquired (Philips Achieva 1.5T scanner, in-plane resolution of the images is 0.1×0.1 mm, and the time needed for each slide was approximately 7 minutes), as shown in **Fig. 11**.

The results for soft tissue apex displacements are reported for Cutometer and aspiration device in **Figs. 12** and **13**. A homogeneous mechanical response of the skin in different face regions is shown by the Cutometer data (see **Fig. 12**). These results are caused by the uniform skin thickness of the regions tested. Measurements performed with the aspiration device (see **Fig. 13**) show a larger variability, probably related to the different thickness of

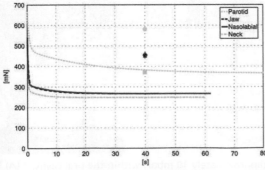

Fig. 9. Comparison of measured (*lines*) and calculated (*symbols*) pull-up forces.

the SMAS layer and the contribution of stiff deeper tissues, such as the masseter muscle and the parotid gland or the bone, or to the more compliant response of deep fat underneath the SMAS in the jaw and the zygomatic region (see **Fig. 11**).

The quantitative analysis for mechanical model parameter determination was based on the detailed anatomic information, used to generate a refined FE model of each measurement location for simulation of the experiments. A tied contact (no sliding, no opening) is assumed between the 2 layers, because it is known that the application of a force, and sometimes even cutting, is necessary to separate the tissue layers (eg, during facelift surgeries). The mechanical properties of the skin were determined from an iterative calculation of the response to the Cutometer experiment, for which the influence of the SMAS is negligible. The simulations of the aspiration measurements were used to characterize the SMAS, because the corresponding skin response was known. Specific constitutive model equations and related parameters are reported by Barbarino and colleagues.[29] In general, the observed response led to higher resistance to deformation for skin and for SMAS, compared with the mechanical parameters used for the simulations discussed earlier. This finding might be related to the nonzero in-vivo stress state of skin and SMAS.

Simulation of Gravimetric Soft Tissue Descent

The comparison of physical observations and simulations reported earlier showed that the FE model provides realistic representation of the mechanical behavior of the face. As a first application of this model, gravimetric soft tissue descent was simulated. The application of gravity forces for the face in the erect position leads to a progressive descent of soft tissue related to loss of stiffness of facial tissue, which is the most commonly held theory of facial aging.[24] Corresponding changes of shape in specific regions of the face are described in the literature, such as the deep nasolabial fold forming as a consequence of gravimetric descent.[24]

Fig. 14 represents the calculated displacement field in the vertical direction caused by long-term gravity loading. As detailed by Barbarino and colleagues,[21] the constitutive model of all soft tissue was modified for these calculations, with a general progressive reduction of stiffness, which is justified at the histologic level by tissue degradation processes.[31,32] Realistic representation of aging effects is a complex matter. Plastic surgery literature describes the overall mechanisms as being related to a reduction of firmness of the

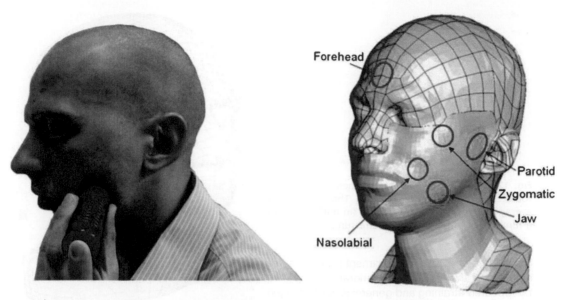

Fig. 10. Suction measurements on the face, with indication of the regions of application.[29]

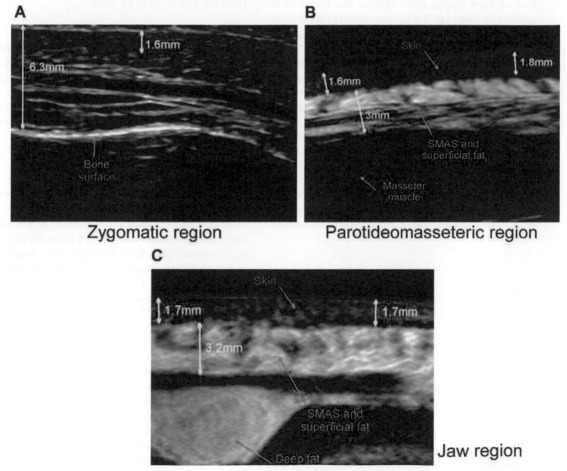

Fig. 11. Ultrasound (*A*) and MRI (*B, C*) images for local analysis of superficial layer configurations.[29] This information was used for the interpretation of local mechanical measurements with Cutometer and aspiration device.

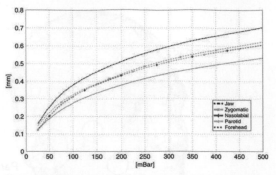

Fig. 12. Measurement results obtained with the Cutometer at different face locations. The curves show average values of tissue elevation (in millimeters) as a function of applied negative pressure.

SMAS and the retaining ligaments, and loss of stiffness of the skin. This deterioration is caused by repeated straining and general loss of collagen and elastin because of actinic damage and solar elastosis. The calculated gravimetric descent might be considered as a highly simplified description of face aging: other effects like increase in volume of deep fat; the accumulation of fat around the eyes, in the cheeks, and under the chin; lengthening of the musculature; laxity of the ligaments; and skeletal resorption[33,34] were not considered in the present model. Because of the limitations of the spatial resolution of the proposed model, the formation of wrinkles and skin folds could not be represented. Given all these limitations, it might be stated that the simulated face aging leads to plausible results: the region of maximum displacement is located at the jowl, between the chin and the masseter muscle; tissue descends also from the middle-cheek region. The modiolus and the upper lip undergo a small displacement compared with the cheek. The calculated displacement

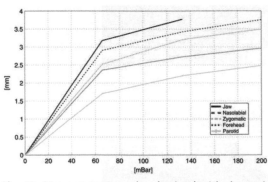

Fig. 13. Measurement results obtained with the aspiration device at different face locations. The curves show average values of tissue elevation (in millimeters) as a function of applied negative pressure.

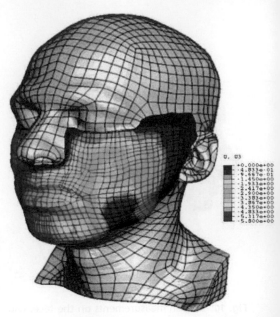

Fig. 14. Calculated soft tissue gravimetric descent.[21] Colors indicate vertical displacement (in millimeters) from the age of 30 to 60 years.

distributions are also in line with expectations concerning fold formation: a deeper nasolabial fold arises because of the pronounced relative displacement (descent) in the cheek region with respect to the tissue around the nose and mouth; the same applies to the vertical fold delimiting chin and cheek regions.

These qualitative considerations are also supported by a quantitative comparison between predicted gravimetric soft tissue descent and observed modification of face shape from a photographic aging database acquired and cataloged by Nkengne and colleagues,[35] based on photos of female volunteers. The photos were divided into age groups and then superposed, resulting in a series of average faces of the age window considered. The face contour was extracted, giving an average age-dependent facial external contour (Fig. 15). The FE results of the aging simulation, with progressive loss of tissue stiffness according to the tissue aging characteristics proposed by Mazza and colleagues,[26] were compared with these data. The magnitude of descent (for a selected point) predicted by the calculation and the calculated face contour transition from young to old agree with the data obtained from the analysis of the photos (see Fig. 15). These results validate the realism of the model prediction, and might be interpreted as a general confirmation of the theory of aging as characterized mainly by soft tissue gravimetric descent.

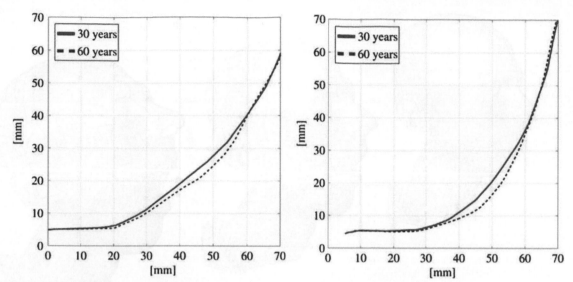

Fig. 15. Modification of facial external contour predicted using the FE model (*left*), and based on averaged photos of volunteers of different age groups (*right*).

DISCUSSION AND SUMMARY

The procedure for generation and validation of an FE model of the face have been described. It was shown that it is possible (1) to use detailed medical images for extracting information on the geometry of all soft tissue parts relevant to the mechanical behavior of the face; (2) to assign specific mechanical properties to all tissues considered representative of their nonlinear force-deformation characteristics; (3) to calculate 3D face deformations associated with the application of distributed or localized loads; (4) to evaluate the predictive capabilities of the proposed model through the comparison with a series of experiments on the face addressing global and local mechanical characteristics of facial soft tissue.

Calculation of gravimetric facial tissue descent provided an example of the application of the model, showing its predictive capabilities but also highlighting the limitations in the representation of a complex process such as facial aging. The representation of the corresponding face aging pattern is realistic. As part of our collaboration with J&J Medical, we are using the FE model to investigate aging-related volume redistribution within the face, as well as the corresponding restoring effect of surgical tissue repositioning procedures. The application of suture devices and supportive medical meshes is simulated to help optimize the design of devices and materials for plastic surgery.

Further potential use of the FE model includes the simulation of physiologic deformation of the face, for instance for the analysis of the mandible's kinematic (**Fig. 16**) for mastication or speech. The corresponding FE calculations can provide information on the distribution of stresses and deformations within soft facial tissue, and thus help understand the influence of each anatomic part on physiologic and pathologic conditions.

In collaboration with colleagues from the Co-Me research program (Swiss National Science Foundation) we use the FE model of the face for simulation of maxillofacial surgery. Barbarino and colleagues[36] present a calculation of the repositioning of maxilla and mandibula. The influence of the specific selection of mechanical model parameters for muscles and superficial layer on the calculated displacement of the outer surface is quantified. These results can provide useful information for the development of patient-specific numerical models for planning surgery. Within the Co-Me collaborative project, the FE model of the face provides benchmark results, thus complementing real preoperative and postoperative data for the validation of computer-based methods for patient-specific surgery simulation.

The results described earlier also highlight current limitations of this modeling technique, regarding the realism of the calculation:

1. The predicted resistance to deformation of facial soft tissue is overestimated. Local measurements of the mechanical behavior of skin and SMAS and parametric investigations on the influence of mesh refinement indicate that

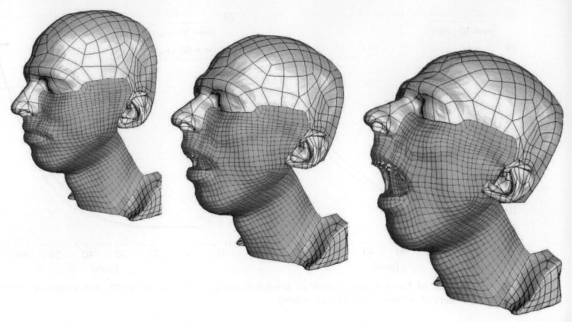

Fig. 16. (*Left* to *right*) Simulation of the backward rotation of the skull.

the stiff response is also associated with the insufficient level of spatial discretization of the present FE mesh.[36]

2. All mechanical measurements showed the significance of time-dependent effects in the mechanical behavior of facial tissue, which were neglected in the present model formulation.

3. The muscles are considered as passive, thus not allowing the investigation of the influence of muscle contraction on tissue response or the simulation of facial expressions.

4. Point 3 also involves simulation of wrinkle formation, which cannot be realized with the present mesh configuration. These problems are investigated in our current work to overcome the associated limitations.

The development of the present FE model involved a cumbersome and time-consuming procedure for the extraction and processing of anatomic data to generate a detailed FE mesh of the face. This approach makes it factually impossible to create individual FE models for patient-specific prediction of surgery outcomes. We are exploring alternative procedures for creating FE meshes of nonhomogeneous tissues based on a location-dependent assignment of material properties, as opposed to the explicit geometric representation of each single organ.

Optimization of the element formulation and numerical integration scheme is necessary to reduce the computation time: most of the simulation described in this article required several hours of computation on a standard computer. The determination of mechanical model parameters for each soft tissue in the patient's face also represents a formidable task, which currently impairs the realization of patient-specific FE simulations. To this end, suction experiments (tissue aspiration or Cutometer) and elastography techniques could provide useful information, without harm to the patient.

The present work shows the feasibility of physically based simulations of facial soft tissue deformation. Our results indicate that numerical simulation techniques might provide useful tools for the planning of esthetic or reconstructive surgery, or for the development of medical devices. This work also highlights significant limitations of the current model and challenging interdisciplinary problems that need to be solved before these tools become available for clinical use.

REFERENCES

1. Shen W, Niu Y, Mattrey RF, et al. Development and validation of subject-specific finite element models for blunt trauma study. J Biomech Eng 2008;130:021022.

2. Snedeker JG, Bajka M, Hug JM, et al. The creation of a high-fidelity finite element model of the kidney for use in trauma research. J Visual Comp Animat 2002;13(1):53–64.

3. Szekely G. Surgical simulators. Minim Invasive Ther Allied Technol 2003;12(1):14–8.

4. Puls M, Ecker TM, Tannast M, et al. The equidistant method: a novel hip joint simulation algorithm for detection of femoroacetabular impingement. Comput Aided Surg 2010;15(4–6):75–82.

5. Cevidanes LH, Tucker S, Styner M, et al. Three-dimensional surgical simulation. Am J Orthod Dentofacial Orthop 2010;138(3):361–71.

6. Terzopoulos D, Waters K. Physically-based facial modeling, analysis, and animation. J Visual Comp Animat 1990;1(2):73–80.

7. Rohrle O, Pullan AJ. Three-dimensional finite element modelling of muscle forces during mastication. J Biomech 2007;40(15):3363–72.

8. Gladilin E, Zachow S, Deuflhard P, et al. Anatomy- and physics-based facial animation for craniofacial surgery simulations. Med Biol Eng Comput 2004; 42(2):167–70.

9. Mollemans W, Schutyser F, Nadjmi N, et al. Predicting soft tissue deformations for a maxillofacial surgery planning system: from computational strategies to a complete clinical validation. Med Image Anal 2007;11(3):282–301.

10. Luboz V, Chabanas M, Swider P, et al. Orbital and maxillofacial computer aided surgery: patient-specific finite element models to predict surgical outcomes. Comput Methods Biomech Biomed Engin 2005;8(4):259–65.

11. Kovacs L, Zimmermann A, Wawrzyn H, et al. Computer aided surgical reconstruction after complex facial burns injuries-opportunities and limitations. Burns 2005;31(1):85–91.

12. Keeve E, Girod S, Kikinis R, et al. Deformable modeling of facial tissue for craniofacial surgery simulation. Comput Aided Surg 1998;3(5):228–38.

13. Meehan M, Teschner M, Girod S. Three-dimensional simulation and prediction of craniofacial surgery. Orthod Craniofac Res 2003;6(1):102–7.

14. Chabanas M, Luboz V, Payan Y. Patient specific finite element model of the face soft tissues for computer-assisted maxillofacial surgery. Med Image Anal 2003;7(2):131–51.

15. Zachow, S, Gladilin, E, Hege, HC, et al. Towards patient specific, anatomy based simulation of facial mimics for surgical nerve rehabilitation. Computer Assisted Radiology and Surgery, Paris: Springer; 2002. p. 3–6.

16. Nazari MA, Perrier P, Chabanas M, et al. Simulation of dynamic orofacial movements using a constitutive law varying with muscle activation. Comput Methods Biomech Biomed Engin 2010;13(4):469–82.

17. Chabanas M, Payan Y, Marecaux C, et al. Comparison of linear and non-linear soft tissue models with post-operative CT scan in maxillofacial surgery. Lect Notes Comput Sci 2004;3078:19–27.

18. Har-Shai Y, Bodner SR, Egozy-Golan D, et al. Mechanical properties and microstructure of the superficial musculoaponeurotic system. Plast Reconstr Surg 1996;98(1):59–70.

19. Mazza E, Papes O, Rubin MB, et al. Simulation of the aging face. ASME J Biomech Eng 2007;129(4):619–23.

20. Lee CF, Chen PR, Lee WJ, et al. Three- dimensional reconstruction and modeling of middle ear biomechanics by high-resolution computed tomography and finite element analysis. Laryngoscope 2006; 116(5):711–6.

21. Barbarino GG, Jabareen M, Trzewik J, et al. Development and validation of a three dimensional finite element model of the face. J Biomech Eng 2009; 131:041006.

22. Ghassemi A, Prescher A, Riediger D, et al. Anatomy of the SMAS revisited. Aesthetic Plast Surg 2003; 27(4):258–64.

23. Ferreira LM, Hochman B, Locali RF, et al. A stratigraphic approach to the superficial musculoaponeurotic system and its anatomic correlation with the superficial fascia. Aesthetic Plast Surg 2006;30(5):549–52.

24. La Trenta G. Aesthetic face & neck surgery. Philadelphia: Saunders; 2004.

25. Rubin MB, Bodner SR. A three-dimensional nonlinear model for dissipative response of soft tissue. Int J Solids Struct 2002;39(19):5081–99.

26. Mazza E, Papes O, Rubin MB, et al. Nonlinear elastic-viscoplastic constitutive equations for aging facial tissues. Biomech Model Mechanobiol 2005; 4(2–3):178–89.

27. Duck FA. Physical properties of tissue: a comprehensive reference book. London: Academic Press; 1990.

28. Barbarino GG, Jabareen M, Mazza E. Experimental and numerical study of the relaxation behavior of facial soft tissue. Proc Appl Math Mech 2009;9:87–90.

29. Barbarino GG, Jabareen M, Mazza E. Experimental and numerical study on the mechanical behaviour of the superficial layers of the face. Skin Res Technol. [Online]. DOI:10.1111/j.16000846.2011.00515.x.

30. Heintz S, Hirsch S, Thelen A, et al. Three-dimensional surface measurement using digital holography with pulsed lasers, advances in medical engineering. Berlin: Springer; 2007. p. 435–40.

31. Craven NM, Watson RE, Jones CJ, et al. Clinical features of photoaged human skin are associated with a reduction in collagen VII. Br J Dermatol 1997;137:344–50.

32. Fleischmajer R, Perlish JS, Bashey RI. Human dermal glycosaminoglycans and aging. Biochim Biophys Acta 1972;279:265–75.

33. Coleman SR, Grover R. The anatomy of the aging face: volume loss and changes in 3-dimensional topography. Aesthet Surg J 2006;26:S4–9.

34. Albert AM, Ricanek K, Patterson E. A review of the literature on the aging adult skull and face: implications for forensic science research and applications. Forensic Sci Int 2007;172(1):1–9.

35. Nkengne A, Bertin C, Stamatas GN, et al. Influence of facial skin attributes on the perceived age of Caucasian women. J Eur Acad Dermatol Venereol 2008;22:982–91.

36. Barbarino GG. Modeling the mechanical behavior of the face. PhD thesis, N. 19551. Zurich: ETH; 2011.

3D Video Analysis of Facial Movements

Manfred Frey, MD*, Chieh-Han John Tzou, MD,
Maria Michaelidou, MD, Igor Pona, MD,
Alina Hold, MD, Eva Placheta, MD,
Hugo B. Kitzinger, MD

KEYWORDS

- 3D video analysis • Facial movements
- Facial paralysis • Gracilis muscle transplantation
- Masseter muscle transposition • Three-dimensional

The exact local extent and degree of facial paralysis as well as their implications on the different functions of the mimetic muscle system, on the aesthetic appearance of the face, and on the patient's sequelae are difficult to assess. The authors' first experiences with the International Muscle Transplant Registry[1] had shown that the traditional scoring systems for facial palsy are not suitable for an exact and scientific evaluation. As a consequence the authors concentrated research on the possibilities of 3-dimensional (3D) measuring of movements in the face during standardized mimic activities initially using a VICON videosystem,[2] and later a digital caliper (Faciometer) developed in tight cooperation with the Laboratory for Biomechanics of the Swiss Federal Institute of Technology, Zurich.[3]

However, from the beginning it was the authors' aim to document the facial movements by taking standardized videos and to quantify the facial movements by computer-assisted 3D analysis of the video film. This idea was realized by a completely new development.[4]

METHODS

The equipment consists in its entirety of a system for taking videos in front of two special mirrors arranged at a sharp angle, a calibration grid, a digital video camera, and a computer workstation. For this system the video is transferred to the hard disk to prepare the selected sequences by an editing program for analysis. When the real image and the two mirror images in all single pictures have been analyzed point by point by the computer, these final data are stored on a compact disk (CD). A visualization program gives easy access to the stored data.

Taking the Video

At first the standardized static and dynamic points to be measured are marked in the face. The 3 static points (tragus points of both sides and the central nose point) define a triangle, to which all dynamic points are related during the facial movements. The definitions of the static and dynamic points are explained further in an article

This work was supported by a grant from the Austrian Ministry for Education, Science and Culture within the project "International Reference Center for Neuromuscular Reconstruction in the Face".

The authors have nothing to disclose.

Division of Plastic and Reconstructive Surgery, Department of Surgery, Medical University of Vienna, Waehringer Guertel 18-20, A-1090 Vienna, Austria

* Corresponding author.

E-mail address: manfred.frey@meduniwien.ac.at

published in 1994.[2] To calibrate the system a calibration grid is brought between the two mirrors and is filmed. Afterwards, the head of the patient is positioned between two mirrors arranged at a sharp angle. By this method a frontal image and side-view mirror images from the left and right side of the patient's face are taken by the camera, including all marked points. All standardized facial movements[2] are now recorded by the video camera 3 times:

1. Maximal lifting of the eyebrows
2. Closing of the eyes as if for sleeping
3. Maximal closing of the eyes
4. Maximal showing of the teeth
5. Maximal closing of the eyes and showing of the teeth at the same time
6. Smiling with showing the teeth
7. Smiling with closed lips
8. Pursing the lips and whistling
9. Pulling the corners of the mouth downwards.

To document the influence of the facial palsy on speech the video with sound track is continued, while the patient counts from 1 to 10 and pronounces his or her name and address.

3D Analysis of the Video

After transferring the digital video film from the camera to the computer picture by picture, all static and dynamic points of the face in the frontal and the two mirror views are marked with the cursor of the mouse in a constant order indicated by the program. The measurement has to be calibrated by doing the same to one picture of the calibration grid and its two mirror images. After this has been done for all standardized facial movements, the data are recorded on a CD.

Visualization of Patient Data

A visualization program gives easy access to the data. The change of the distance over time of any 2 standardized points can be shown on a graph for each of the standardized movements and for both sides of the face. An exact measurement can be performed at each phase of the movement. Parallel to this a video clip of this movement can be reviewed, or the picture of the resting face and the picture of the maximum of this movement can be seen. A qualitative documentation in the video clip occurs in parallel with a quantitative measurement.

By way of 2-dimensional (2D) graphs, the movement of each dynamic point is visualized for each of the movements. The movement of all points can be shown 3-dimensionally at the same time and for each of the standardized facial movements.

Changes in speech can also be observed on the acoustic track by comparison of the recordings during the different video sessions.

RESULTS

The design of the mirror system has been shown to be suitable for children as well as for different sizes of adults. The dimensions and the angle between the two mirrors has never limited the possibility to have the frontal view and both mirror images of the face on the same picture.

The algorithm to reconstruct the 3D points used is a modified Tsai algorithm.[5] This algorithm compensates the lens distortion but not the distortion of the mirrors. If 2 points with a distance of 50 mm are measured, the accuracy of the distance is better than $\pm$ 0.25 mm. If the distance is smaller, the accuracy is even better. The reproducibility of a point is better than $\pm$ 0.2 mm.

DISCUSSION

Most techniques to document and measure facial movements developed during the past 10 years are not able to give a detailed insight into the actual function of the facial muscles.[1] Even in recent reports on the functional outcome of large series of free muscle transplantation for facial paralysis, the authors' documentation system was not used for functional assessment although it was published as early as 1994.[2,6–10] Information indicates that the authors were the first to use 3D tracing of skin surface markers to analyze facial movements for the first time; this technique was published in 1992[1] followed by a more extensive description in 1994.[2] At that time the authors also developed the Faciometer, an electronic caliper system for easy clinical application. This simple instrument for 3D measurements fulfilled an important role during standardized quantification of facial paralysis and its improvement by surgical treatment within the International Registry for Neuromuscular Reconstructions in the Face.[3] Because of disadvantages, including the necessary contact with the skin of the patient, the patient-fatiguing process of measuring, the missing possibility of later data analysis, and the missing correlate to the quality of the facial movements, the authors pursued further development and refinement of the system.

The new mirror system was the great breakthrough, because it was the basis for 3D analysis of a video. Instead of multiple cameras, the two mirrors add two perspectives of the moving face. The frontal view of the face together with the two mirror images on one video film are not only used for 3D measurements of the different standardized facial movements, but also give an insight into the quality of the facial movements from 3 different views at the same time. A very complex computer program has been developed for analysis of the videos.[4]

Visualization of the analyzed data is easy and quick for all movements recorded. The movement of a selected single point in the paralyzed side of the face can be displayed on a 2D graph (x,y; x,z; or y,z axes) and compared with the corresponding point on the healthy side. The changes of the distance between any 2 points documented can be shown on a graph for any of the facial movements. Selecting a representative distance for each of the facial movements is important.[2] In the authors' opinion this kind of presentation, together with pictures of the resting position and position of maximum movement, seems to be ideal for publication of a functional result for a patient. A video clip of every movement can be reviewed and stopped at any point in time during the movement, to be studied in more detail. 3D graphs of the displacement of all registered points during a selected facial movement give a good survey on the dynamics of the face, the degree of asymmetry, and on synkinesis eventually initiated by this facial movement.

CLINICAL EXPERIENCE
Decision-Making Process with the Help of 3D Video Analysis, Part One: Dynamic Reconstruction of Eye Closure by Muscle Transposition or Functional Muscle Transplantation?

Using the aforementioned technique the authors performed the first quantitative study of 3D preoperative and postoperative eyelid movements in patients treated for facial paralysis.[11] Between February 1998 and April 2002, 44 patients were treated for facial palsy, including reconstruction of eye closure. Temporalis muscle transposition to the eye was used in 34 cases, and a regionally differentiated part of a free gracilis muscle transplant after double cross-face nerve grafting was used in 10 cases. Patients' facial movements were documented by the authors' video-analysis system preoperatively and 6, 12, 18, and 24 months postoperatively. For this comparative study, only the data of patients with preoperative and 12-month postoperative measurements were included (**Figs. 1–4**).

In the 27 patients with a final result after temporalis muscle transposition for eye closure, the distance between the upper and lower eyelid points during eye closing (as for sleep) was reduced

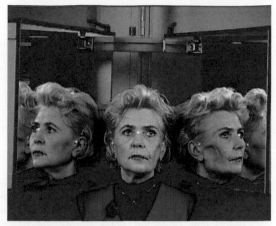

Fig. 1. A 48-year-old patient with left-sided complete and irreversible facial palsy after wide excision of a squamous cell carcinoma infiltrating the parotid gland and zygomatic bone, before the functional reconstruction: resting position of the face as positioned between the two mirrors.

from 10.33 ± 2.43 mm (mean ± SD) preoperatively to 5.84 ± 4.34 mm postoperatively on the paralyzed side, compared with 0.0 ± 0.0 mm preoperatively and postoperatively on the contralateral healthy side. In the resting position, preoperative valuesfor the paralyzed side changed from 15.11 ± 1.92 mm preoperatively to 13.46 ± 1.94 mm postoperatively, compared with 12.17 ± 2.02 mm preoperatively and 12.05 ± 1.95 mm postoperatively on the healthy side. In the 9 patients with a final result after surgery using a part of the

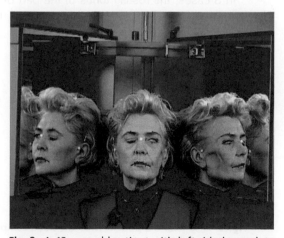

Fig. 2. A 48-year-old patient with left-sided complete and irreversible facial palsy after wide excision of a squamous cell carcinoma infiltrating the parotid gland and zygomatic bone, before the functional reconstruction: the face as seen at the end point of the movement "closing the eyes like for sleep."

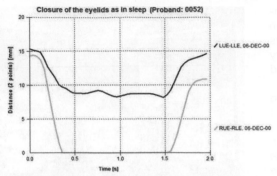

Fig. 3. A 48-year-old patient with left-sided complete and irreversible facial palsy after wide excision of a squamous cell carcinoma infiltrating the parotid gland and zygomatic bone, before the functional reconstruction: the course of motion "closing the eyes like for sleep" demonstrated 2-dimensionally as distance of the upper to the lower eyelid point during the time. The green curve represents the healthy right eye and the blue curve represents the paralyzed left eye. The extent of the preoperative lagophthalmus can be read directly off the curve, and reaches in this case 8.29 mm.

free gracilis muscle transplant reinnervated by a zygomatic branch of the contralateral healthy side through a cross-face nerve graft, eyelid closure achieved was from 10.21 ± 2.72 mm during rest to 1.68 ± 1.35 mm when closed, compared with 13.70 ± 1.56 mm to 6.63 ± 1.51 mm preoperatively. The average closure for the healthy side was from 11.20 ± 3.11 mm to 0.0 ± 0.0 mm preoperatively and from 12.70 ± 1.95 mm to 0.0 ± 0.0 mm postoperatively (**Figs. 5–8**).

In 3 cases, the resting tonus of the part of the gracilis muscle transplant around the eye had

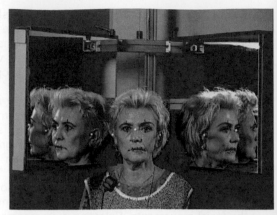

Fig. 5. The same patient 16 months after reconstruction of the ocular sphincter by a territorially differentiated gracilis muscle transplant innervated by 2 separate cross-face nerve grafts, during the movement "closing the eyes like for sleep": resting position of the face as positioned between the two mirrors.

increased to an extent that muscle weakening became necessary. Temporalis muscle transposition and free functional muscle transplantation for reanimation of the eye and mouth at the same time are reliable methods for reconstructing eye closure, with clinically adequate results. Detailed analysis of the resulting facial movements led to an important improvement in the authors' operative techniques within the last few years, thus enabling the number of secondary operative corrections to be significantly reduced. These qualitative and quantitative studies of the

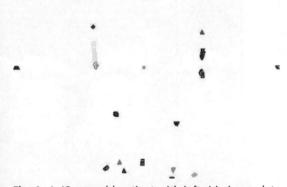

Fig. 4. A 48-year-old patient with left-sided complete and irreversible facial palsy after wide excision of a squamous cell carcinoma infiltrating the parotid gland and zygomatic bone, before the functional reconstruction: the excursion of all marked points of the face during the same movement are demonstrated in a 3D graph of the whole face.

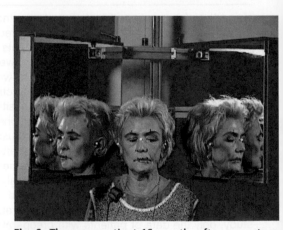

Fig. 6. The same patient 16 months after reconstruction of the ocular sphincter by a territorially differentiated gracilis muscle transplant innervated by 2 separate cross-face nerve grafts, during the movement "closing the eyes like for sleep": the face as seen at the end point of the movement "closing the eyes like for sleep."

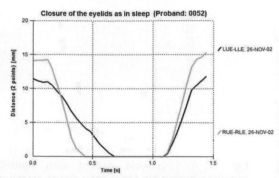

Fig. 7. The same patient 16 months after reconstruction of the ocular sphincter by a territorially differentiated gracilis muscle transplant innervated by 2 separate cross-face nerve grafts, during the movement "closing the eyes like for sleep": the course of motion "closing the eyes like for sleep" is demonstrated 2-dimensionally as distance of the upper to the lower eyelid point during the time. The blue curve represents the healthy right eye and the green curve represents the paralyzed left eye. The extent of eyelid closure is for both eyes complete, and the width of the eye fissure reaches at both sides 0 mm at the end point of motion.

reconstructed lid movements by 3D video analysis support the clinical concept of temporalis muscle transposition being the first-choice method in adult patients with facial palsy. In children, free muscle transplantation is preferred for eye closure, so as not to interfere with the growth of the face by transposition of a masticatory muscle. In addition, a higher degree of central plasticity in children might be expected.

Decision-Making Process with the Help of 3D Video Analysis, Part Two: Reconstruction of a Smile with Muscle Transposition or Muscle Transplantation?

In two other studies the authors tried to quantify the average of the functional recovery of the smile after muscle transposition[12] as well as after muscle transplantation.[13] Muscle transplantation is performed in their department by free gracilis muscle transplantation either as a single graft for the mouth or as a territorially differentiated graft for the mouth and the eye. Muscle transposition is performed by means of the masseter muscle.

The study of masseter transposition for smile reconstruction included 8 patients with final results.[12] The low number of patients resulted from the authors' priority for free functional muscle transplantation, and their indication for muscle transposition to the mouth being restricted to patients older than 60 years or to patients with limited life expectancy.

In this group of patients static asymmetry of the mouth corner improved from 14.17 ± 5.26 mm preoperatively to 5.38 ± 3.23 mm postoperatively. The index of dynamic symmetry improved from −0.17 ± 0.25 preoperatively to 0.18 ± 0.19 postoperatively. This result means that postoperatively, the amplitude of motion on the reconstructed side reached 18% ± 19% that of the amplitude on the healthy side, whereas preoperatively a shift of the paralyzed mouth corner toward the healthy side occurred.

The final results of 31 patients with irreversible unilateral facial paralysis treated by gracilis muscle

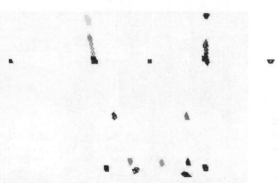

Fig. 8. The same patient 16 months after reconstruction of the ocular sphincter by a territorially differentiated gracilis muscle transplant innervated by 2 separate cross-face nerve grafts, during the movement "closing the eyes like for sleep": the excursion of all marked points of the face during the same movement is demonstrated in a 3D graph of the whole face. Upper and lower lid point meet at the end point of motion at both eyes, and no synkinesia is observed.

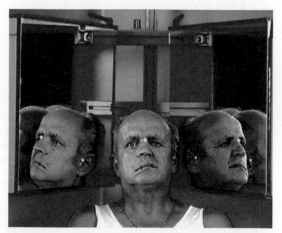

Fig. 9. A 53-year-old patient with right-sided complete irreversible facial palsy due to resection of a cholesteatoma of the right middle ear, during the movement "smiling with showing of the teeth" before the functional reconstruction: resting position of the face as positioned between the two mirrors.

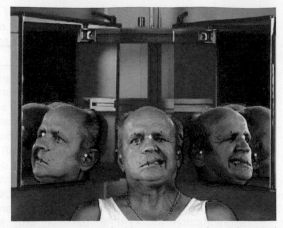

Fig. 10. A 53-year-old patient with right-sided complete irreversible facial palsy due to resection of a cholesteatoma of the right middle ear, during the movement "smiling with showing of the teeth" before the functional reconstruction: the face as seen at the end point of the movement "smiling with showing of the teeth."

transplantation between 1997 and 2006 were documented by 3D video analysis and published 2008.[13] Twenty-two patients had reinnervation completed by a single cross-face nerve graft and a free gracilis muscle graft for reconstruction of

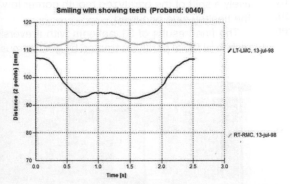

Fig. 11. A 53-year-old patient with right-sided complete irreversible facial palsy due to resection of a cholesteatoma of the right middle ear, during the movement "smiling with showing of the teeth" before the functional reconstruction: the course of motion "smiling with showing of the teeth" is demonstrated 2-dimensionally as distance of the mouth corner to the tragus in the course of time. The blue curve represents the distance of the healthy left mouth corner from the left tragus and the green curve represents the distance of the paralyzed right mouth corner from the right tragus. The preoperative excursion of motion reaches 14.02 mm on the left side, whereas the excursion on the right side follows a nonanatomic pattern and reaches −2.61 mm.

Fig. 12. A 53-year-old patient with right-sided complete irreversible facial palsy due to resection of a cholesteatoma of the right middle ear, during the movement "smiling with showing of the teeth" before the functional reconstruction: the excursion of all marked points of the face during the same movement is shown in a 3D graph.

the smile, and 9 patients had been treated with 2 cross-face nerve grafts followed by a territorially differentiated gracilis muscle transplant for reconstruction of the smile and eye closure. Smiling with showing of teeth, maximal showing of teeth, and closing of eyes as in sleep were analyzed in detail (**Figs. 9–12**).

In the group of patients with the gracilis muscle graft for smile reconstruction alone, static asymmetry was reduced from 12.19 ± 8.73 mm preoperatively to −1.84 ± 7.67 mm at 18 months postoperatively. Smile amplitude increased from 9% to 60% of that on the healthy side in 10 incomplete facial palsies of this group, and

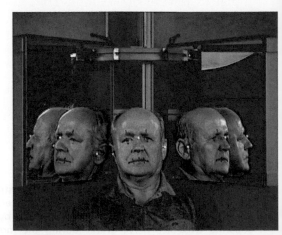

Fig. 13. The same patient 4.5 years after reconstruction of the smile with a free gracilis muscle transplant innervated by a cross-face nerve graft, during the movement "smiling with showing of the teeth": resting position of the face as positioned between the two mirrors.

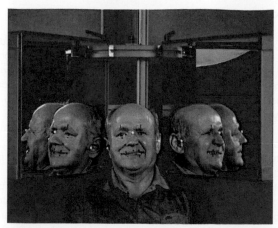

Fig. 14. The same patient 4.5 years after reconstruction of the smile with a free gracilis muscle transplant innervated by a cross-face nerve graft, during the movement "smiling with showing of the teeth": the face as seen at the end point of the movement "smiling with showing of the teeth."

from 0% to 62% in 8 functionally successful muscle grafts among 11 patients with complete lesions.

When the free gracilis muscle transplant had been used for smile reconstruction and for functional reconstruction of the eye sphincter at

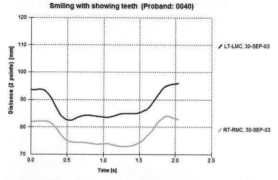

Fig. 15. The same patient 4.5 years after reconstruction of the smile with a free gracilis muscle transplant innervated by a cross-face nerve graft, during the movement "smiling with showing of the teeth": the course of motion "smiling with showing of the teeth" is demonstrated 2-dimensionally as distance of the mouth corner to the tragus in the course of time. The blue curve represents the distance of the healthy left mouth corner from the left tragus, and the green curve represents the distance of the paralyzed right mouth corner from the right tragus. The amplitude of motion on the healthy left side reaches 11.46 mm and on the reconstructed right side 9.03 mm. The curves show a parallel course, due to the emotional coupling of both sides of the mouth through the cross-face nerve transplant.

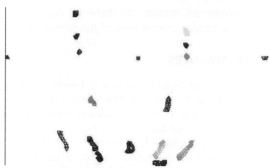

Fig. 16. The same patient 4.5 years after reconstruction of the smile with a free gracilis muscle transplant innervated by a cross-face nerve graft, during the movement "smiling with showing of the teeth": the excursion of all marked points of the face during the same facial movement is demonstrated in a 3D graph. No pathologic synkinesia is observed.

the same time, static asymmetry improved from 7.24 ± 12.64 mm to −5.36 ± 9.07 mm; the overcorrection was intentional. Both smile movement and eye closure were improved in 8 of the 9 patients studied; one patient recovered for eye closure alone. Smile amplitude reached 68% ± 43% of that on the normal side. Lagophthalmus improved from 7.21 ± 3.59 mm to 1.38 ± 2.49 mm. All improvements were statistically significant ($P \leq .05$) (Figs. 13–16).

SUMMARY

The authors found out that static asymmetry can be improved by all 3 methods equivalently. Muscle transplantation provides significantly larger amplitude of motion than muscle transposition, and greater improvement in the dynamic symmetry of the face. Nevertheless, the dynamic improvement obtained by muscle transposition renders this concept superior to static reconstruction procedures alone. The additional gracilis muscle segment for reconstruction of the ocular sphincter does not negatively influence the perioral muscle function. Overall, muscle transplantation is superior to muscle transposition. Nonetheless, muscle transposition can be applied with good results in the elderly patient, who does not qualify for the larger microsurgical procedure for reconstruction.

3D video analysis provided an exact quantitative documentation of the degree of facial palsy preoperatively and the reconstructed movements on the originally paralyzed side of the face. The option of viewing a video clip of the same facial analyzed movement allows simultaneous quantitative and qualitative comparisons of functional results.

REFERENCES

1. Frey M, Sing D, Harii K, et al. Free muscle transplantation for treatment of facial palsy. First experiences with the International Muscle Transplant Registry. Eur J Plast Surg 1991;14:212.
2. Frey M, Jenny A, Giovanoli P, et al. Development of a new documentation system for facial movements as a basis for the International Registry for Neuromuscular Reconstruction in the Face. Plast Reconstr Surg 1994;93:1334–9.
3. Giovanoli P, Frey M, Stuessi E. The improvement of facial paralysis assessment by the use of the faciometer. In: Frey M, Giovanoli P, editors. Proceedings of the 4th International Muscle Symposium. Zurich (Switzerland): March 23–25, 1995.
4. Frey M, Giovanoli P, Gerber H, et al. 3-D analysis of facial movements by video analysis—a new method to assess the quantity and the quality of the smile. Plast Reconstr Surg 1999;104:2032–9.
5. Tsai R. An efficient and accurate camera calibration technique for 3D machine vision. Proceedings of IEEE Conference on Computer Vision and Pattern Recognition. Miami Beach (FL): 1986.
6. Terzis JK, Noah ME. Analysis of 100 cases of free-muscle transplantation for facial paralysis. Plast Reconstr Surg 1997;99:1905–21.
7. Ueda K, Harii K, Asato H, et al. Neurovascular free muscle transfer combined with cross-face nerve grafting for the treatment of facial paralysis in children. Plast Reconstr Surg 1998;101:1765–73.
8. Cacou C, Greenfield BE, Richards R, et al. Studies of co-ordinated lower facial muscle function by electromyography and surface laser scanning techniques. In: Frey M, Giovanoli P, editors. Proceedings of the 4th International Muscle Symposium. Zurich (Switzerland): March 23–25, 1995.
9. Johnson PC, Brown H, Kuzon WM, et al. Simultaneous quantification of facial movements: the maximal static response assay of facial nerve function. Ann Plast Surg 1994;32:171–9.
10. Bajaj-Luthra A, Mueller T, Johnson PC. Quantitative analysis of facial motion components: anatomic and nonanatomic motion in normal persons and in patients with complete facial paralysis. Plast Reconstr Surg 1997;99:1894–902.
11. Frey M, Giovanoli P, Tzou CH, et al. Dynamic reconstruction of eye closure by muscle transposition or functional muscle transplantation in facial palsy. Plast Reconstr Surg 2004;114:865–75.
12. Michaelidou M, Tzou CH, Gerber H, et al. The combination of muscle transpositions and static procedures for reconstruction in the paralyzed face of the patient with limited life expectancy or who is not a candidate for free muscle transfer. Plast Reconstr Surg 2009;123:121–9.
13. Frey M, Michaelidou M, Tzou CH, et al. Three-dimensional video analysis of the paralyzed face reanimated by cross-face nerve grafting and free gracilis muscle transplantation: quantification of h functional outcome. Plast Reconstr Surg 2008;122:1709–22.

Custom-Made, 3D, Intraoperative Surgical Guides for Nasal Reconstruction

Babar Sultan, MD, Patrick J. Byrne, MD*

KEYWORDS

- Nasal reconstruction • 3D technology • Anaplastology
- Intraoperative guide • Three-dimensional

The reconstruction of total or subtotal nasal defects can be an extremely daunting task. It is essential to abide by the principles of nasal subunit anatomy and the 3 layers of reconstruction: vascularized inner lining flaps, rigid framework, and the external skin lining.[1] The ideal is to reapproximate the original functional and aesthetic characteristics. The 3-dimensional (3D) nature of the nose requires careful attention to lifelike dimensions and surface contour while guarding against scar contracture and asymmetric healing. The accurate recreation of the 3D anatomy of the nose is fairly straightforward in most nasal defects created by skin cancer resections and trauma, because most defects spare the majority of the nose, such as the contralateral side. Thus there exists a visible 3D reference. The challenge is vastly greater in subtotal and particularly total nasal defects. When the entire nose (including the nasal septum) is removed, it is very difficult to envision accurately the 3D anatomy, including the accurate relationship of the nasal structures to the surrounding facial anatomy. Various strategies have been proposed to navigate the small margin of error for successful outcomes. The authors present their use of an intraoperative surgical guide for reconstruction of full-thickness, complex nasal defects, created by 3D laser surface scanning and rapid prototyping (RP). This guide increases the ease and accuracy of creating the subsurface framework and highlights the increasing role of technology in surgical advancement. The development of this sterile, translucent template requires the multidisciplinary team of a surgeon and anaplastologist in close cooperation with the patient.

ANAPLASTOLOGY

An anaplastologist specializes in the prosthetic rehabilitation of absent or disfigured aesthetically critical portions of the body such as the ear and nose.[2] Certification in anaplastology is provided by the Board for Certification in Clinical Anaplastology (BCCA), and requires studies in the arts and sciences. Specifically photography, illustration, sculpture, superficial anatomy, and polymer science are emphases of study. The authors' institution has a facial prosthetics clinic staffed by a certified clinical anaplastologist (CCA) in which one can provide prostheses as an alternative to surgical reconstruction for total nasal defects. Patients with full-thickness complex nasal defects are referred by the senior author to the CCA in the

---

The authors have nothing to disclose.
Department of Otolaryngology-Head and Neck Surgery, Johns Hopkins School of Medicine, 6th Floor, 601 North Caroline Street, 6252, Baltimore, MD 21287, USA
* Corresponding author.
E-mail address: pbyrne2@jhmi.edu

Facial Plast Surg Clin N Am 19 (2011) 647–653
doi:10.1016/j.fsc.2011.07.008

Johns Hopkins Department of Art as Applied to Medicine for consultation. The CCA, in careful consultation with the patient and through use of predefect photographs, constructs a model of the patient's original nose using wax (**Fig. 1**). This model is approved by both the surgeon and the patient, and a duplicate is formed. At this point, the senior surgeon defines the subunits of the nose and the outer perimeter (**Fig. 2**). The model is then sent to Direct Dimensions, Inc (Owings Mills, MD) for creation of the intraoperative surgical guide.

CREATION OF THE TRANSLUCENT 3D INTRAOPERATIVE GUIDE
Direct Dimensions, Inc

Direct Dimensions, Inc (DDI) has expertise in the application of geometric measurement technology. Employing techniques in data measurement, inspection, and reverse engineering, DDI can digitally "clone" a 3-dimensional product.

3D Data Acquisition

There are multiple ways to collect 3D data, but two of the most common methods are laser scanning and digitizing. During laser scanning, surface data are captured by a camera sensor mounted in the laser scanner recording accurate dense 3D points in space. This noncontact-based method of acquisition includes subtypes such as laser

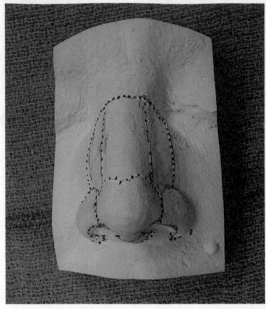

Fig. 2. After the wax model is approved by the patient and surgeon, a duplicate is made and the nasal subunits and outer perimeter are defined.

line, patch, and spherical. The surface laser scanner used for the authors' nasal prostheses is from Perceptron Laser Scanning Systems (Plymouth, MI). The machinery for surface laser scanning costs approximately $80,000, and requires a year of training and experience to operate it effectively.

Digitizing involves contacting a probe on various points on the surface of the object to collect 3D information. Unlike laser scanning, which collects a large area of points at one time, digitizing allows one to record individual data points. This method is more accurate for defining the geometric form of an object rather than organic freeform shapes. Recently, photo-image–based systems are being used more frequently in 3D scanning.

3D Data Analysis

Digital modeling is the process of creating a computer model of an object that exactly replicates the form of the object. The surface laser scanner produces 3D point cloud data, and using PolyWorks software (Inovmetric Software, Inc, Quebec City, QC, Canada), a 3D polygonal model is created. A polygonal model is a faceted model consisting of many triangles formed by connecting the points within the cloud data. This software costs approximately $15,000, and requires 2 years of training and experience to operate effectively.

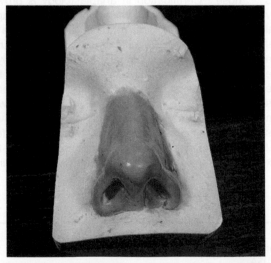

Fig. 1. The certified clinical anaplastologist, in careful consultation with the patient and using predefect photographs, constructs a model of the patient's original nose using wax.

Rapid Prototyping

The digital 3D model is divided into vertical thirds and offset from the external surface contour. Because the intraoperative guide is only supposed to approximate the subsurface framework, there is reduction in height to accommodate for the eventual placement of the paramedian forehead flap. The top third is often left unaltered, the middle third is offset by 1 mm, and the bottom third is offset 1.5 to 2 mm. These parameters may be subject to change, given unique elements of the defect and individual variability in skin thickness. Once the surgeon and anaplastologist approve of the digital model, a rapid prototype is made of a semitransparent resin material. The machine that produces the rapid prototype retails for approximately $80,000, and requires 3 months of training and experience to operate effectively. During surgical reconstruction, to be discussed later, it has been found that it is easier to use a translucent guide as opposed to a semitransparent guide (**Fig. 3**). To do this, a negative is made of the semitransparent mold and a 1.5 mm thick thermoforming clear baseplate is then vacuformed over the negative model. Trimming is done as necessary, and openings are made for the nostril. The template is sterilized for intraoperative use with cold sterilization (using iodine solution; STERRAD Sterilization Systems, Advanced Sterilization Products, Miami, FL). The overall cost for an individual nasal intraoperative guide is approximately $1100, broken down as follows: $250 for laser scanning, $650 for software analysis, and $250 for production of the rapid prototype.

SURGICAL RECONSTRUCTION

Reconstruction is guided by recreating the 3 layers of the nose: vascularized inner lining flaps, rigid

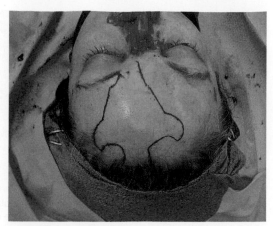

Fig. 4. The paramedian forehead flap is primarily used to form the external skin lining, as shown outlined in this patient.

framework, and the external skin lining with respect for nasal subunits. As mentioned earlier, the paramedian forehead flap is used to form the external skin lining (**Fig. 4**). Aluminum foil is used to create the template for the forehead flap, which is done by molding the foil over the model nose and then flattening the template into 2 dimensions onto the forehead (**Fig. 5**). The inner lining of the reconstructed nose has to be well vascularized, and the method is guided by patient anatomy. Reconstructive methods commonly used by the authors' group include septal mucosa flaps, tunneled galeal flaps, nasal turn-in flaps, or free tissue transfer. The intraoperative guide is used to guide the

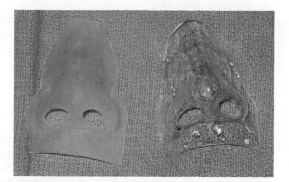

Fig. 3. On the left is a rapid prototype made of a semitransparent resin material from the digital model. During surgical reconstruction, it is easier to use a translucent guide (*right*) as opposed to a semitransparent guide.

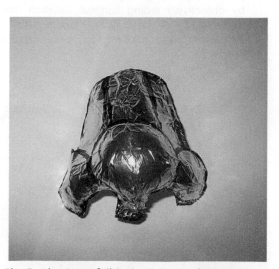

Fig. 5. Aluminum foil is draped over the intraoperative nasal guide and then flattened over the forehead to have the appropriate dimensions for the paramedian forehead flap.

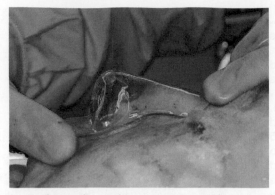

Fig. 6. The sterile nasal intraoperative guide is placed over the defect to guide the construction of the rigid framework.

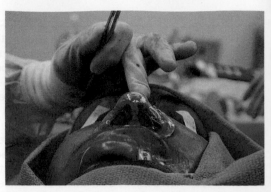

Fig. 8. The nasal intraoperative guide is used throughout the procedure to ensure the accuracy of the width and projection of the rigid framework.

construction of the rigid framework (**Fig. 6**). Cartilage is harvested from the rib and ear, and a stable L-shaped strut is constructed, which can be shaped as a caudal septal extension graft or an open framework L-shaped strut. The nasal tip is then constructed starting at the nasal base (**Fig. 7**). The surgical template guides the surgeon regarding the patient's unique needs for projection and dimension (**Fig. 8**), including how the nose relates to the rest of the facial structures (its orientation in space, rotation, and so forth). In addition, the use of the translucent guide is then used to create the fine detail of the nasal tip. Additional layers of cartilage micrografts are used to fill in the surgical template while ensuring the framework is structurally sound. The use of the intraoperative guide greatly enhances patient care by objectively aiding surgical decision making, decreasing the difficulty of creating the rigid framework, and allowing for more predictable outcomes.

CASE EXAMPLES

The authors have used the intraoperative nasal guide in 3 patients. Patient 1 is a 26-year-old man who had extensive trauma to the face from shrapnel, specifically the nose, with loss of the entire septum and cartilaginous framework. **Fig. 9** shows has preoperative and postoperative appearance. He has good projection and width, but the skin thickness from the paramedian forehead flap is prominent. This outcome led the authors to reduce the height of the nasal guide to accommodate for the eventual placement of the paramedian forehead flap.

Patient 2 is a 32-year-old woman who presented after a rhinectomy and total septectomy, with resection of the upper lateral cartilages and midline nasal bones, due to squamous cell carcinoma of the septum. The rigid framework is vascularized by a tunneled galeal frontalis flap and nasal turn-in flaps (**Fig. 10**).

Patient 3 is a 54-year-old woman who presented with a nasal defect secondary to resection for an adenosquamous carcinoma of the vestibule of the nose (**Fig. 11**).

All 3 patients are pleased with their appearance and are breathing well. The intraoperative nasal guide was extremely helpful in providing the positive functional and cosmetic outcome.

ADVANCED TECHNOLOGY AND RECONSTRUCTIVE SURGERY

New, advanced technology is being increasingly used in the preoperative and intraoperative planning of facial surgery. Surface scanners have been used in reconstruction after complex facial burn injuries and reconstructive rhytidectomy.[3,4] The use of a 3D radiologic viewer in the preoperative period with rhinoplasty patients was found to

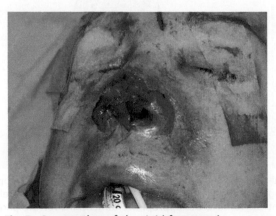

Fig. 7. Construction of the rigid framework.

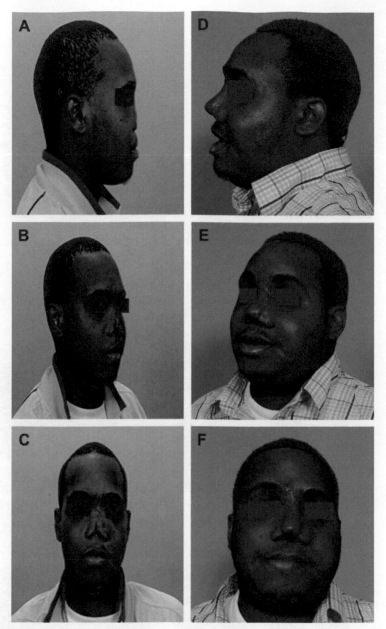

Fig. 9. Preoperative (*A–C*) and postoperative (*D–F*) appearance of patient 1. The skin thickness from the paramedian forehead flap is prominent.

show a reduction in postoperative surgical corrections, reduction in surgical time for the functional intervention, a higher rate of improvement in nasal function, a higher percentage of postoperative satisfaction, and reduced costs.[5] Craniofacial surgery requires significant preoperative preparation to best manipulate the skull, facial bones, mandible, and the overlying soft tissue. A method has been presented for interactive computer-assisted surgery planning and visualization.[6] This technique is based on a patient's preoperative imaging data obtained from 3D computed tomography and a photo-realistic model of the soft-tissue appearance obtained by a laser surface scanner.

There have also been multiple reports of surgeons attempting to use intraoperative templates to increase the accuracy and ease of nasal reconstruction. Aquaplast has been used to better approximate skin replacement,[7] and silicone and

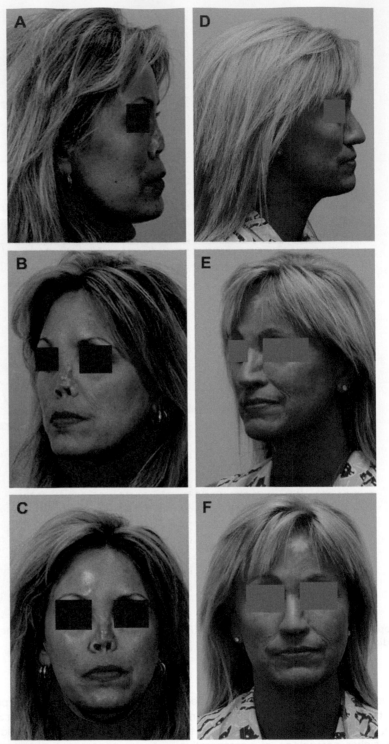

Fig. 10. Reconstruction of patient 2 secondary to rhinectomy and total septectomy, with resection of the upper lateral cartilages and midline nasal bones. (*A–C*) Preoperative; (*D–F*) postoperative.

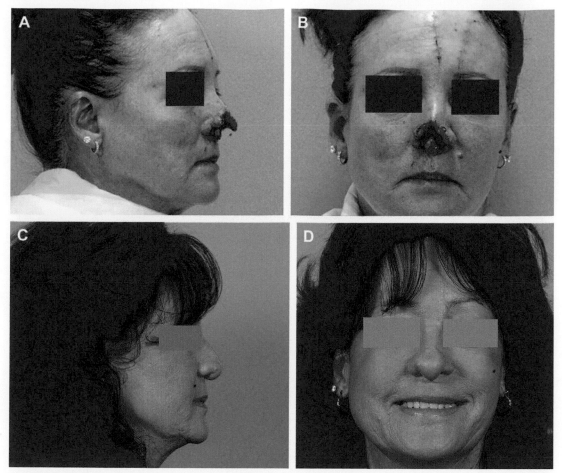

Fig. 11. Reconstruction of patient 3 secondary to resection of an adenosquamous carcinoma of the vestibule. (*A, B*) Preoperative; (*C, D*) postoperative.

bone wax has been used to help with cartilaginous reconstruction.[8]

SUMMARY

The endeavor of creating an intraoperative nasal guide requires a multidisciplinary approach involving the surgeon, patient, and anaplastologist, with close collaboration with the engineers at DDI. This process results in improved patient outcomes by increasing the accuracy of width and projection while aiding greatly in approximating the patient's original fine details and contours. The introduction of new technologies into the preoperative and operative arena plays a great role in improving surgical ease and patient satisfaction.

REFERENCES

1. Burget GC, Menick FJ. The subunit principle in nasal reconstruction. Plast Reconstr Surg 1985;76(2):239–47.

2. Federspil PA. Craniofacial prostheses for facial defects. HNO 2010;58(6):621–31 [in German].

3. Kovacs L, Zimmermann A, Wawrzyn H, et al. Computer aided surgical reconstruction after complex facial burn injuries—opportunities and limitations. Burns 2005; 31(1):85–91.

4. Wettstein R, Kalbermatten DF, Rieger UM, et al. Laser surface scanning analysis in reconstructive rhytidectomy. Aesthetic Plast Surg 2006;30(6):637–40.

5. Moscatiello F, Herrero Jover J, Gonzalez Ballester MA, et al. Preoperative digital three-dimensional planning for rhinoplasty. Aesthetic Plast Surg 2010;34(2): 232–8.

6. Meehan M, Teschner M, Girod S. Three-dimensional simulation and prediction of craniofacial surgery. Orthod Craniofac Res 2003;6(Suppl 1):102–7.

7. Murrell GL, Burget GC. Aesthetically precise templates for nasal reconstruction using a new material. Plast Reconstr Surg 2003;112(7):1855–61.

8. Manavbasi I, Agaoglu G. Silicon template for nasal tip graft. Ann Plast Surg 2006;56(2):226.

This page intentionally left blank

The Use of 3D Imaging Tools in Facial Plastic Surgery

Michael R. Markiewicz, DDS, MPH, MD[a],
R. Bryan Bell, DDS, MD[a,b,c],*

KEYWORDS

- Frameless stereotaxy • Surgery • Computer-assisted
- Orbit • Orbital fractures • Navigation • Maxillofacial surgery
- Imaging • Three-Dimensional • Surgery • Plastic • 3-D

Despite the use of sound surgical technique, some outcomes in facial plastic surgery may be viewed as suboptimal to clinician and patient. Recently, there has been an explosion of 3-D imaging tools that have made their way from the research bench to clinical bedside, in an effort to assist surgeons in achieving optimal functional and esthetic results. The innovation of computer-aided design and computer-aided modeling (CAD/CAM) software, initially implemented in neurosurgery and radiology procedures, and the easy acquisition and transfer of Digital Imaging and Communications in Medicine (DICOM) data has facilitated the development of various proprietary software programs for use in the craniomaxillofacial skeleton. Contemporary software allows surgeons to analyze patients by performing 3-D measurements and to manipulate deformed or missing anatomy by mirror imaging, segmentation, or insertion of unaltered or ideal skeletal constructs. The virtual reconstruction may be transferred to reality (the patient) by using custom stereolithographic models (SLMs), implants, cutting jigs, or occlusal splints that are constructed using a CAD/CAM process, or through image-guided surgery in the

form of intraoperative navigation (frameless stereotaxy) performed to the idealized virtual image. Finally, the accuracy of the surgical reconstruction may be confirmed using modern portable intraoperative CT scanners. Third-party service providers have made this technology available and accessible to most surgeons.

Computer-aided surgery can be divided into 4 phases:

1. Data acquisition phase, in which all clinical information, anthropometric measurements, and bite registrations are obtained
2. Planning phase, in which CT data are imported into a proprietary software program for the purposes of virtual planning before surgery
3. Surgical phase, which is performed using CAD/CAM-derived SLMs, guide stents, occlusal splints, and/or intraoperative navigation
4. Assessment phase, in which the accuracy of the treatment plan transfer is evaluated using intraoperative (or postoperative CT imaging).

Recently, basic and patient-oriented research has demonstrated efficacy of this approach in (1) head and neck/skull base surgery; (2) maxillomandibular

---

Funding support: research supported in part by the Stryker Craniomaxillofacial.

Financial disclosures: the authors have no financial disclosures to declare.

a Department of Oral and Maxillofacial Surgery, Oregon Health and Science University, Mail code SDOMS, 611 SW Campus Drive, Portland, OR 97239, USA

b Oral, Head and Neck Cancer Program, Providence Cancer Center, Providence Portland Medical Center, Portland, OR 97213, USA

c Trauma Service/Oral and Maxillofacial Surgery Service, Legacy Emanuel Medical Center, Portland, OR 97227, USA

* Corresponding author. 1849 Northwest Kearney, Suite 300, Portland, OR 97209.

E-mail address: bellb@hnsa1.com

Facial Plast Surg Clin N Am 19 (2011) 655–682
doi:10.1016/j.fsc.2011.07.009

reconstructive surgery; (3) orbital surgery (**Fig. 1**), and (4) orthognathic/craniofacial surgery (**Fig. 2**). The purpose of this article is to describe the authors' approach to craniomaxillofacial surgery and how 3-D analysis and virtual surgery have affected the workflow process at their institution.

DATA ACQUISITION

Data acquisition occurs in the form of

- Quantifying the clinical deformity or problem through clinical examination
- Obtaining all necessary anatomic bite registrations and/or dental models
- Acquiring a CT scan of the patient, with the DICOM data to be imported into the appropriate planning software.

The clinical information necessary for computer planning depends on the clinical application. In head and neck surgery, for example, very specific information regarding the particular pathologic diagnosis (benign vs malignant), injury, hard and soft tissue involvement, and the extent of the planned surgical resection or reconstruction should be documented, but it is generally not necessary to obtain bite registrations. In contrast, computer-aided surgical simulation in orthognathic surgery requires registration of centric relation

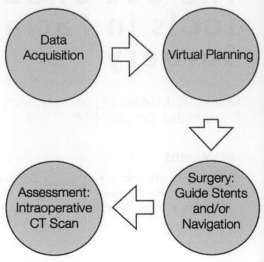

Fig. 2. Example workflow diagram of the use of 3-D software, in which preoperative surgical planning and surgical stents are used. Example of this process is in orthognathic surgery or head and neck tumor reconstruction, in which 3-D data points are obtained from the patient preoperatively; virtual surgery with maxillomandibular movements or FFOF insertion performed for orthognathic and tumor reconstructive surgery, respectively; and postoperative CT is taken to assess the final outcome.

before CT imaging, registration of natural head position, laser scanning of plaster dental models, and high-quality facial photography, in addition to accurate anthropometric data.

Once the clinical evaluation is completed and presurgical records have been obtained, the CT scan is completed using the standard scanning algorithm, matrix of 512 × 512 at 0.625-mm slice thickness, 25 cm or lesser field of view, 0° gantry tilt, and 1:1 pitch. The CT images are then transferred to the appropriate surgical planning software in DICOM format.

Surface imaging, or scanning, is a technique in which a laser or other capturing device is used to replicate the 3-D surface of soft tissue, bones, or even dental cast. These data can then be imported digitally into a computer software program. Advantages compared with 3-D reconstruction of CT data include the lack of exposure to radiation and general anesthesia, particularly in the pediatric patient population.[1] Surface scanning software imports individual points on the face, and then combines them in the X, Y, and Z axes rendering a 3-D representation of the soft-tissue skeleton. Therefore, the scans resolution is limited by the number of points in can imported into its data set, which is increasing with the development of higher-resolution laser acquisition software.

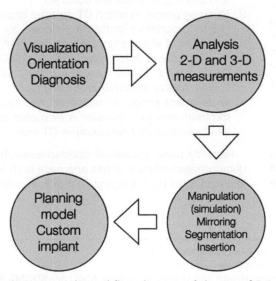

Fig. 1. Example workflow diagram of the use of 3-D software, in which mirroring and custom implants are used. Example of this process is in complex orbital reconstruction, in which the deformity (enophthalmos) is diagnosed, preoperative 3-D measurements are obtained, the unaffected orbit is mirrored to the affected side, and a custom implant designed using CAD/CAM techniques is used to restore the defect to preoperative conditions.

Facial surface acquisition devices are classified as either coordinate measurement machines, range imaging, moire, stereophotogrammetry, and position tracking devices. Recently, surface imaging devices have shown accuracy in the submillimeter range when compared with their real-life representations,[2,3] becoming especially popular in the field of craniofacial/cleft lip and palate surgery where precision is crucial for flap design and movement. One group in particular has rigorously developed and tested a 3-D laser scanner for acquisition of the surface anatomy in the cleft/lip and palate population.[2–4] The patient is scanned at a set distance (ie, 1 mm) as controlled by a tape measure fixed to the camera. The patient's facial surface then reflects the distorted light of the laser, which is then captured by a charged-coupled distributor camera and converted into distance information using triangulation principles. The system then captures geometric points on a scatter plot. Using a software program, the scatter plot is then transferred into surface information via a software program, which can then manipulate the surfaces texture and color rendering an accurate representation of the soft tissue profile of the patient.

PREOPERATIVE PLANNING

Surgical stimulation and manipulation of the 3-D facial skeleton using data derived from CT datasets can now be performed on several software systems.[5–8] The planned surgery derived from preoperative surgical simulation can then be combined with intraoperative navigation to implement the plan, check its accuracy, and modify it if

needed.[9–15] The simplest, yet most studied and effective, way to perform hard tissue reconstruction is by mirroring the images of the opposite, unaffected side of the facial skeleton, to the affected side of the face using a variety of software programs. Virtual software allows segmentation of the area of interest and either virtual manipulation or reconstruction of a patient's native anatomy, such as in congenital craniofacial defects, or insertion of implants into the virtual field, such as in traumatic or postablative reconstruction.

In the case of maxillomandibular reconstruction, the jaws can be virtually analyzed for horizontal, vertical, and sagittal discrepancies; 3-D measurements are obtained; and osteotomies are made, segmented, and manipulated in the X, Y, and Z axes and a virtual surgery can be undertaken in minutes. Furthermore, the resultant virtual outcome can then be transformed into an SLM to show the clinician and patient the final planned result. Patient-specific implants can be derived or implants can be prebent before surgery based on this idealized model. For complex orbital reconstruction, not only can implants be inserted and adapted into the virtual field but also plates can be constructed using the digital data derived from virtual hardware adaption.

Several CAD/CAM programs are currently available to the craniomaxillofacial surgeon (**Table 1**). Although all have their advantages and drawbacks, several offer the specific feature of back-converting data from the software's proprietary language to standard DICOM format. This allows the virtual data and subsequent work done in one software system to be transferred to another. The purpose

Table 1
Commercially available 3-D imaging software

Software Program	Cost (Estimates May Vary)
Amira (Visage Imaging GmbH, Berlin, Germany)	$4800 (base package)
Analyze (AnalyzeDirect, Inc, Overland Park, Kansas)	$5000
iNtellect Cranial Navigation System (Stryker, Freiburg, Germany)	NA
iPlan (BrainLab, Westchester, Illinois)	$30,000 (planning station and software)
Maxilim (Medicim, Bruges, Belgium)	NA
Mimics (Materialise, Leuven, Belgium)	NA
SurgiCase CMF (Materialise, Leuven, Belgium)	$6500.00
SimPlant OMS (Materialise Dental, Leuven, Belgium)	NA
Voxim (IVS Solutions, Chemnitz, Germany)	$20,000 (Voxim basics)
3dMD (Atlanta, Georgia)	NA
Alma3D (Alma IT Systems, Barcelona, Spain)	NA
ImageJ (National Institutes of Health, Boston, Masssachusetts)	Free (http://rsbweb.nih.gov/ij/)

of this may be to use components of several software systems that are unique to each or to display and teach via presentation at other workstations not loaded with the original software used to do a virtual procedure. In addition, the data set may be transferred into a navigation system, to guide the accurate placement of osteotomies, bone grafts, flaps, or implant placement.

SURGERY

Virtual surgical planning in and of itself is useful as an educational and teaching instrument by allowing 3-D analysis of the clinical problem and visualization of idealized digital manipulations. Without the ability to transfer the virtual plan into reality, however, it remains just that: an educational tool. The incorporation of CAD/CAM technology into the head and neck work flow process at our institution has allowed replicating the virtual plan in patients and theoretically positively affecting functional and esthetic treatment outcomes, reducing operating times, and improving quality.

The preoperative virtual plan is transferred to the patient in 1 of 3 ways, depending on the clinical problem. Reconstruction of the mandible and the inset of microvascular bone flaps may be facilitated by using virtually reconstructed or idealized SLMs, guide stents, and cutting guides. In the maxilla and midface, the cutting guides are augmented by intraoperative navigation, which is also used to aid in orbital reconstruction and skull base surgery. Orthognathic surgery is facilitated by the use of intermediate and final occlusal splints designed based on the virtual reconstruction.

Stereolithographic Modeling

Developed and refined in the later part of the twentieth century,[7,16–18] SLMs are 3-D representations of the craniomaxillofacial skeleton. Using a variety of manufacturing techniques and materials, they are a direct representation of a patient's CT data set. Early on, SLMs were milled from 2-D CT data. These models were useful as an adjunct in preoperative planning and helpful in getting a general view of the craniomaxillofacial skeleton, but by no means were taken for an exact representation of a patient's hard tissues. With the advent of high-resolution, however, CT the resultant accuracy of SLMs has increased immensely. Current manufacturing protocols fabricate models that are highly accurate and are fabricated with a photocurable monomer hardened by lasers.[19] SLMs may assist surgeons in preoperative planning

and intraoperative bony reconstruction.[19–21] These models offer an unprecedented level of accuracy and variations of these techniques continue to be developed and used today.[22]

The utility of SLMs is in the preoperative staging of facial surgery patients. There has been an abundance of studies demonstrating their efficacy in the preoperative stages of maxillomandibular reconstruction including anteroposterior jaw positioning, guiding plate adaptation, maxillomandibular contouring, and craniofacial and dental implant placement.[23,24] SLMs are used in orthognathic surgery and distraction osteogenesis and give surgeons a once unobtainable 3-D view of the maxilla and mandible, allowing precise visualization of the pitch, row, and yaw of planned maxillomandibular movement and vector plane in distraction osteogenesis.[25] Craniofacial surgery has also reaped the benefits of SLMs using them in the preoperative planning of craniofacial recontouring and skeletal segment repositioning.[26] Likewise, preoperative planning using SLMs in head and neck tumor reconstruction has been implemented in the reconstruction of oncologic defects by aiding preoperative plate adaptation, planned tumor resection, and custom implant and osteocutaneous flap placement.[27] The reconstruction of complex orbital defects secondary to trauma or tumor ablation has significantly benefited from SLMs. SLMs allow surgeons to visualize deep into the bony orbit and to adapt stock implants or construct custom plates to the intricate anatomy of the orbit. Bell and Markiewicz[28] demonstrated the use of SLMs on a cohort of patients with complex secondary traumatic defects and found SLMs extremely useful in reducing intraoperative plate adaptation and bone graft recontouring.

The drawbacks of SLMs lie in their poor representation of the midface and possibly the orbit where the thin walls of these areas of the facial skeleton may be misrepresented by lower-resolution CT and may not be as accurately represented as other craniomaxillofacial structures. Therefore, it is pivotal that patients receive high-resolution CT when SLMs are implemented. One area of poor representation of the facial skeleton that cannot be ameliorated by high-resolution CT are the occlusal surfaces of the dentition. This becomes critical in the preoperative planning of the orthognathic surgery and distraction osteogenesis patient. Recently, Xia and colleagues[29] circumvented this dilemma by digitally substituting laser scans of the teeth of plaster models for the low-resolution teeth of the CT, thereby allowing the surgeon to making accurate movements of the jaws and to digitally fabricate highly accurate intraoperative and final occlusal stents.

Intraoperative Navigation

Intraoperative navigation software programs import a DICOM CT data set and allow surgeons real-time confirmation of their position within the craniomaxillofacial skeleton. Intraoperative navigation has 3 key components:

1. Localizer, which is the camera or device that tracks the movements of the
2. Surgical probe, which is the actual position of the patient currently on the operating table
3. CT scan data set, which is projected and confirms the position of the probe within the patient to the preoperative 3-D image.

A patient's position in space is maintained by the tracking system via the placement of fiducial markers on stable and reliable anatomic points on the patient. The fiducial markers may be invasive and fixed, or noninvasive. In the invasive technique, the fiducial markers are secured into the patient's facial skeleton with screws via small incisions into the scalp or by the use of a custom splint that is adapted precisely to the patient face. When using these types of fiducial markers, the patient's head must be immobilized by attaching it to a Mayfield headrest. Noninvasive, surface fiducial markers are now commercially available in the form of individual adhesive markers or light-emitting diode (LED) mask. This technique is much quicker and far less invasive than the fixed techniques and offers more mobility of the patient during surgery. Disadvantages of the noninvasive technique include if the mask is in the operating zone, such as when a coronal flap is used. In this instance, the fixed technique must be used. A third, yet more time-consuming method is the markerless technique, where a set of points on the patients face are scanned and correlated with the CT data set. The position of the surgical probe relative to the patient is determined by the computer using the local rigid body concept for

Box 2
Indications for intraoperative navigation

Complex septoplasty/rhinoplasty

Facial implant placement

Head and neck tumor resection

Skull base surgery

Complex craniofacial/orthognathic surgery

Temporomandibular joint surgery

Foreign body removal

Complex orbital reconstruction

Maxillomandibular reconstruction

Cranial reconstruction

which there must be at least 3 registration points (fiducial markers).[30] A registration process is then undertaken in which the navigation software integrates the spatial information from the headset, surgical probe, and fiducial markers and the end result is alignment of the Cartesian coordinates of the actual patient in the X, Y, and Z planes onto the computer monitor in comparison with the preoperative CT data set.

Tracking systems have changed dramatically in recent years. Older navigation systems use electromagnetic fields that are superimposed over the operative site tracking the surgical probe, which may be by itself, or attached to an instrument of the surgeon's choice. These systems, however, carried the disadvantage of interference from the metallic surgical instruments used during an operation. More recent systems use an optical tracking system design, similar to the current motion activated gaming systems available today for the public. They rely on LEDs or reflective spheres that are tracked by the optical systems.

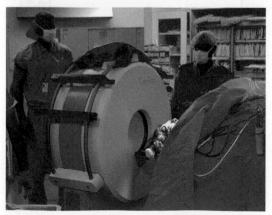

Fig. 3. Example of use of an intraoperative CT in the operating room.

Optical tacking systems can be divided into 2 categories, active and passive trackers. Active trackers are equipped with battery-powered LEDs attached to the surgical probe. These probes can be placed anywhere in the body with a high degree of accuracy. Passive optical tacking systems have reflectors on the surgical probe instead of LEDs and have the advantage of not needing electrical wires or batteries attached to the probe making for a lighter probe with more flexible maneuverability. The major disadvantage of passive optical tacking systems, however, is that artificial light sources, such as operating room lights, may interfere with tracking.

Initially developed for neurosurgical[31–33] and endoscopic sinus surgical procedures,[34] intraoperative navigation is used for a variety of facial surgery procedures, including complex orbital repair,[28] head and neck oncologic surgery,[35] and craniofacial surgery.[36] Intraoperative navigation

Table 2
Subjects treated with computer guided tumor ablation and reconstruction

	Diagnosis		Computer Planning	Intraoperative Navigation	Margins	Follow-Up
1.	Melanoma max gingiva		+	+	−	23 mo
2.	Basosquamous cell ca midface		+	+	−	22 mo
3.	SCC hard palate mucosa		+	+	−	16 mo
4.	SCC L max sinus		+	+	+	12 mo
5.	SCC R max gingiva		+	+	−	12 mo
6.	SCC L max sinus		+	+	−	5 mo
7.	ORN maxilla		+	+	NA	4 mo

Abbreviations: ca, carcinoma; max, maxilla; ORN, osteoradionecrosis; SCC, squamous cell carcinoma.

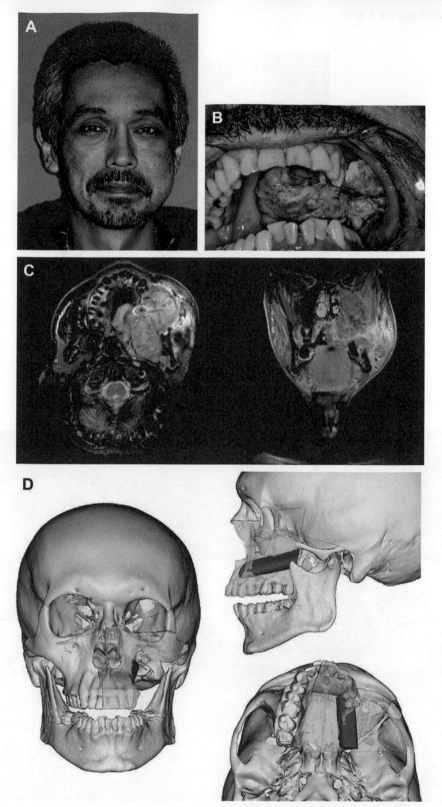

Fig. 4. A patient with squamous cell carcinoma that invaded the maxillary sinus (*A–C*). Preoperative surgical simulation was performed, as was insetting of the virtual FFOF (*D, E*). Steriolithographic models were then constructed of the final virtual bony reconstruction (*F*). Cutting jigs were then made via CAD/CAM techniques to clinically replicate the precise virtual osteotomies of the FFOF (*G, H*). Tumor resection and inset of the FFOF was carried with the aid of surgical navigation (*I*). The surgical defect that would be difficult to reconstruct using conventional FFOF inset techniques (*J*). Using surgical navigation, the FFOF was placed in the same position as planned virtually in the preoperative period (*K, L*). (*M*) A final frontal view of the patient 2 months postoperatively (*N*).

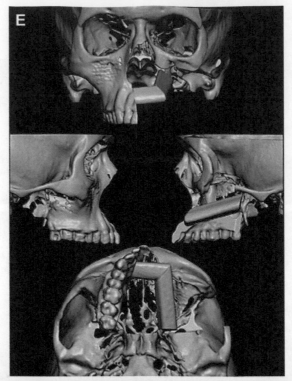

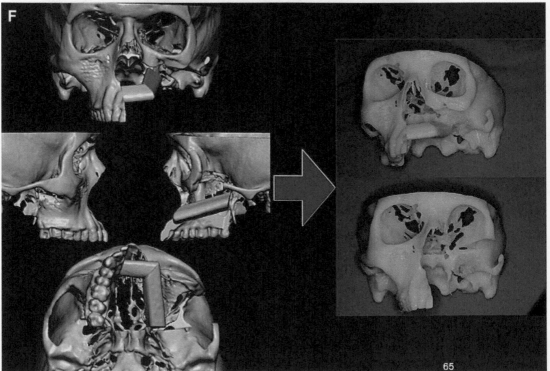

Fig. 4. (continued)

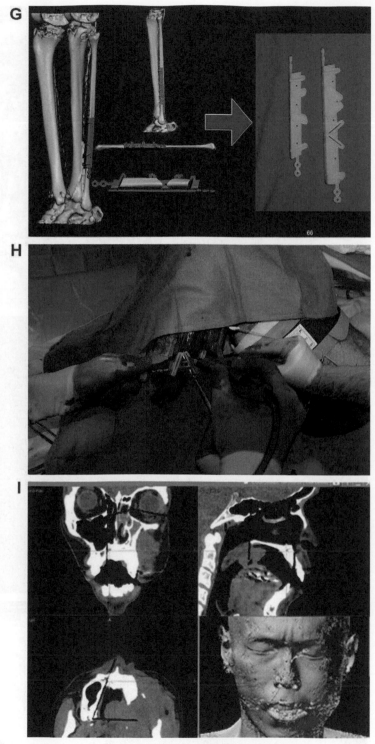

Fig. 4. (*continued*)

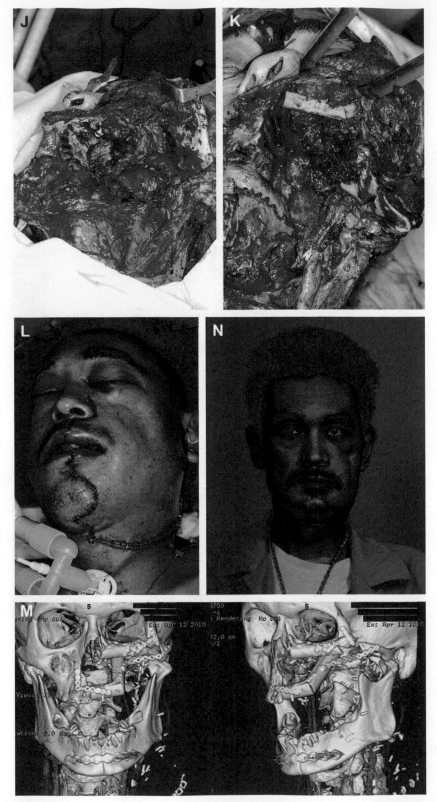

Fig. 4. (*continued*)

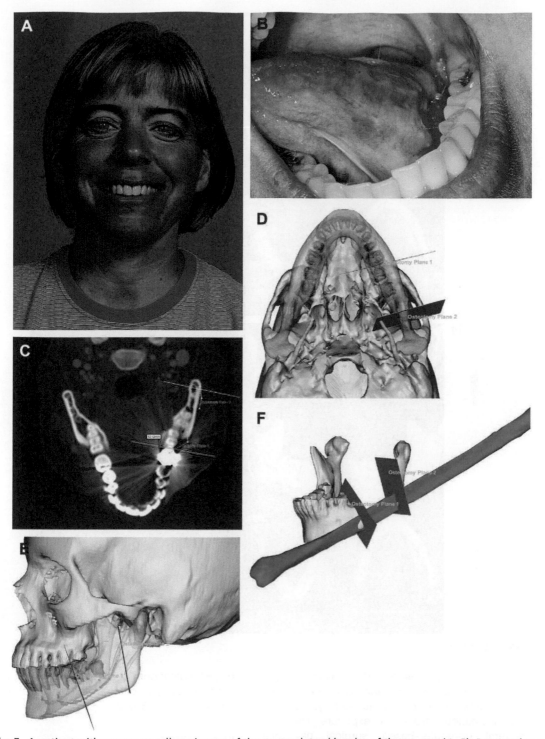

Fig. 5. A patient with squamous cell carcinoma of the posterolateral border of the tongue (*A*, *B*). Proposed mandibulectomy segments in the 2-D (*C*) and 3-D (*D*, *E*) views are displayed. The virtual fibula is inserted into ideal the ideal position chosen by the surgeon (*F*). Virtual cutting jigs are fabricated to replicate the virtual osteotomies of the mandible and fibula (*G*). A reconstruction plate is then contoured to the virtual mandible and graft (*H*). A reconstruction plate is fashioned to the SLM in the preoperative period (*I*). Cutting jigs are applied to the native mandible intraoperatively to replicate the virtual osteotomies performed in the preoperative period (*J*, *K*, *L*), and the preformed reconstruction plate is applied to the mandible and FFOF (*M*). Frontal (*N*) and occlusal (*O*) views of the patient 2 months postoperatively.

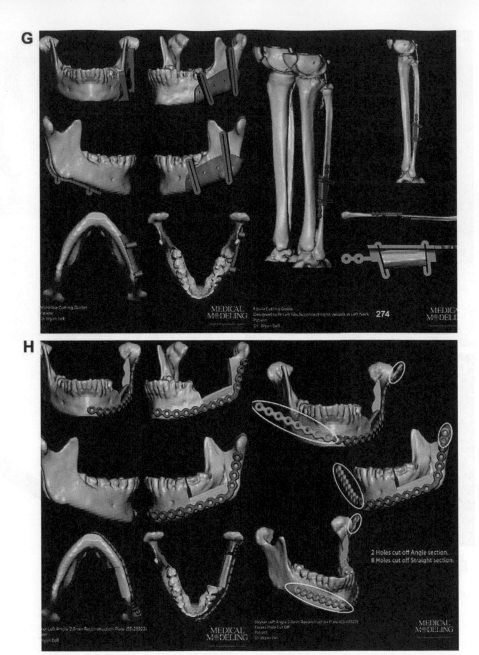

Fig. 5. (continued)

offers the advantage of virtual visualization of a patient's anatomy and access to areas of the facial skeleton that once required larger incisions and increased hard tissue exposure. There are several computer-based surgical navigation systems available for use in facial surgery (**Box 1**). Using frameless stereotaxy, which literally means, *touching a point in space*, these programs allow precise location of anatomic landmarks or implants to with a margin of error of 1 mm to 2 mm when compared with the projected CT in the operating room.[37,38] There are several evidence-based indications for intraoperative navigation in the facial surgery patient, which are elaborated in further detail in **Box 2**.

EVALUATION

Once the virtual plan has been transferred to the patient by performing osteotomies or insetting grafts, flaps, or implants, the accuracy of the surgery is assessed (when appropriate) using a portable CT scanner. Available at many tertiary care facilities with an active neurosurgical

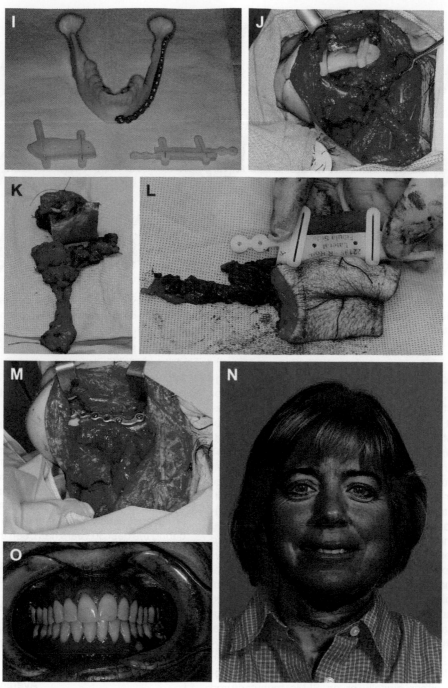

Fig. 5. (*continued*)

presence, intraoperative CT assessment allows for any revision to occur before the patient leaving the operating room. This is particularly useful in orbital reconstruction, where the surgical access is limited and the relationship of the orbital implant relative to the orbital apex and critical medial and inferior bulges is unclear.

CLINICAL OUTCOMES
Head and Neck/Skull Base Surgery

3-D imaging in the form of intraoperative CT (**Fig. 3**) scanning has several benefits in head and neck oncologic surgery, originally reported in skull base surgery.[39] Batra and colleagues[39] found that the use of intraoperative CT in the resection

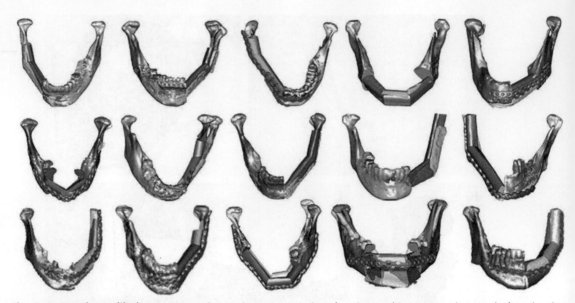

Fig. 6. Series of mandibular reconstructions using preoperative planning and intraoperative surgical navigation. The pink shaded areas represent the planned postoperative position of the mandible. The green shaded areas of the mandible represent the actual postoperative position of the mandible.

of sinonasal and skullbase tumors offered advantages, such as evaluating the extent of tumor resection and margin confirmation and subsequent additional tumor resection, dissection of the ethmoid partitions, frontal stent placement, and frontal bone drilling. Preoperative 3-D CT imaging and intraoperative navigation has been shown an effective way to outline the margins of tumor resection in other areas of the craniomaxillofacial skeleton.[30,32,40–42] Intraoperative navigation allows full visualization of the tumor using minimal exposure and morbidity to uninvolved tissues. Surgical resection of tumors of the pterygomaxillary fossa, skull base, infratemporal fossa, paranasal sinuses, and temporomandibular joint complex[35,43,44] may be performed with increased maneuverability yet with the ability to virtually visualize and defer from involvement of adjacent vital structures without necessarily exposing the overlying tissues. Preoperative 3-D planning also affords surgeons the ability to perform osteotomies, either digitally or on SLMs manufactured from the CT data.

An audit of the authors' early experience in a series of patients with locoregionally advanced malignant tumors involving the midface and anterior skull base documented favorable functional and esthetic results in all patients. All but one patient with extensive disease had a negative resection margin. All patients (including the patient with a positive margin) remain without evidence of disease at a minimum of 1-year follow-up (**Table 2**).

Additional outcomes assessments as well as cost-benefit analyses are necessary in the future.

Palatomaxillary and Mandibular Reconstruction

Tumor resection and severe trauma often render loss of continuity of the maxillomandibular complex, causing significant functional and esthetic defect. Perhaps the most significant advancement in reconstruction of the midface and mandible during the past 30 years has been the development of microvascular osteocutaneous flaps, specifically, the fibular osteocutaneous free flap (FFOF).[45,46] Considered by many centers the gold

Table 3
Differences in planned and actual outcomes in subjects undergoing free fibula flap reconstruction

Category	Average (mm)	Std Dev (mm)
Registration quality	0.83	0.81
FFOF/native junctions	3.89	1.96
Mandibular width at gonions	4.91	3.91
Mandibular width at condyles	3.1	2.46
Mandible cuts	1.49	1.30
FFF segment lengths	2.27	2.46

Abbreviation: Std dev, standard deviation.

standard for reconstruction of large hard tissue defects of the head and neck region, the FFOF not only offers surgeons the ability to restore defects to original levels of preablative and pretraumatic skeletal dimensions but also serves as a foundation to restore the dentition via the use of the endosseous dental implants.[47–51]

Rigid fixation and reconstruction plates offer the advantage of recreation of the shape of the native mandible by bending the plate to the contour of the mandible before tumor resection. Tthis process is time consuming, however, and unless multiple osteotomies are performed, clinical outcomes may not portray the preoperative mandibular shape of a patient. The increasing numbers of un-needed osteotomies of the FFOF adds to the complexity of the procedure and the risk of adjacent soft tissue and vascular damage. In addition, in situ plate bending may not be applicable for tumors that invade neighboring soft tissues.

SLMs developed from 3-D preoperative imaging allow surgeons to assess the contour of the maxillomandibular complex by removal of the external deformation left by the tumor creating ideal anatomic surfaces. In addition to transverse assessment of the jaws, sagittal relationships of the jaws may be assessed for proper anteroposterior positioning. Traditional FFOF reconstruction is often inadequate in the sagittal plan for appropriate maxillomandibular relationships, making dental implant reconstruction difficult due to overprojectin or underprojection of the reconstructed

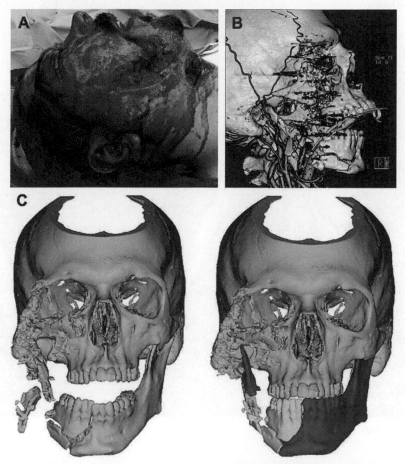

Fig. 7. A patient who suffered complex craniomaxillofacial soft and hard tissue injuries after a shotgun blast to the face (*A*, *B*). 3-D virtual planning was used to manipulated the comminuted orbital, midface, and mandible segments into ideal position (*C*, *D*). An SLM was then fabricated from the virtual reconstruction and a reconstruction bar was adapted (*E*). The preformed reconstruction bar was then adapted to the native mandible intraoperatively (*F*). Using preoperative planning and surgical navigation, postoperative plate placement was confirmed (*G*). Preoperative planning was then used to realign the midface segments into ideal position (*H*) and intraoperative surgical navigation was used to confirm placement compared with the preoperative plan (*I*). (*J*) Depicts the planned virtual outcome and SLMs were fabricated from the planned surgery (*K*). Postoperative positioning was confirmed (*L*). (*M*) The patient 2 months after his initial surgery.

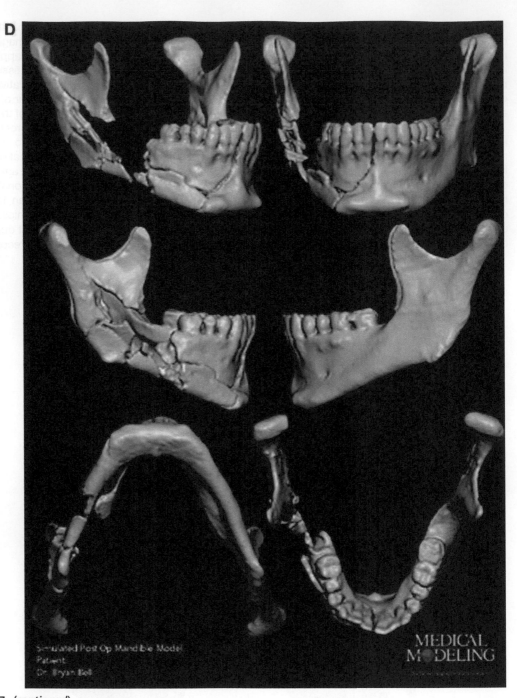

Fig. 7. (*continued*)

mandible. SLMs developed from 3-D imaging allow for precise plate bending and maxillomandibular relationships allowing for ideal immediate dental implant placement at the time of FFOF inset in the maxilla and mandible.[47,52]

Using data from preoperative CT datasets, CAD/CAM software offers surgeons a way to virtually perform tumor resection, make custom implants, and perform osteotomies on the 3-D FFOF, inset the FFOF, and generate custom guide stents to reproduce osteotomies in the operating room.[53,54] In the preoperative period, a CT of the fibula is obtained (**Figs. 4** and **5**). This can be segmented to produce the bony part of the FFOF and imported

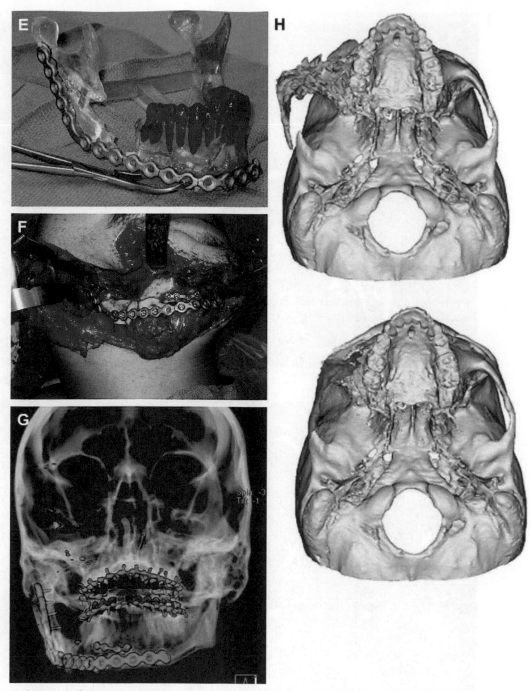

Fig. 7. (*continued*)

into the virtual environment. Using preoperative planning software, ideal position and angle of osteotomy cuts are made by a surgeon, and final inset of the fibula is made to fit the precise dimensions of the virtual tumor resection defect. Using CAD/CAM technology, the data are exported and custom guide stents can be fabricated so virtual cuts can be precisely reproduced during the actual surgery.

Final position of the FFOF in relation to the native maxilla or mandible is then confirmed using intraoperative navigation by comparing actual movements with the preoperative CT data present on the monitor in the operating room Additionally, dental implants may be placed into the FFOF in the exact positions planned in the preoperative planning stages. Early outcomes of the authors'

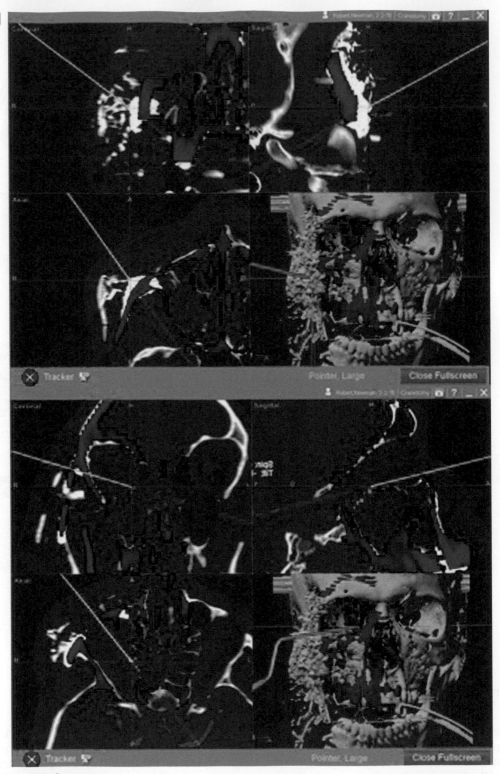

Fig. 7. (*continued*)

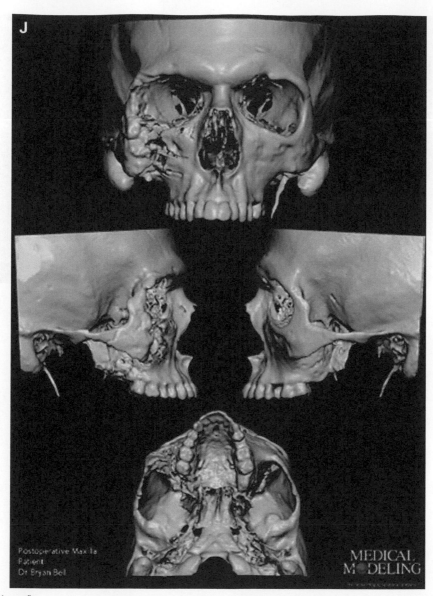

Fig. 7. (*continued*)

own series of patients undergoing mandibular reconstruction after tumor resection have shown promising results with regards to the difference between planned and actual postoperative outcomes (**Fig. 6, Table 3**). Additionally, the authors' have used the techniques (described previously) for use in the reconstruction of complex traumatic craniomaxillofacial defects (**Fig. 7**).

Posttraumatic Cranio-orbital Reconstruction

Despite the use of traditional reconstructive principles, lasting functional and esthetics complications, such as enophthalmos, inaccurate globe projection, and vertical and horizontal dystopia, may persist after orbital reconstruction of post-traumatic, and postablative defects.[55] This is especially true in traumatic injury leading to the shattered orbit or tumor resection with margins spanning multiple orbital walls.

In these defects, it is especially difficult to obtain previous orbital dimensions due to lack of reliable bony landmarks to guide the placement of bony plates and implants. Specific areas of difficulty are re-establishing proper orbital contour, volume, and the ethmoidal and antral bulges of the medial and inferior floors respectively, as well as plate adaptation around the orbital apex. Not only has

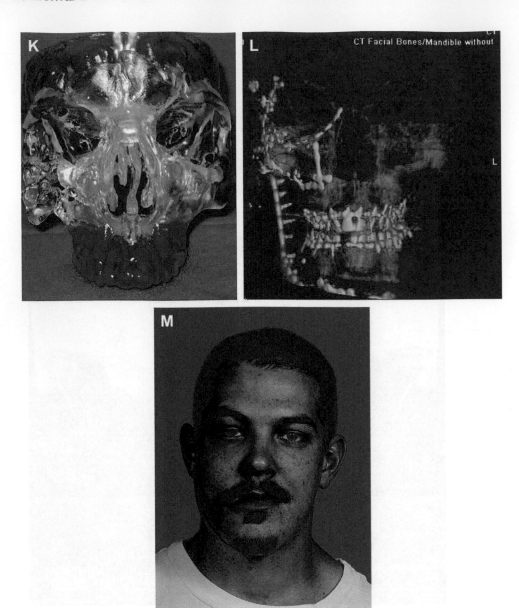

Fig. 7. (*continued*)

3-D imaging assisted preoperative planning of orbital defects but also intraoperative navigation has allowed increased precision of traditional reconstructive techniques leading to a decrease in orbital volume and subsequent decrease in enophthalmos and more favorable position of the globe (**Fig. 8**).[56,57]

A novel study by Ploder and colleagues[58,59] attempted to assess the accuracy of the 3-D CT and the software program, Analyze, in measuring the volume of fracture defect and tissue herniation into the maxillary sinus of orbital floor fractures. Using human cadaver skulls, fractures defects were manually created with an osteotome, and

herniation of the orbital contents was simulated with silicone impression material. Both fracture size and volume of silicone were assessed by direct measurement, 3-D CT volumetric measurement, and measurement using Analyze software. Both 3-D CT and analyze showed a significant linear correlation with direct measurements. A subsequent study by Ploder and colleagues[60] found a direct correlation between both the size of the fracture and degree of enophthalmo, and the orbital volume and enophthalmos.

Gellrich and colleagues[56] used 3-D imaging in a study of subjects with increased enophthalmos and decreased globe projection secondary to

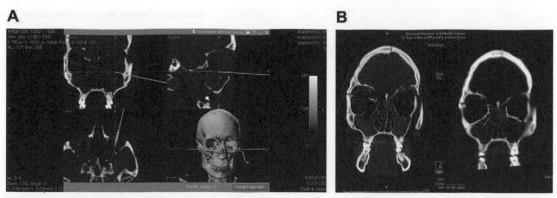

Fig. 8. (*A*) Use of intraoperative navigation to confirm real-time position within the orbit. (*B*) Intraoperative plate placement after severe blowout fractures is aided via the use of intraoperative navigation.

posttraumatic orbital deformities. In their landmark study, the investigators mirrored the unaffected orbit to the affected, traumatized orbit using 3-D preoperative image software. Using this as their

goal orbital dimensions, the subjects then underwent orbital reconstruction using intraoperative navigation. Navigation guidance was used to confirm plate placement of grafts at the goal

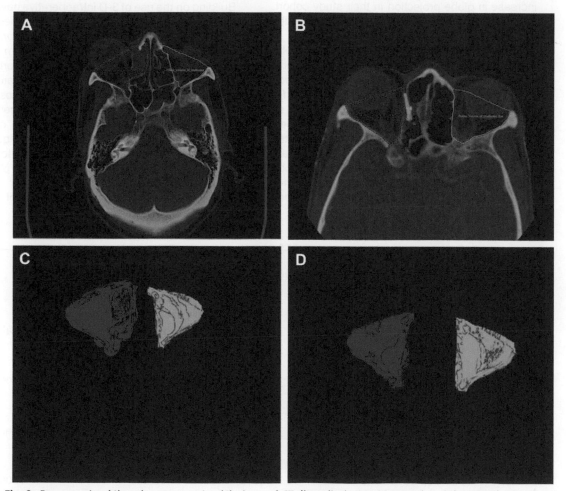

Fig. 9. Preoperative (*A*) and postoperative (*B*) views of CT slices displaying increased and decreased orbital area respectively. 3D rendering of preoperative (*C*) and postoperative (*D*) orbital volume in a patient undergoing intra-operative navigation-assisted orbital reconstruction.

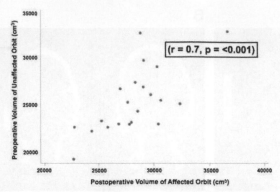

Fig. 10. Scatter plot showing a linear relationship of preoperative planned and actual postoperative orbital volume of patients after intraoperative navigation guided orbital reconstruction.

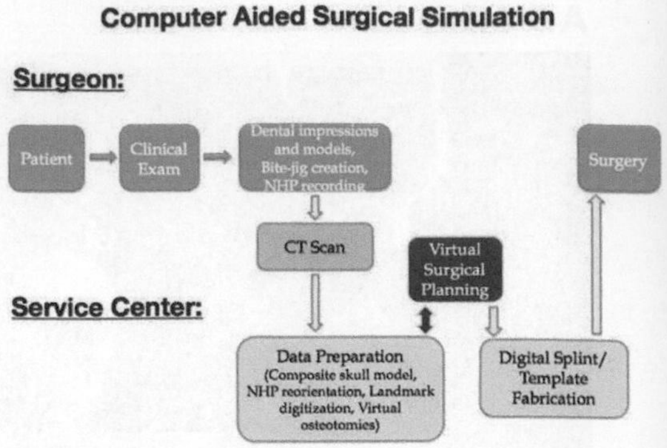

Fig. 11. Flow diagram displaying a protocol for computer-assisted orthognathic surgery. NHP, natural head position.

dimensions set preoperatively. The investigators found a significant decrease in orbital volume and increase in globe projection in their study cohort. Markiewicz and colleagues[61] performed a similar study, using the imaging software Analyze, to assess the change in orbital volume and globe projection in a cohort of subjects with not only defects secondary to trauma, but tumor ablation as well.[28,61] Additionally, they used the SLMs for preoperative graft contouring before surgery as well as confirming graft placement using intraoperative navigation. They found similar results to the study by Gellrich and colleagues with a significant decrease in orbital volume and increase in globe projection (**Figs. 9,10, Table 4**). In addition, they found a significant, linear correlation between

goal and actual orbital volume and globe projection measurements after orbital reconstruction.

Building on the use of 3-D intraoperative navigation, several protocols have been developed to build custom plate's specific to a patient's orbital defects.[62–64] Using an SLM derived from CT data, a plaster layer may be adapted to the orbital defect of the SLM and contoured to the anatomy of the orbit.[62] Using conventional techniques for denture fabrication, the plaster is then immersed in stone and burnt out leaving a template cast. Using traditional dental crown casting techniques, commercially annealed titanium is casted into the stone template making a custom titanium plate. Another protocol developed by Metzger and colleagues[64] removes the SLM stage of the

Table 4
Change in orbital volume and globe projection in subjects undergoing computer-assisted orbital reconstruction

Absolute Δ in preoperative and postoperative orbital volume excess			
	Mean (cm³)	Standard error (cm³)	P Value
Preoperative orbital volume excess	1.2	1.3	NA
Postoperative orbital volume excess	−1.3	6.6	NA
Absolute Δ in preoperative and postoperative orbital volume excess	5.1	1.2	<0.001[a]
Absolute Δ in preoperative and postoperative globe projection excess			
	Mean (mm)	Standard error (mm)	P Value
Preoperative globe projection excess	−0.12	0.7	NA
Postoperative globe projection excess	2.4	0.5	NA
Absolute Δ in preoperative and postoperative globe projection excess	4.1	1186.0	<0.001[a]

[a] p value is for matched pairs t test.

previously described technique. In their unique protocol, a custom plate is made virtually to the contours of the patient's orbit and transported directly to a template machine for fabrication of a custom titanium mesh.

Cranial Reconstruction

Traditionally, reconstruction of cranial defects has been performed by the use of autogenous bone or alloplastic materials, such as titanium mesh; acrylics, such as polymethylmethacrylate[65]; ceramics, such as hydroxyapatite[66]; or high-performance thermoplastics, such as porous high-density polyethylene or polyetheretherketone.[67] Traditionally, success rates have varied and are inversely correlated with the size of the size of the defect.[68] The choice of material depends on the size and location of the defect, the quality and quantity of soft tissue

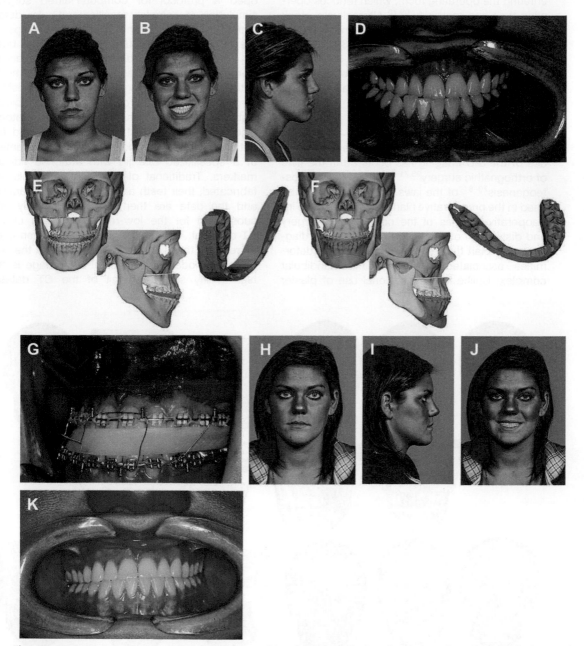

Fig. 12. Preoperative photographs of a patient with a hemimandibular elongation, class III malocclusion and facial asymmetry (*A–D*). Virtual osteotomies are performed and the segments are manipulated within the software program (*E–F*). CAD/CAM generated intermediate splint (*G*). Postoperative photographs show restoration of the patient's midline, a more esthetic profile and functional occlusal relationship (*H–K*).

coverage, the proximity to the paranasal sinuses, the presence or absence of infection, and the experience of the surgeon with a particular material.

Preoperative 3-D CT imaging can be a valuable adjunct to assess the size and shape of the cranial defect. Using CAD/CAM software technology, custom titanium implants can virtually constructed and milled from preoperative CT data. This offers the ability to have a well-adapted implant before entering the operating room, which reduces operating time and morbidity.[69,70] Alternatively, stock plates and implants can be adapted in the preoperative period to SLMs created from 3-D CT data sets. In this instance, the SLM not only allows the surgeon to visualize the full extent of the defect but also to reduce operating time by adapting the plate in the preoperative period.[70]

Orthognathic Surgery

Perhaps the most innovative advancement in the use of the 3-D imaging has occurred in the field of orthognathic surgery[25,71–78] and distraction osteogenesis[79–81] of the jaws. 3-D imaging can be used in the preoperative planning as well as the intraoperative stages of the orthognathic surgery and distraction osteogenesis being used to diagnose and plan the treatment of congenital deformities associated with the maxillomandibular complex. Unlike in the traditional use of plaster

models, skeletal maxillofacial defects of pitch, roll, and yaw can be assessed virtually. Using novel software programs, osteotomy cuts for maxillary, mandibular, and chin movements can be either performed virtually on the digital maxillofacial skeleton or on SLMs derived from 3-D CT datasets.

Perhaps the most work in this area has been performed by Xia and Gateno, who have developed a protocol for computer-aided surgical simulation of complex maxillomandibular deformities.[29,76,77,79,82,83] The rate-limiting steps in previous computer-simulated protocols has been the low-quality reproduction of patient's occlusion by CT that is needed for intricate movements of the jaws and obtaining the natural head position of the patient. To circumvent this roadblock, Gateno and colleagues[77] developed a protocol where during the initial preoperative period the patient undergoes a facial CT using the placement of a specialized bite jig with attached fiducial markers. Traditional plaster dental models are fabricated, their teeth are surface laser scanned, and the data are then imported digitally and substituted for the low-resolution teeth of the CT data set. The fiducial markers are then used to register the digital dental models to the 3-D CT skull model. The resultant 3-D image is the high-quality skeletal detail of the CT dataset

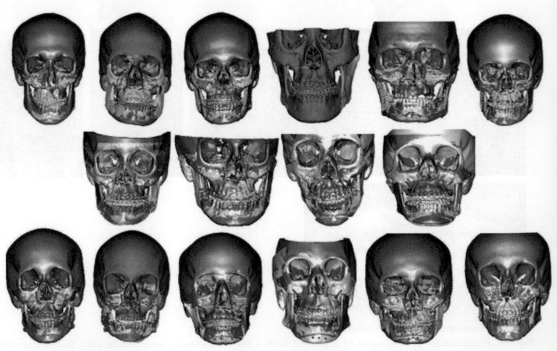

Fig. 13. Series of mandibular reconstructions using preoperative planning and intraoperative surgical navigation. The pink shaded areas represent the planned postoperative position of the mandible. The green shaded areas of the mandible represent the actual postoperative position of the mandible.

Table 5
Differences in planned and actual outcomes in subjects undergoing computer assisted orthognathic surgery

Procedure	Category	Average (mm)	Std Dev (mm)
Orthognathic	Midface registration quality	0.92	0.59
	Mandible registration quality	0.93	0.63
	LeFort triangle	2.54	0.99
	Distal mandible triangle	1.17	0.66
	[Averaged occlusal patients]	1.83	1.08
	Chin triangle	5.82	3.41

combined with the accurate rendering of the laser-scanned dental models. To obtain the natural head position of the patient, gyroscopic measurements are taken and used to orient the CT data set in the appropriate 3-D space. Next, using a 3-D software planning program, such as SimPlant OMS (Materialise Dental, Leuven, Belgium), as in lateral cephalometric analysis in traditional orthognathic surgery planning, the dentofacial is quantified, virtually using anthropometric measurements. Unlike in traditional lateral cephalometric analysis, however, which is limited to the sagittal plane, 3-D imaging software programs allow planning in the transverse and coronal planes as well. Lastly, the surgery is then either simulated on an SLM or, more commonly, virtually using the planning software (**Figs. 11, 12**). Osteotomy cuts are made, and the virtual segmentalization of the maxilla, mandible, and chin is performed. The proposed movements are then made in concordance with planned measurements. Any inaccuracies of the proposed surgical plan can be changed for alternative movements. Intermediate and virtual splints are then made using a CAM/CAM technique based on intermediate and final positions of the virtual surgery. In addition, if the surgeon prefers, cutting guides can be made using a CAD/CAM technique to be used in the operating room that aid in replicating the osteotomies made during the virtual procedure. Early outcomes of the authors' patients undergoing computer-assisted orthognathic surgery have shown marginal difference in planned and actual postoperative outcomes (**Fig. 13, Table 5**).

SUMMARY

The advent of 3-D imaging has ushered in a new era of diagnosis and treatment planning for complex craniomaxillofacial problems. The preliminary results using various computer-aided surgical simulation systems by which the virtual plan is transferred to the patient are promising. It seems that use of these systems has educational value, reduces operating room time, and may provide more accurate reconstructions than were previously not easily obtainable. Additional studies are needed to compare functional and esthetic results with similar cohorts treated without virtual planning and thorough cost-benefit analysis.

REFERENCES

1. Riphagen JM, van Neck JW, van Adrichem LN. 3D surface imaging in medicine: a review of working principles and implications for imaging the unsedated child. J Craniofac Surg 2008;19(2):517–24.
2. Schwenzer-Zimmerer K, Boerner BI, Schwenzer NF, et al. Facial acquisition by dynamic optical tracked laser imaging: a new approach. J Plast Reconstr Aesthet Surg 2009;62(9):1181–6.
3. Schwenzer-Zimmerer K, Chaitidis D, Berg-Boerner I, et al. Quantitative 3D soft tissue analysis of symmetry prior to and after unilateral cleft lip repair compared with non-cleft persons (performed in Cambodia). J Craniomaxillofac Surg 2008;36(8):431–8.
4. Schwenzer-Zimmerer K, Chaitidis D, Boerner I, et al. Systematic contact-free 3D topometry of the soft tissue profile in cleft lips. Cleft Palate Craniofac J 2008;45(6):607–13.
5. Altobelli DE, Kikinis R, Mulliken JB, et al. Computer-assisted three-dimensional planning in craniofacial surgery. Plast Reconstr Surg 1993;92(4):576–85 [discussion: 586–7].
6. Girod S, Keeve E, Girod B. Advances in interactive craniofacial surgery planning by 3D simulation and visualization. Int J Oral Maxillofac Surg 1995; 24(1 Pt 2):120–5.
7. Vannier MW, Marsh JL, Warren JO. Three dimensional CT reconstruction images for craniofacial surgical planning and evaluation. Radiology 1984; 150(1):179–84.
8. Bohner P, Holler C, Hassfeld S. Operation planning in craniomaxillofacial surgery. Comput Aided Surg 1997;2(3–4):153–61.
9. Zizelmann C, Gellrich NC, Metzger MC, et al. Computer-assisted reconstruction of orbital floor

based on cone beam tomography. Br J Oral Maxillo-fac Surg 2007;45(1):79–80.

10. Pham AM, Rafii AA, Metzger MC, et al. Computer modeling and intraoperative navigation in maxillofacial surgery. Otolaryngol Head Neck Surg 2007;137(4):624–31.

11. Bell RB. Computer planning and intraoperative navigation in cranio-maxillofacial surgery. Oral Maxillo-fac Surg Clin North Am 2010;22(1):135–56.

12. Bell RB, Weimer KA, Dierks EJ. Computer planning and intraoperative navigation for palatomaxillary and mandibular reconstruction with fibular free flaps. J Oral Maxillofac Surg 2011;69(3):724–32.

13. Gregoire C, Adler D, Madey S, et al. Basosquamous carcinoma involving the anterior skull base: a neglected tumor treated using intraoperative navigation as a guide to achieving negative margins. J Oral Maxillofac Surg 2011;69(1):230–6.

14. Markiewicz MR, Bell RB, Arce K, et al. Computer aided maxillofacial surgery. Otorinolaringologia 2010;60(2).

15. Bell RB, Chen J. Frontobasilar fractures: contemporary management. Atlas Oral Maxillofac Surg Clin North Am 2010;18(2):181–96.

16. Hemmy DC, David DJ, Herman GT. Three-dimensional reconstruction of craniofacial deformity using computed tomography. Neurosurgery 1983;13(5):534–41.

17. Gillespie JE, Isherwood I. Three-dimensional anatomical images from computed tomographic scans. Br J Radiol 1986;59(699):289–92.

18. Bill JS, Reuther JF, Dittmann W, et al. Stereolithography in oral and maxillofacial operation planning. Int J Oral Maxillofac Surg 1995;24(1 Pt 2):98–103.

19. Klein HM, Schneider W, Alzen G, et al. Pediatric craniofacial surgery: comparison of milling and stereolithography for 3D model manufacturing. Pediatr Radiol 1992;22(6):458–60.

20. Lambrecht JT, Brix F. Individual skull model fabrication for craniofacial surgery. Cleft Palate J 1990;27(4):382–5 [discussion: 386–7].

21. Sinn DP, Cillo JE Jr, Miles BA. Stereolithography for craniofacial surgery. J Craniofac Surg 2006;17(5):869–75.

22. Chang PS, Parker TH, Patrick CW Jr, et al. The accuracy of stereolithography in planning craniofacial bone replacement. J Craniofac Surg 2003;14(2):164–70.

23. Kleinman A, Leyva F, Lozada J, et al. Loma Linda guide: a stereolithographically designed surgical template: technique paper. J Oral Implantol 2009;35(5):238–44.

24. Kim SH, Kang JM, Choi B, et al. Clinical application of a stereolithographic surgical guide for simple positioning of orthodontic mini-implants. World J Orthod 2008;9(4):371–82.

25. Mavili ME, Canter HI, Saglam-Aydinatay B, et al. Use of three-dimensional medical modeling methods for precise planning of orthognathic surgery. J Craniofac Surg 2007;18(4):740–7.

26. Hidalgo HM, Romo GW, Estolano RT. Stereolithography: a method for planning the surgical correction of the hypertelorism. J Craniofac Surg 2009;20(5):1473–7.

27. Ekstrand K, Hirsch JM. Malignant tumors of the maxilla: virtual planning and real-time rehabilitation with custom-made R-zygoma fixtures and carbon-graphite fiber-reinforced polymer prosthesis. Clin Implant Dent Relat Res 2008;10(1):23–9.

28. Bell RB, Markiewicz MR. Computer-assisted planning, stereolithographic modeling, and intraoperative navigation for complex orbital reconstruction: a descriptive study in a preliminary cohort. J Oral Maxillofac Surg 2009;67(12):2559–70.

29. Xia JJ, Gateno J, Teichgraeber JF, et al. Accuracy of the computer-aided surgical simulation (CASS) system in the treatment of patients with complex craniomaxillofacial deformity: a pilot study. J Oral Maxillofac Surg 2007;65(2):248–54.

30. Schramm A, Gellrich NC, Schmelzeisen R. Navigational surgery of the facial skeleton. Berlin: Springer; 2007.

31. Smith JS, Quinones-Hinojosa A, Barbaro NM, et al. Frame-based stereotactic biopsy remains an important diagnostic tool with distinct advantages over frameless stereotactic biopsy. J Neurooncol 2005;73(2):173–9.

32. Barnett GH, Miller DW, Weisenberger J. Frameless stereotaxy with scalp-applied fiducial markers for brain biopsy procedures: experience in 218 cases. J Neurosurg 1999;91(4):569–76.

33. Brinker T, Arango G, Kaminsky J, et al. An experimental approach to image guided skull base surgery employing a microscope-based neuronavigation system. Acta Neurochir (Wien) 1998;140(9):883–9.

34. Freysinger W, Gunkel AR, Bale R, et al. Three-dimensional navigation in otorhinolaryngological surgery with the viewing wand. Ann Otol Rhinol Laryngol 1998;107(11 Pt 1):953–8.

35. Gregoire C, Adler D, Madey S, et al. Basosquamous carcinoma involving the anterior skull base: a neglected tumor treated using intraoperative navigation as a guide to achieve safe resection margins. J Oral Maxillofac Surg 2011;69(1):230–6.

36. Taub PJ, Narayan P. Surgical navigation technology for treatment of pneumosinus dilatans. Cleft Palate Craniofac J 2007;44(5):562–6.

37. Marmulla R, Niederdellmann H. Computer-assisted bone segment navigation. J Craniomaxillofac Surg 1998;26(6):347–59.

38. Luebbers HT, Messmer P, Obwegeser JA, et al. Comparison of different registration methods for

surgical navigation in cranio-maxillofacial surgery. J Craniomaxillofac Surg 2008;36(2):109–16.

39. Batra PS, Kanowitz SJ, Citardi MJ. Clinical utility of intraoperative volume computed tomography scanner for endoscopic sinonasal and skull base procedures. Am J Rhinol 2008;22(5):511–5.

40. Schramm A, Gellrich NC, Gutwald R, et al. Indications for computer-assisted treatment of cranio-maxillofacial tumors. Comput Aided Surg 2000; 5(5):343–52.

41. Schramm A, Suarez-Cunqueiro MM, Barth EL, et al. Computer-assisted navigation in craniomaxillofacial tumors. J Craniofac Surg 2008;19(4):1067–74.

42. To EW, Yuen EH, Tsang WM, et al. The use of stereotactic navigation guidance in minimally invasive transnasal nasopharyngectomy: a comparison with the conventional open transfacial approach. Br J Radiol 2002;75(892):345–50.

43. Schmelzeisen R, Gellrich NC, Schramm A, et al. Navigation-guided resection of temporomandibular joint ankylosis promotes safety in skull base surgery. J Oral Maxillofac Surg 2002;60(11):1275–83.

44. Lubbers HT, Jacobsen C, Konu D, et al. Surgical navigation in cranio-maxillofacial surgery: an evaluation on a child with a cranio-facio-orbital tumour. Br J Oral Maxillofac Surg 2010. [Epub ahead of print].

45. Hidalgo DA. Fibula free flap: a new method of mandible reconstruction. Plast Reconstr Surg 1989;84(1):71–9.

46. Wei FC, Santamaria E, Chang YM, et al. Mandibular reconstruction with fibular osteoseptocutaneous free flap and simultaneous placement of osseointegrated dental implants. J Craniofac Surg 1997; 8(6):512–21.

47. Odin G, Balaguer T, Savoldelli C, et al. Immediate functional loading of an implant-supported fixed prosthesis at the time of ablative surgery and mandibular reconstruction for squamous cell carcinoma. J Oral Implantol 2010;36(3):225–30.

48. Papadopulos NA, Schaff J, Sader R, et al. Mandibular reconstruction with free osteofasciocutaneous fibula flap: a 10 years experience. Injury 2008; 39(Suppl 3):S75–82.

49. Hundepool AC, Dumans AG, Hofer SO, et al. Rehabilitation after mandibular reconstruction with fibula free-flap: clinical outcome and quality of life assessment. Int J Oral Maxillofac Surg 2008; 37(11):1009–13.

50. Garrett N, Roumanas ED, Blackwell KE, et al. Efficacy of conventional and implant-supported mandibular resection prostheses: study overview and treatment outcomes. J Prosthet Dent 2006; 96(1):13–24.

51. Chiapasco M, Biglioli F, Autelitano L, et al. Clinical outcome of dental implants placed in fibula-free flaps used for the reconstruction of maxillomandibular defects following ablation for tumors or

osteoradionecrosis. Clin Oral Implants Res 2006; 17(2):220–8.

52. Sclaroff A, Haughey B, Gay WD, et al. Immediate mandibular reconstruction and placement of dental implants. At the time of ablative surgery. Oral Surg Oral Med Oral Pathol 1994;78(6):711–7.

53. Hirsch DL, Garfein ES, Christensen AM, et al. Use of computer-aided design and computer-aided manufacturing to produce orthognathically ideal surgical outcomes: a paradigm shift in head and neck reconstruction. J Oral Maxillofac Surg 2009; 67(10):2115–22.

54. Leiggener C, Messo E, Thor A, et al. A selective laser sintering guide for transferring a virtual plan to real time surgery in composite mandibular reconstruction with free fibula osseous flaps. Int J Oral Maxillofac Surg 2009;38(2):187–92.

55. Hammer B, Kunz C, Schramm A, et al. Repair of complex orbital fractures: technical problems, state-of-the-art solutions and future perspectives. Ann Acad Med Singapore 1999;28(5):687–91.

56. Gellrich NC, Schramm A, Hammer B, et al. Computer-assisted secondary reconstruction of unilateral posttraumatic orbital deformity. Plast Reconstr Surg 2002;110(6):1417–29.

57. Yu H, Shen G, Wang X, et al. Navigation-guided reduction and orbital floor reconstruction in the treatment of zygomatic-orbital-maxillary complex fractures. J Oral Maxillofac Surg 2010;68(1):28–34.

58. Ploder O, Klug C, Backfrieder W, et al. 2D- and 3D-based measurements of orbital floor fractures from CT scans. J Craniomaxillofac Surg 2002; 30(3):153–9.

59. Ploder O, Klug C, Voracek M, et al. A computer-based method for calculation of orbital floor fractures from coronal computed tomography scans. J Oral Maxillofac Surg 2001;59(12):1437–42.

60. Ploder O, Klug C, Voracek M, et al. Evaluation of computer-based area and volume measurement from coronal computed tomography scans in isolated blowout fractures of the orbital floor. J Oral Maxillofac Surg 2002;60(11):1267–72 [discussion: 1273–4].

61. Markiewicz MR, Dierks EJ, Bell RB. The effectiveness and reliability of computer assisted orbital surgery in restoring orbital dimensions in post-traumatic and post-ablative defects paper presented at: American Association of Oral and Maxillofacial Surgeons Annual Meeting. Chicago, IL, September 30, 2010.

62. Lieger O, Richards R, Liu M, et al. Computer-assisted design and manufacture of implants in the late reconstruction of extensive orbital fractures. Arch Facial Plast Surg 2010;12(3):186–91.

63. Metzger MC, Schon R, Zizelmann C, et al. Semiautomatic procedure for individual preforming of titanium meshes for orbital fractures. Plast Reconstr Surg 2007;119(3):969–76.

64. Metzger MC, Schon R, Schulze D, et al. Individual preformed titanium meshes for orbital fractures. Oral Surg Oral Med Oral Pathol Oral Radiol Endod 2006;102(4):442–7.

65. Sahoo N, Roy ID, Desai AP, et al. Comparative evaluation of autogenous calvarial bone graft and alloplastic materials for secondary reconstruction of cranial defects. J Craniofac Surg 2010;21(1):79–82.

66. Ducic Y. Titanium mesh and hydroxyapatite cement cranioplasty: a report of 20 cases. J Oral Maxillofac Surg 2002;60(3):272–6.

67. Lethaus B, Poort Ter Laak M, Laeven P, et al. A treatment algorithm for patients with large skull bone defects and first results. J Craniomaxillofac Surg 2011;39(6):435–40.

68. Grant GA, Jolley M, Ellenbogen RG, et al. Failure of autologous bone-assisted cranioplasty following decompressive craniectomy in children and adolescents. J Neurosurg 2004;100(2 Suppl Pediatrics): 163–8.

69. Chim H, Schantz JT. New frontiers in calvarial reconstruction: integrating computer-assisted design and tissue engineering in cranioplasty. Plast Reconstr Surg 2005;116(6):1726–41.

70. Solaro P, Pierangeli E, Pizzoni C, et al. From computerized tomography data processing to rapid manufacturing of custom-made prostheses for cranioplasty. Case report. J Neurosurg Sci 2008;52(4): 113–6 [discussion: 116].

71. Metzger MC, Hohlweg-Majert B, Schwarz U, et al. Manufacturing splints for orthognathic surgery using a three-dimensional printer. Oral Surg Oral Med Oral Pathol Oral Radiol Endod 2008;105(2):e1–7.

72. Swennen GR, Mommaerts MY, Abeloos J, et al. The use of a wax bite wafer and a double computed tomography scan procedure to obtain a three-dimensional augmented virtual skull model. J Craniofac Surg 2007;18(3):533–9.

73. Olszewski R, Villamil MB, Trevisan DG, et al. Towards an integrated system for planning and assisting maxillofacial orthognathic surgery. Comput Methods Programs Biomed 2008;91(1):13–21.

74. Noguchi N, Tsuji M, Shigematsu M, et al. An orthognathic simulation system integrating teeth, jaw and face data using 3D cephalometry. Int J Oral Maxillofac Surg 2007;36(7):640–5.

75. Papadopoulos MA, Christou PK, Athanasiou AE, et al. Three-dimensional craniofacial reconstruction imaging. Oral Surg Oral Med Oral Pathol Oral Radiol Endod 2002;93(4):382–93.

76. Xia J, Ip HH, Samman N, et al. Computer-assisted three-dimensional surgical planning and simulation: 3D virtual osteotomy. Int J Oral Maxillofac Surg 2000;29(1):11–7.

77. Gateno J, Xia J, Teichgraeber JF, et al. A new technique for the creation of a computerized composite skull model. J Oral Maxillofac Surg 2003;61(2):222–7.

78. Santler G. The Graz hemisphere splint: a new precise, non-invasive method of replacing the dental arch of 3D-models by plaster models. J Craniomaxillofac Surg 1998;26(3):169–73.

79. Gateno J, Teichgraeber JF, Xia JJ. Three-dimensional surgical planning for maxillary and midface distraction osteogenesis. J Craniofac Surg 2003; 14(6):833–9.

80. Robiony M, Salvo I, Costa F, et al. Virtual reality surgical planning for maxillofacial distraction osteogenesis: the role of reverse engineering rapid prototyping and cooperative work. J Oral Maxillofac Surg 2007;65(6):1198–208.

81. Ploder O, Kohnke R, Klug C, et al. Three-dimensional measurement of the mandible after mandibular midline distraction using a cemented and screw-fixated tooth-borne appliance: a clinical study. J Oral Maxillofac Surg 2009;67(3):582–8.

82. Gateno J, Xia JJ, Teichgraeber JF, et al. Clinical feasibility of computer-aided surgical simulation (CASS) in the treatment of complex craniomaxillofacial deformities. J Oral Maxillofac Surg 2007;65(4):728–34.

83. Xia JJ, Gateno J, Teichgraeber JF. New clinical protocol to evaluate craniomaxillofacial deformity and plan surgical correction. J Oral Maxillofac Surg 2009;67(10):2093–106.

3D Volume Assessment Techniques and Computer-Aided Design and Manufacturing for Preoperative Fabrication of Implants in Head and Neck Reconstruction

Ashish Patel, DDS, MD[a], David Otterburn, MD[b],
Pierre Saadeh, MD[b], Jamie Levine, MD[b],
David L. Hirsch, DDS, MD[c,*]

KEYWORDS

- Three dimensional volumetric analysis
- Craniomaxillofacial surgery • Computer-aided design
- Head and neck reconstruction • Virtual surgical planning

Three dimensional (3D) facial analysis and virtual surgical simulation has revolutionized the way surgeons diagnose, treat, and reconstruct head and neck diseases and defects. In our modern computer era, digital planning has been the standard in architectural design, engineering, and biomedical fabrication; this trend has recently made an impact on clinical medicine and surgery. In all aspects of surgery, proper planning facilitates more predictable operations and operative results, but prior to the use of virtual planning, much of this relied on inaccurate surgical models, intraoperative trial and error, and 2-dimensional (2D) imaging. This process increases operative time, operator frustration, and postoperative inaccuracies.

The goal of this article is to illustrate the ease with which virtual surgery and computer-assisted design can be integrated into one's armamentarium, and benefit the surgeon and the patient with more precise surgical planning, decreased operating time, and creation of accurate postoperative results compared with traditional craniomaxillofacial surgical treatment planning. At their institution, the authors have reliably achieved excellent results in corrective surgery of the jaws, maxillofacial trauma, temporomandibular joint reconstruction, skull base surgery, jaw reconstruction, head and neck oncologic surgery, and postablative reconstruction. For the 90+ cases the authors have virtually planned and completed, the cost has ranged from 2000 to 4000 dollars per case depending on the amount of templates and implants fabricated. These techniques have become the authors' preferred method for complex craniomaxillofacial surgery and reconstruction.

CORRECTIVE JAW SURGERY

Orthognathic surgery is widely used in the correction of craniomaxillofacial deformities. There is

The authors have nothing to disclose.

[a] Division of Oral and Maxillofacial Surgery, New York University Langone Medical Center, 462 First Avenue, Suite 5 South, New York, NY 10016, USA
[b] Department of Plastic and Reconstructive Surgery, New York University Langone Medical Center, 560 First Avenue, Suite TH169, New York, NY 10016, USA
[c] Division of Oral and Maxillofacial Surgery, Department of Plastic and Reconstructive Surgery, New York University Langone Medical Center, 560 First Avenue, Suite TH169, New York, NY 10016, USA
* Corresponding author. Manhattan Maxillofacial Surgery, 366 Fifth Avenue, Suite 709, New York, NY 10001.
E-mail address: davidlhirsch@yahoo.com

Facial Plast Surg Clin N Am 19 (2011) 683–709
doi:10.1016/j.fsc.2011.07.010
1064-7406/11/$ – see front matter © 2011 Published by Elsevier Inc.

Case 1. Class III Skeletal Malocclusion with Vertical Maxillary Excess

Fig. 3 shows a 17-year-old otherwise healthy female referred for surgical correction of a skeletal class III occlusion and vertical maxillary excess.

Initial steps in treatment planning as already described call for acquiring a high-resolution CT while the patient wears an interocclusal record with an acrylic facebow (see **Fig. 1**A), and measuring natural head position with a gyroscopic attachment to the facebow bite jig (see **Fig. 1**B). After acquisition of the CT scan (see **Fig. 2**A), the laser scanned dental models are integrated into the radiographic data and the planning phase can begin. The head position as measured by the gyroscope allows for calibration of the 3D movements in the virtual software, and cephalometric landmarks can be marked and referenced. The central condylar hinge axis is virtually applied to the mandible and assists in accurate autorotation (see **Fig. 2**B). The surgical movements are then planned via Internet meeting with the surgeons and biomedical engineer from the modeling company.

Lefort I and sagittal split osteotomies are performed virtually, and the correction of the midline discrepancies, vertical excess, and prognathism are completed. Correction of yaw, pitch, and roll are confirmed by numerical leveling of the 3 axes compared with the preoperative gyroscopic facebow measurements. The osteotomized bony segments are color coded (**Fig. 4**), and can be moved in all 3 planes of the space with the computer mouse. Once the ideal virtual surgery is performed, the plan is submitted and the modeling phase can begin. The modeling company (Medical Modeling Inc, Golden, CO) fabricates stereolithographic models of the skull as well as intermediate (**Fig. 5**A) and final (see **Fig. 5**B) occlusal splints. In the surgical phase, the osteotomies are performed as planned: Lefort I followed by application of the intermediate splint and maxillomandibular fixation (MMF), and microplate fixation to the vertical facial buttresses. Once the maxilla is fixated, the MMF is released and the mandibular sagittal split osteotomies are performed, placed into final occlusion with the final occlusal splint, and the mandibular segments are fixated with sagittal plates and screws. The desired occlusion and skeletal changes were successfully achieved (**Fig. 6**).

The fourth and final stage of computer-assisted surgery may be the most important. The evaluation phase begins in the postoperative period, and allows the surgeon to compare the predicted results with the actual outcome. Clinically the correction of this patient's vertical maxillary excess, midface deficiency, and mandibular prognathism is evident (**Fig. 7**), but does it correlate with the virtual surgery and treatment plan? A postoperative CT is acquired and sent to the modeling company. This CT scan is rendered into a 3D image and overlaid against the 3D image of the treatment plan. Here, the surgeon can see how accurate the planned movements are reflected in the actual result. The overlay is color-shaded to provide a visual representation of the accuracy, thus allowing the surgeon to identify both anatomic areas of error and the cause of these inaccuracies.

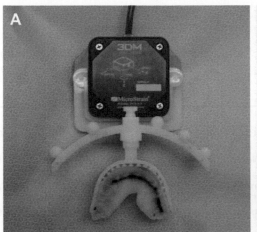 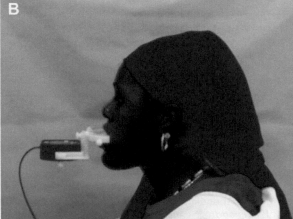

Fig. 1. (*A*) Facebow bite jig. (*B*) Natural head position with gyroscopic attachment to facebow bite jig.

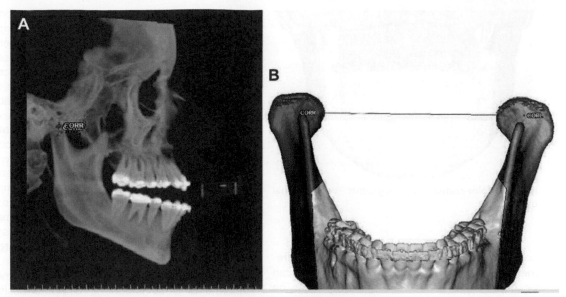

Fig. 2. Computed tomography scan with facebow in place (*A*), virtual condylar hinge axis applied (*B*).

a rich history of preoperative planning and evolution of surgical techniques dating back to the 1800s and, for the most part, the basis of these procedures has not changed in the last several decades. Traditional planning for correction of skeletal facial deformities is complex, and requires several sets of patient data to establish the correct

diagnosis and treatment plan. Facial and intraoral photographs, lateral cephalogram, orthopantomogram, and articulated dental casts are necessary to begin this process. After evaluating the aforementioned data, most surgeons digitally or manually trace the lateral cephalogram and plan sagittal maxillomandibular movements based on

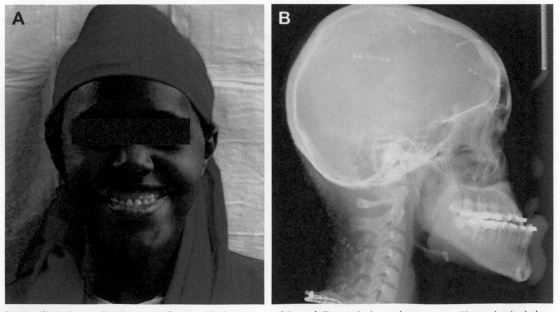

Fig. 3. Clinical examination reveals mandibular prognathism, dolicocephaly, and excess maxillary gingival show on smiling (*A*). Her lateral cephalogram is significant for a skeletal class III sagittal pattern and hyperdivergent mandible (*B*).

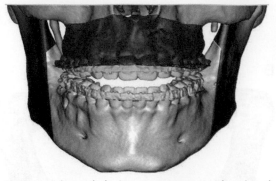

Fig. 4. Color-coded jaw segments with virtual osteotomies.

correction of predefined cephalometric measurements. Correction of yaw and roll, however, can be much more difficult and generally relies on precise dental cast mounting, clinical examination, and facial/intraoral photographs. After determining the amount of correction of the maxilla and mandible in all 3 planes, "surgery" on the dental models is performed to replicate the intraoperative repositioning of the jaws, and interocclusal splints are fabricated with acrylic. These splints are essential in repositioning the jaws, especially when maxillary and mandibular surgeries are performed together, but their accuracy is dependent on several factors. Because most of these movements are in the 1- to 10-mm range, small errors

and discrepancies in each step of the workup can compound and lead to inaccurate and unpredictable final results. Facebow records, interocclusal records, deformation of dental impression material, inaccurate mounting, shrinkage of acrylic splints, inaccurate placement of line markings, and small discrepancies in model surgery all lead to some degree of error, rendering the exact measurements in movement planning not totally predictive of the end result.[1] Facebow records rely on the arc of rotation of the mandible when transferred, but the hinge axis is connected to the maxillary arm of dental articulators. Complex facial asymmetries are nearly impossible to correct in 2D planning, and many times[2] asymmetries are induced, due to the compounding of small errors throughout the planning and model surgery process.

In an operation whereby planning in millimeter increments is so important, computer-assisted virtual surgery proves to be a valuable asset in producing more predictable results. By eliminating several sources of error, one can plan more precisely and achieve more accurate movements. The first step in this process involves acquisition of the appropriate data set. Noncontrast maxillofacial computed tomography (CT) is acquired while the patient occludes in maximum intercuspation. To ensure an accurate transfer of the patient's occlusion to the radiographic data, a facebow bite jig is fabricated by impressing the dentition with hard-set acrylic. When set, this model provides an

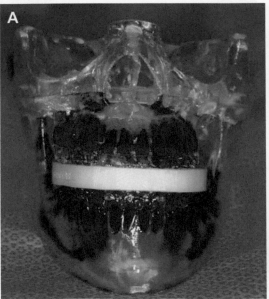
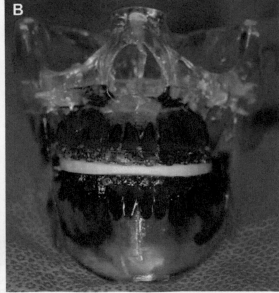

Fig. 5. Stereolithographic model of skull with intermediate (*A*) and final (*B*) occlusal splints.

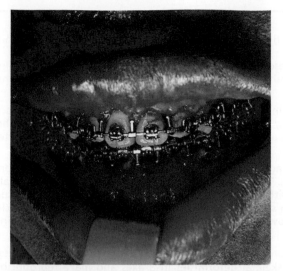

Fig. 6. Final occlusion after completion of the maxillary and mandibular osteotomies.

accurate representation of the patient's bite. The patient is sent to the CT scanner with the jig in place and 1-mm cuts or high-resolution CT is acquired (see **case 1, Figs. 1**A and **2**A). A gyroscope is then attached to the facebow jig to measure the natural head position, yaw, pitch, and roll, thus replacing the need for facebow transfer and dental cast articulation. The CT scan, along with traditional gypsum maxillary and mandibular dental models, is sent to the desired modeling company. The dental casts are laser scanned and digitally merged into the maxillofacial CT to allow for accurate representation of the dentition without scatter artifact. Treatment planning is completed via the software using the 3D facial reconstructions of the CT scan. Accurate correction of yaw, pitch, and roll as well as midline correction and facial heights can be completed in all 3 planes of space. Using plain cephalometric films as in traditional orthognathic treatment

A

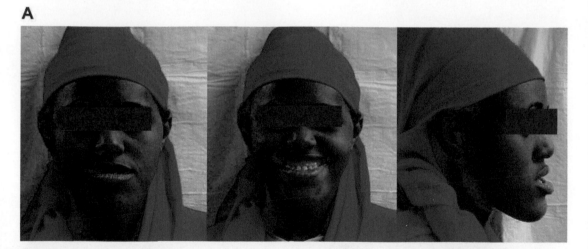

B

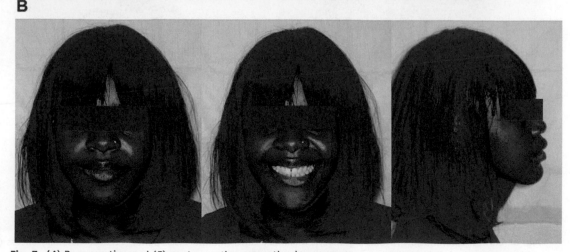

Fig. 7. (A) Preoperative and (B) postoperative corrective jaw surgery.

CASE 2. COMPLEX FACIAL ASYMMETRY

A 32-year-old woman with a history of right-sided mandibular condylar hyperplasia presents with a chief complaint of facial asymmetry (Fig. 8).

After acquisition of the appropriate data as described previously, the Web meeting with 3D imaging takes place. Preoperative facial skeletal relationships with soft-tissue overlays are analyzed in all planes (Fig. 9).

The osteotomies are planned (Fig. 10A, B), and in this case a malar implant was virtually constructed to correct the left-sided orbitozygomatic deficiency (see Fig. 10C). The modeling phase consisted of fabrication of intermediate and final occlusal splints as well as the custom planned cheek implant, all fitted to the stereolithographic model (see Fig. 10D).

In the surgical phase, the Lefort I and bilateral sagittal split osteotomies are performed as planned, and fixated using the intermediate and final splints. The left-sided malar implant is introduced transorally and fits precisely over the malar prominence without rocking or moving, and is secured with titanium screws through the premilled screw holes. After stable fixation of the maxilla and mandible, the occlusion is noted to be class I as planned. Fig. 11 shows postoperative correction of maxillary cant, midline, vertical excess, and orbitozygomatic deficiency.

In the authors' experience, virtual treatment planning provides very accurate and predictable results in orthognathic surgery. The ability to visualize skeletal deformities in 3 axes and make reproducible submillimeter movements allows the surgeon to attain the desired outcome. In addition, virtual planning saves a significant amount of preoperative time, as many of the steps in traditional planning have no utility in this model.

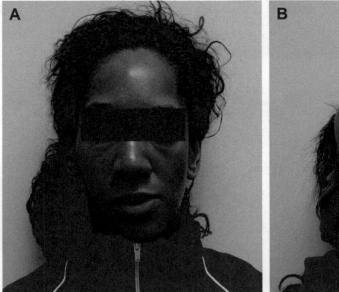
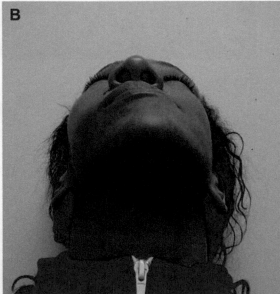

Fig. 8. Clinical examination reveals significant maxillary cant, midline discrepancy, vertical maxillary excess (*A*), orbitozygomatic deficiency, and mandibular asymmetry (*B*).

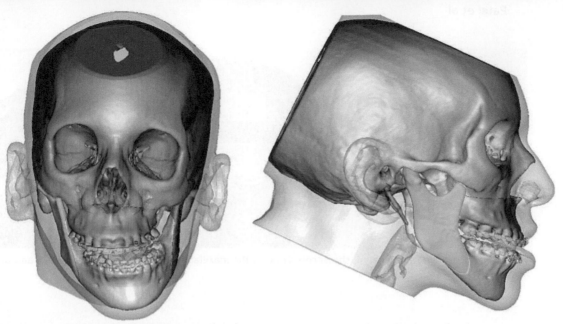

Fig. 9. Preoperative hard and soft tissue overlay.

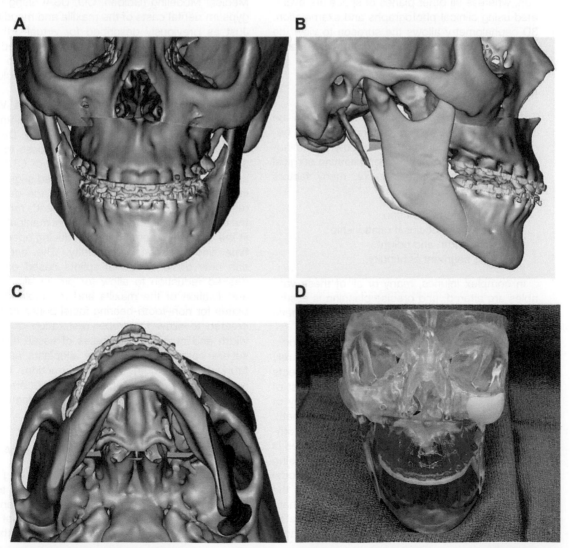

Fig. 10. (*A*, *B*) Frontal and sagittal views of 3D virtual osteotomies. (*C*) Virtual malar implant. (*D*) Model with occlusal splint and cheek implant.

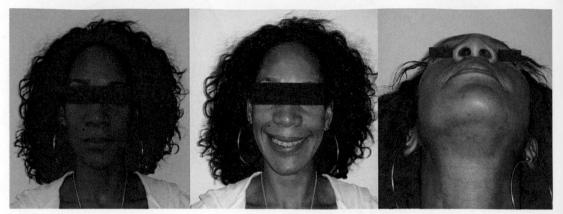

Fig. 11. Postoperative facial analysis shows correction of the maxillary cant, midline, vertical excess, and orbito-zygomatic deficiency.

planning only allows for two dimensional correction, whereas all other planes of space are evaluated using clinical photographs and examination. 3D cephalometry allows the surgeon to view the skeletal defects in relation to the entire facial skeleton.

MAXILLOFACIAL TRAUMA

Treating complex maxillofacial trauma can be challenging even to experienced surgeons because of severe distortion of anatomy, comminution, and tissue avulsion. When planning surgical correction of a traumatic injury, many factors must be considered:

- Status of the dentition
- Preexisting occlusal relationship
- Facial width and height
- Bone segment continuity.

In complex injuries, many or all of these variables are altered, and precise planning is essential for a favorable functional and aesthetic outcome.[3]

There are several approaches to complex trauma described in the surgical literature, and many rely on reduction and fixation of mandibular defects to serve as the template for reducing the rest of the facial bone fractures. Unfortunately many of these complex injuries involve avulsion of teeth, alveolar process fractures, and mandibular comminution; accurate reduction of these fractures is technically difficult. Preoperative planning using dental casts and premade splints based on model surgery may be helpful but only addresses the tooth-bearing bony segments; this is where computer-assisted virtual surgery is beneficial in planning these operations. CT scan of the facial skeleton is acquired in 1-mm cuts, and is sent to Medical Modeling (Golden, CO, USA) along with gypsum dental casts of the maxilla and mandible. Just as previously described for virtual orthognathic surgery, the casts are laser scanned by the modeling company and matrixed into the maxillofacial CT to provide accurate occlusal anatomy for splint fabrication.

Planning of the surgery starts with a Web meeting between the surgical team and biomedical engineer from the modeling company. During the meeting, all participants have access to the 3D reconstructions of the combined CT/laser scan, and can manipulate the fractured segments in the virtual environment to obtain the desired result. This "virtual reduction" significantly reduces the amount of trial-and-error segment manipulation in the operating room, thereby reducing operating time and associated morbidity. The engineer can now design occlusal splints based on the desired reduction to allow for proper alignment and fixation of the maxilla and mandible. Templates for non–tooth-bearing facial bones can be created to allow for proper restoration of facial width and projection. In cases of tissue loss or severe comminution, custom alloplasts can be fabricated to aid in the reconstruction. These surgical guides and alloplastic implants are sent to the surgical team, sterilized, and implemented intraoperatively.

TEMPOROMANDIBULAR JOINT/SKULL BASE

The key to a successful operation involving the temporomandibular joint (TMJ) or base of skull is exposure and access. Because of the density of vital structures in this area, care must be taken to avoid inadvertently damaging these

CASE 3. PANFACIAL TRAUMA WITH TISSUE AVULSION

A 39-year-old woman taxicab passenger was hit by an 18-wheeler and suffered a traumatic brain injury as well as multiple facial fractures including frontal sinus, right orbital roof, right zygomatic arch, naso-orbitoethmoid, comminuted LeFort III, palatal, and right mandibular parasymphysis fractures. Her initial management included frontal craniectomy by the neurosurgery team to relieve brain edema.

The planning phase begins with acquiring high-resolution maxillofacial CT images and dental models. These images are sent to the modeling company, and a composite merged 3D reconstruction is created (**Figs. 12** and **13**). The bony injuries are analyzed in all planes and virtual reduction of the fractures is performed according to the surgeon's preference—in this case top down, outside in. Volumetric and linear analysis of reduced segments is easily computed by the virtual software to aid in establishing symmetry, facial widths, and facial heights. In complex panfacial trauma, much of this trial-and-error process is completed intraoperatively, resulting in increased operating time and inability to evaluate the final repairs until postoperative imaging is acquired. Using virtual surgery this can take place preoperatively, and the ideal reduction and fixation can be planned to submillimeter increments.

Once the fractures are successfully virtually reduced, planning for replacing lost tissue is addressed. The right orbital bony avulsion is virtually reconstructed with a planned bone graft from the anterior iliac crest (**Fig. 14**A). To successfully recreate the planned surgery, several guides and splints are manufactured in the modeling phase of the virtual surgery. A frontal bandeau guide is fabricated to allow for correction of the upper facial width (see **Fig. 14**B). Bilateral lateral orbital guides are manufactured to reestablish orbitomalar width, projection, and contour (see **Fig. 14**C). A bone graft template is fabricated to mimic the planned corticocancellous block graft for the right orbit (**Fig. 15**C), and occlusal splints are created to establish the correct maxillomandibular relations in the sagittal and axial planes (see **Fig. 14**D).

In the surgical phase, all of the fractures are exposed and the operation is performed as planned, using the prefabricated templates and guides to ensure correct positioning of the fractured facial bones (see **Fig. 15**A–C). Tactile feedback of the guides and templates as they "snap" into place allows the surgeon to verify appropriate application. The guides are secured to healthy bone segments with screws using the premade screw holes, and are designed to not interfere with placement of osteosynthesis plates. The fractured segments are then reduced to fit flush against the guides and secured appropriately. In this case, after reduction and fixation of all fractures and application of the orbital bone graft (see **Fig. 15**D), a titanium mesh was contoured and applied to the craniectomy site and a monocortical calvarial bone graft was harvested from the parietal bone to create a dorsal nasal strut. In a second operation, the titanium mesh was replaced with a custom-fabricated titanium calvarial implant (**Fig. 16**).

In the evaluation phase, a postoperative high-resolution CT scan is obtained and sent to the modeling company. This image is superimposed against the virtual treatment plan, and volumetric analysis is completed by the biomedical engineer using the virtual software. Deviation of the actual results compared with the virtual plan is measured in 3 planes of space, and a set of color-coded matrixed images are created and sent to the surgeon. Using color gradients, it is easy to identify areas of success and error in order to identify potential causative sources and correct them in future operations (**Fig. 17**).

when manipulating the area of interest. Precise positioning of allografts and alloplasts in reconstructing the joints is essential to restoring mandibular and occlusal function. Traditionally, reconstructing a TMJ has been performed as a 2-stage operation. Initially, a gap arthroplasty is performed and postoperative CT is acquired to aid in the custom fabrication of a TMJ prosthesis (although custom-fabricated TMJs can be done in one stage). Once fabricated, a second operation is required for adaptation of the custom joint prosthesis. Recently, intraoperative

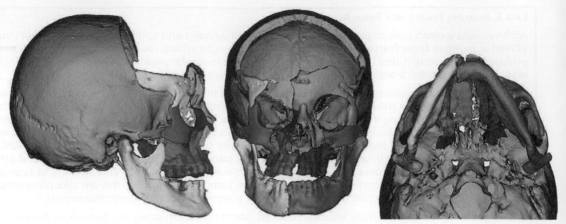

Fig. 12. Each fractured bony segment is color coded for ease of navigation and virtual manipulation.

navigation has been used in these procedures to prevent middle cranial fossa insult and to reduce the risk of neurovascular tissue damage.[4] By combining techniques of computer-assisted design and virtual planning/fabrication with intraoperative navigation, a safe single-stage operation can be provided and the virtual plan intraoperatively confirmed.

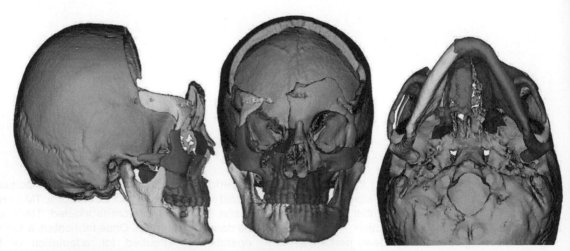

Fig. 13. Virtual reduction of bony segments and restoration of orthognathic relationships.

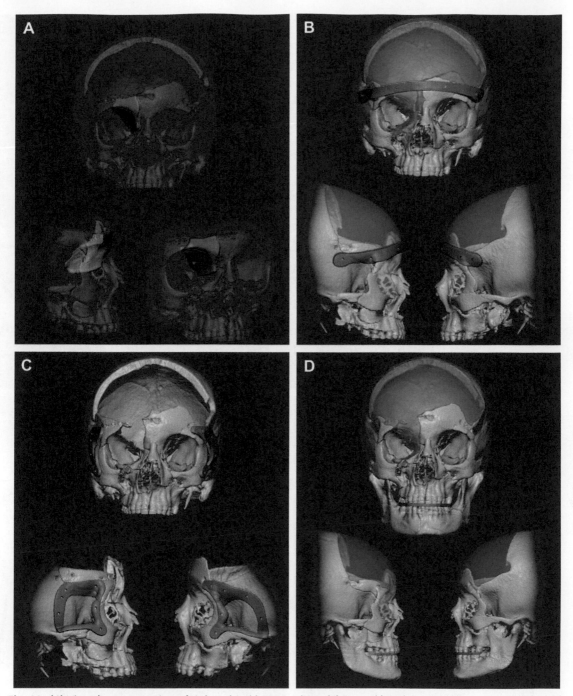

Fig. 14. (*A*) Virtual reconstruction of right orbital bony avulsion (*B*) Frontal bandeau guide for upper facial width correction (*C*) Bilateral lateral guides for orbitomalar width, projection, and contour (*D*) Occlusal splints for maxillo-mandibular relation.

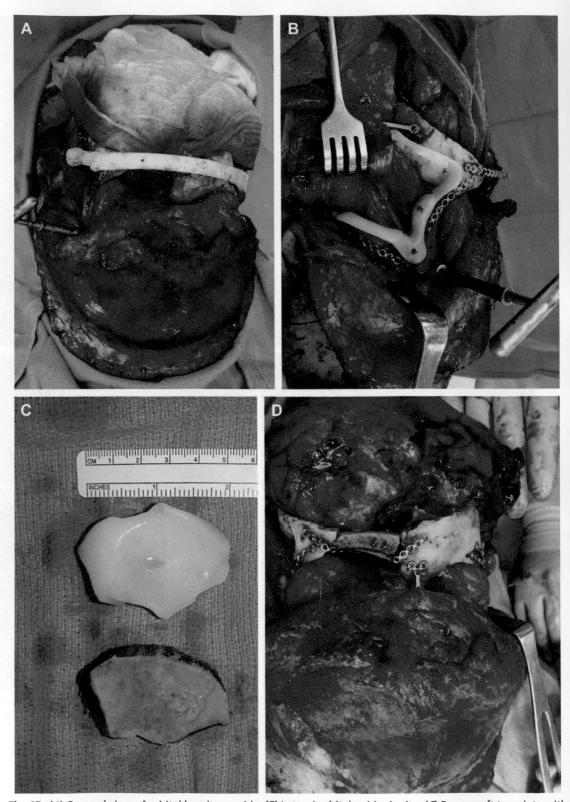

Fig. 15. (*A*) Coronal view of orbital bandeau guide. (*B*) Lateral orbital guides in situ. (*C*) Bone-graft template with corticocancellous anterior iliac crest block. (*D*) Coronal view of orbital bandeau with bone graft in place.

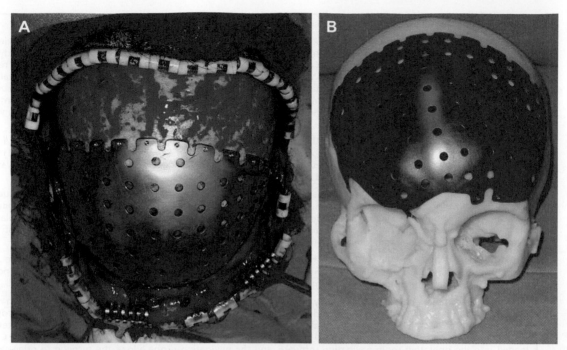

Fig. 16. Custom cranial implant (KLS Martin LP, Jacksonville, FL, USA) on model (*B*), in situ (*A*).

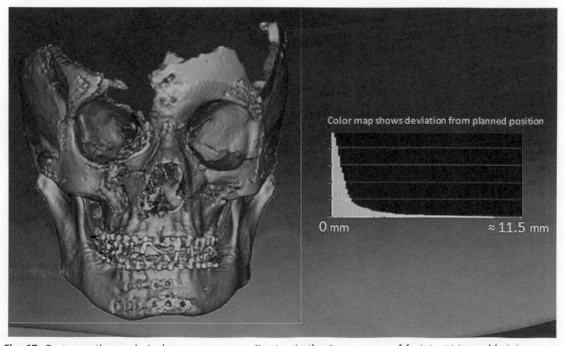

Color map shows deviation from planned position

0 mm   ≈ 11.5 mm

Fig. 17. Postoperative analysis shows accurate replication in the 1-mm range of facial widths and heights.

Case 4. Hard-Tissue Neoplasm with Alloplastic Reconstruction

A 44-year old otherwise healthy man presented with right-sided preauricular enlargement for 6 months and maximal interincisal opening (MIO) of 10 mm. Noncontrast face CT at an outside hospital showed a right mandibular condylar ossified mass extending to the base of skull. Computed tomographic angiography (CTA) revealed the intimate relationships of the infratemporal vasculature to the tumor (**Fig. 18**A). The internal carotid artery passes just medial to the osteochondroma and contacts it briefly, the right posterior auricular artery is draped over the posterior aspect of the mass, and a prominent accessory meningeal artery ascends medially to the mass, contacting it before it enters the foramen ovale. Based on clinical and radiographic findings, the preliminary diagnosis of osteochondroma was made.

To resect the tumor and primarily reconstruct the mandible and TMJ, virtual surgical planning was used. The neck/face CTA with 1-mm cuts and maxillomandibular stone dental casts were sent to the modeling company and uploaded into the virtual software. 3D rendering was completed and a stereolithographic model including the vascular anatomy was fabricated (Medical Modeling Inc) (see **Fig. 18**B).

Surgical resections were designed via Web meeting (**Fig. 19**A), and reconstruction of the joint was created virtually using a stock TMJ prosthesis merged into the virtual 3D rendering (see **Fig. 19**B). By manipulating the osteotomies and ramal and glenoid fossa components of the stock prostheses in the software, ideal positioning of the joint replacement was possible and dental occlusion was maintained. This process allows for a one-stage ablative and reconstructive operation without compromising functional outcome.

Cutting guides for the mandible and glenoid fossa as well as drill guides for the TMJ prosthesis screw holes were designed based on the virtual surgery (**Fig. 20**). A final occlusal splint was also fabricated to maintain ideal mandibular position after resection of the condylar component of the osteochondroma.

Because of the complex anatomy and proximity of the tumor to nerves and blood vessels, intraoperative navigation was planned in addition to the virtual surgical workup. The bulk of the infratemporal component of the osteochondroma was planned to be excised in segments, given the constrictive nature of the anatomy. Preoperatively, selective arterial embolization was performed by interventional radiology. In the ablative phase of the operation, the preoperative CT is loaded into the operating room navigation software, and the navigation probe allows the surgeon to orient and localize 3-dimensionally on the scan (**Fig. 21**A, B). Frameless stereotaxy was used to ensure that the tumor was removed completely without violating vessels and nerves of the infratemporal fossa. Once the tumor was resected using the cutting guides, the virtually planned TMJ reconstruction was loaded into the navigation software. This action allows the surgeon to safely apply the drill guides and TMJ prosthesis as well as localize each screw hole before placement, using the navigation probe to ensure accurate implementation of the virtual plan (see **Fig. 21**C–E). Maxillomandibular fixation was applied using the occlusal splints, and the TMJ prosthesis was fixated via the planned screw holes (**Fig. 22**). After applying the prosthesis and releasing the MMF, the patient was noted to have an intraoperative MIO of 25 mm.

In evaluating the virtual plan a postoperative CT was sent to the modeling company, and a color-coded overlay of the plan and actual result was digitally created (**Fig. 23**).

A   B

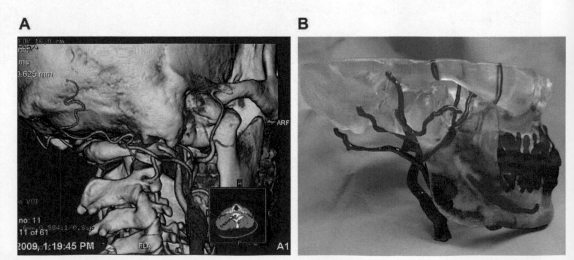

Fig. 18. (*A*) Computed tomographic angiogram showing infratemporal vasculature to tumor. (*B*) 3D stereolithographic model with vascular anatomy.

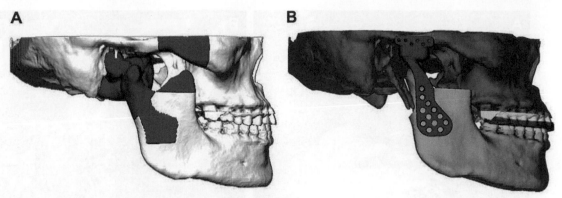

Fig. 19. (*A*) Surgical resection virtual design (*B*) 3D rendering of reconstruction with virtual temporomandibular joint prosthesis.

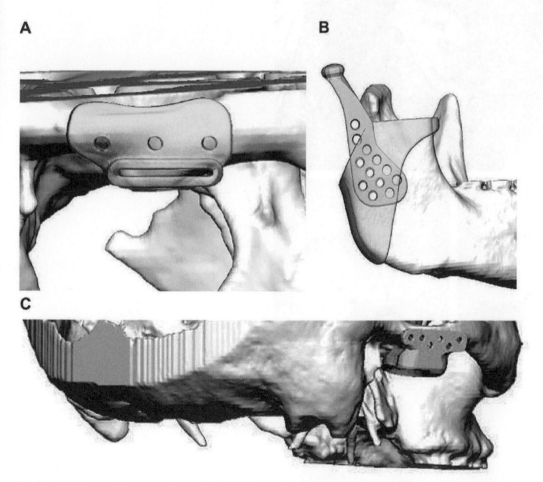

Fig. 20. (*A*) Planned fossa cutting guide. (*B*) Planned ramus cutting guide with prosthesis overlay. (*C*) Planned fossa prosthesis.

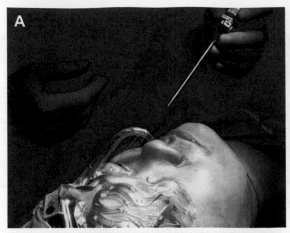

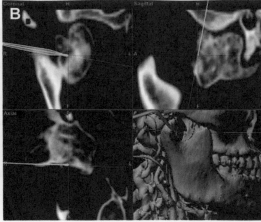

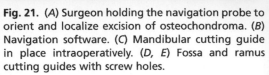

Fig. 21. (*A*) Surgeon holding the navigation probe to orient and localize excision of osteochondroma. (*B*) Navigation software. (*C*) Mandibular cutting guide in place intraoperatively. (*D*, *E*) Fossa and ramus cutting guides with screw holes.

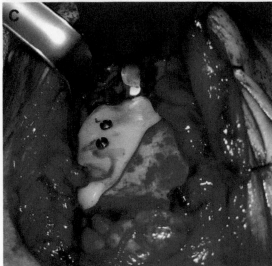

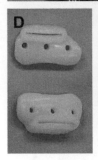

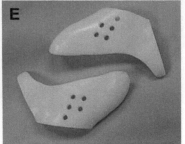

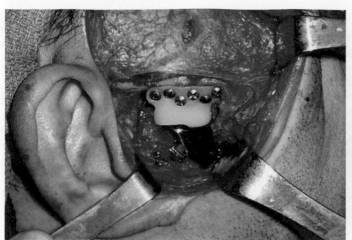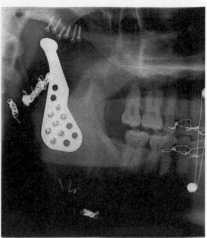

Fig. 22. Fixation of splints and prosthesis intraoperatively and radiographically.

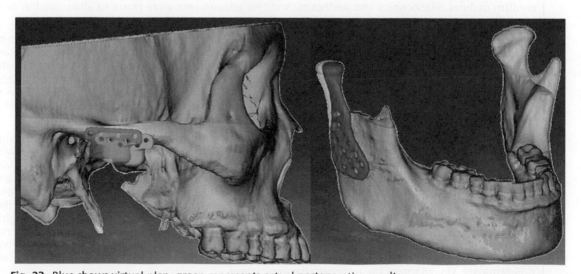

Fig. 23. Blue shows virtual plan, green represents actual postoperative result.

JAW RECONSTRUCTION

Many traumatic craniomaxillofacial injuries involve damage to the dentition and supporting bony structures, and successful reconstruction should include restoration of dental arch form and function. Endosseous implant therapy is the gold standard for tooth replacement given its high success rate, longevity, and durability. Because of the nature of the operation, free-handing the surgical placement of implant fixtures can be unreliable. In cases where multiple implants are planned to support a fixed dental prosthesis, it is imperative to obtain parellelism and recreate dental arch form to create a functional and aesthetically acceptable final reconstruction. Using virtual surgery the ideal diameter, shape, length, and number of fixtures can be planned, all while creating ideal angulations and avoiding damage to neurovascular structures.

CASE 5. POSTTRAUMATIC SKELETODENTAL RECONSTRUCTION

The patient was a 32-year old man, 6 months status post open reduction and internal fixation of a comminuted mandibular symphysis fracture and right subcondylar fracture as well as closed reduction of a left subcondylar and coronoid process fracture sustained during a motor vehicle accident. At the time of his initial injury, several maxillary and mandibular teeth were fractured and avulsed, and all nonrestorable teeth were extracted during the repair of his mandibular fractures.

On examination, the patient's lower face was noted to be widened and was missing multiple teeth. Seven maxillary endosseous implants had been placed in the interim. High-resolution maxillofacial CT along with maxillary and mandibular dental casts were sent to the modeling company to start the surgical planning phase. During the Web meeting, the first step was to establish preinjury mandibular width to create ideal orthognathic relationships for final dental reconstruction. A mandibular midline osteotomy was planned and the left mandibular segment was positioned medially, virtually to seat the condyle in the glenoid fossa and correct for the lingual cortical splaying from initial internal fixation (**Fig. 24**). Endosseous dental implants were planned to restore all missing mandibular teeth (with the exception of third molars). Dimensions of stock implants were imported into the software and placed virtually. Bone-layer transparency and translucency could be controlled easily with the computer mouse so that correct angulations, interimplant distances, bony contact, and proximity to the inferior alveolar nerve could be assessed (**Fig. 25**). Dental restorations were added to the virtual implant surgery to confirm occlusal relationships and aesthetics, and fine adjustments were made to allow for the most ideal fixture placement.

Once the plan was submitted, a mandibular osteotomy cutting guide stabilized to a preosteotomy occlusal splint (**Fig. 26**A), and a final occlusal splint (see **Fig. 26**B) were fabricated. A clear acrylic implant drill guide with metal couplings was designed and manufactured to precisely fit over the mandibular alveolus and remaining teeth (nSequence, Reno, NV, USA) (see **Fig. 26**C). Angulations and exact diameters of the implant osteotomy drills were incorporated into the surgical template to allow the surgeon to replicate the virtual surgery. A stereolithographic model of the facial skeleton was also fabricated so that the reconstruction plate could be prebent to the mandible.

During the actual operation the anterior mandible was exposed transorally, and the mandibular cutting guide was applied and locked into the mandibular dentition. The osteotomy was completed with a sagittal saw and the cutting guide was removed. To replicate the treatment plan, the patient was placed in maxillomandibular fixation with the occlusal splints. The mandible was rigidly fixated and the MMF was released. At this point, the implant drill template was applied to the mandibular alveolus and "snapped" into place over the existing dentition. There was no need to create a mucoperiosteal flap because the position of the implants was preplanned. The guide was designed to fit the correct surgical drill for each implant, and the depth of each osteotomy was replicated by following the depth markings on each drill. The 7 osteotomies were created using a flapless technique, and each implant fixture was driven into its respective site. **Fig. 27** shows implant fixtures in place through use of a surgical implant drill template. **Fig. 28** shows the postoperative radiograph.

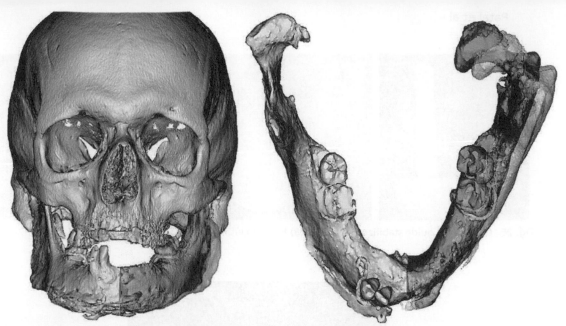

Fig. 24. Virtual positioning and planning of mandibular midline osteotomy.

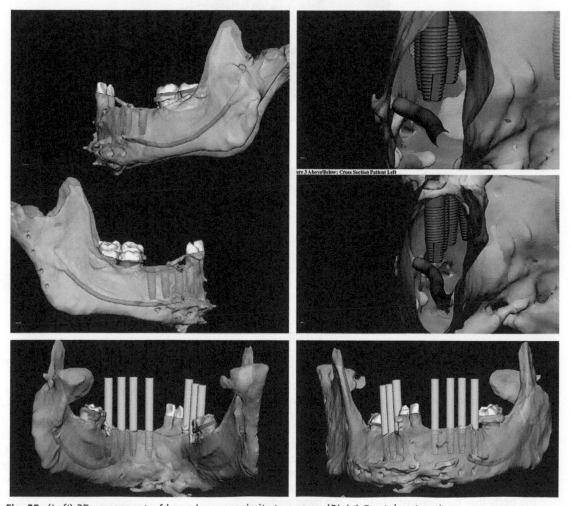

Fig. 25. (*Left*) 3D assessment of bone layer proximity to nerves. (*Right*) Dental restorations.

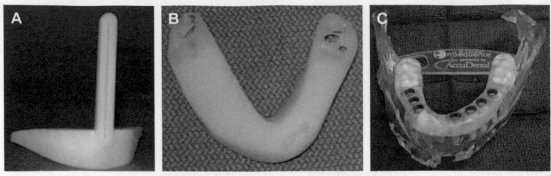

Fig. 26. (*A*) Cutting guide stabilized to splint. (*B*) Final occlusal splint. (*C*) Acrylic implant drill guide.

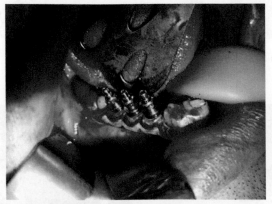

Fig. 27. Implant fixtures in place through surgical implant drill template.

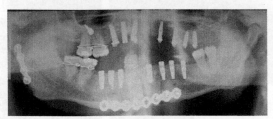

Fig. 28. Postoperatively, it is evident based on radiographic imaging that there is parellelism between the mandibular implant fixtures.

POSTABLATIVE RECONSTRUCTION

Reconstruction of head and neck ablative defects is difficult because many different factors have to be considered. Functionally there are airway, digestive, and speech considerations, while aesthetically there are static and active considerations. Physiologically there are digestive enzymes, high bacterial load, and sheer stresses caused by the constant motion of powerful muscles; therefore, of all the areas in the body that surgeons reconstruct, the head and

neck is the most demanding and also the most rewarding.

As mentioned previously, the cohort of patients with head and neck pathology tend to be some of the most debilitated patients, thus making accurate and efficient surgery a necessity to treat these patients well. The use of 3D modeling to preoperatively plan these surgeries allows for precise extirpative osteotomies, excellent modeling of reconstructive plates, and exact contouring of osteotomies of donor flaps. This

Case 6. Double-Barrel Lateral Segment

This first case for postablative reconstruction demonstrates the possibilities of obtaining good aesthetic outcomes with appropriate functional outcomes. The patient was a 40-year-old man with stage IV squamous cell carcinoma. His preoperative workup, including a CT scan, was consistent with an advanced malignancy of the right mandibular alveolus. Significant bony disruption was noted on the right body of his mandible (**Fig. 29**). Mandibular osteotomies were planned on the 3D reconstructions of the CT scan. Note that generous margins are used to assure that the osteotomies are adequate on the day of surgery (**Fig. 30**).

A CTA of the lower extremity is received to plan accurate osteotomies on the fibula in order to recreate the shape and angles of the native mandible. Stock fibula data can also be used, but does not provide the precision required in complex mandibular reconstruction. This stage is one of the most critical parts of the reconstructive process. By maximizing the chance of 100% bone-to-bone coaptation, one can increase bony healing. The intricate 3D geometry of the mandible, coupled with the triangular-shaped fibula, leads to a complex geometry. It is possible to perform adequate reconstructions without the use of 3D modeling; however, it is difficult to duplicate the predictability of a good result, and the speed and reliability, without using virtual surgery (**Fig. 31**).

To ensure that the osteotomies are performed in the correct planes, cutting guides are created that limit the human variability. These guides are applied to the mandible and secured with screws (**Fig. 32**). Similar guides are also used on the fibula, after care is taken to strip the needed periosteum and to protect the vascular pedicle (**Fig. 33**).

The bending of the reconstruction plate is planned concomitantly with the reconstruction. The bar sets the height of the vascularized bone graft and is therefore important for the positioning of implants. In lateral defects that involve dentition, there is a dichotomy between what is best for aesthetics and what is best for dentition. Dental implants work best when the bony stock is just below where the tooth roots would lie in a normal mandible. However, as the fibula is typically only of 2 cm width, this will not provide the shape or width of a normal lateral mandibular angle. By double barreling, or turning a piece of the neomandible down to fill in that angle, the fibula may be used to accomplish both goals. **Fig. 34** demonstrates this well. It should also be noted that the reconstruction plate is placed at the caudal boarder of the fibula bone graft to ensure that the locking screws placed to hold the fibula to the plate do not interfere with the endosseous implants. Position of the mental nerve is also noted in **Fig. 34**, and the reconstruction plate is positioned to avoid impingement of the nerve. Locking plates and monocortical screws are used on the flap, while bicortical locking screws are used on the native mandible. The most proximal and distal screw holes on the native mandible are planned to coincide with screw holes placed for securing the cutting guides; this allows precise adaptation of the prebent reconstruction plate while maintaining the preoperative orthognathic relationship of the mandibular segments. The double-barrel segment is fixated with monocortical miniplates.

3D virtual surgical preoperative planning helps only when it can be well implemented in the operating room. The critical part of all procedures is relying on hard anatomic markers to position the cutting jigs and to be able to keep in plane while performing the osteotomies. The saw can damage the cutting guides, so this last point is not insignificant.

On the day of surgery, the extirpation is performed as planned with the use of the cutting guides (**Fig. 35**). The guides designed for the mandibular angle and parasymphysis have obvious points of reference, and once secured with screws their use is straightforward. The central cutting guide can be positioned based on dentition if available, giving another stable anatomic marker to ensure the planned result. A sagittal saw is used to complete the mandibular osteotomies through the slots of the cutting guides, and the cutting-guide screw holes on the remaining native mandible are then used for reference points for the proximal and distal ends of the plate.

At their institution the authors use the fibula osteocutaneous flap for almost all their reconstructions (**Fig. 36**). The authors prefer its minimal donor site morbidity along with its plasticity. No other flap allows for a long pedicle, reliable skin and muscle flap, and the convenience of intraoperative positioning and ability for a simultaneous 2-team approach. The authors routinely take a skin paddle, even if the oral mucosa could be primarily closed, for 3 reasons:

1. The skin paddle allows the extirpative surgeons to re-resect margins they had not planned without the fear of compromising the reconstruction, or the need for a second flap

2. The skin paddle allows for another method of flap monitoring

3. The skin paddle brings healthier tissue into the oral cavity, and in the authors' hands decreases fistula rate

Occlusion is maintained following extirpation with use of the reconstruction plate and maxillomandibular fixation. The fibula flap is then placed into the recipient site, as planned preoperatively. This normally involves the vascular pedicle exiting posteriorly. The bony pieces should align well on the plate and be easily secured in place. The skin paddle is draped into the oral cavity, usually with the septum covering the reconstruction plate. Note that in **Fig. 37**, because of the double barreling the skin paddle was brought into the oral cavity posteriorly, therefore not draping over the plate. Revascularization can then be performed and the surgical site closed.

A panoramic plain film or CT scan is obtained before discharge (**Fig. 38**). Once the patient has recovered from the initial surgery, endosseous implants can be placed (**Fig. 39**).

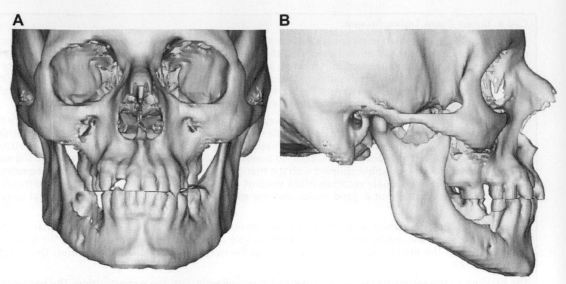

Fig. 29. (*A, B*) Preoperative CT scan identifying right mandibular body tumor invasion.

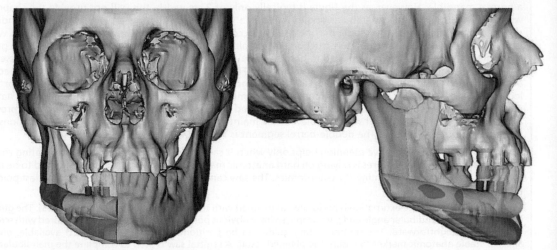

Fig. 30. Planned osteotomies in transparent green, with a superimposed image of the planned reconstruction with double-barreled fibula and osteointegrated implants.

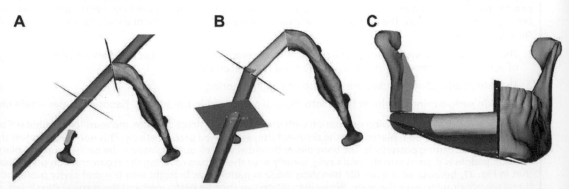

Fig. 31. Planned fibula osteotomies demonstrating the multiple plane angles (*A, B*) to ensure good coaptation including the double-barreled segment (*C*).

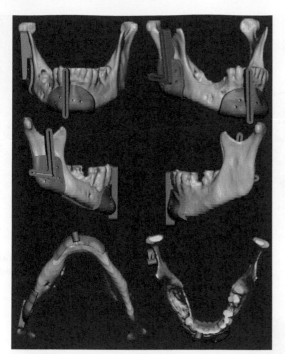

Fig. 32. Mandibular cutting guides.

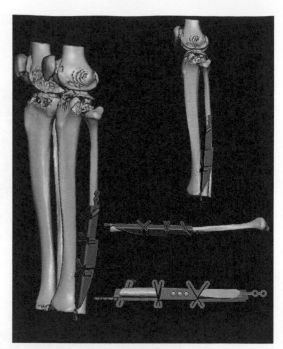

Fig. 33. Fibula cutting guides.

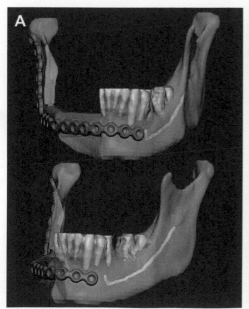

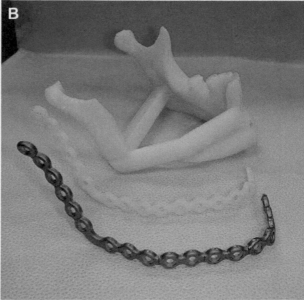

Fig. 34. (*A*) Planning and positioning of the reconstruction bar on 3D modeling software. (*B*) Prebent plate using manufactured neomandible model.

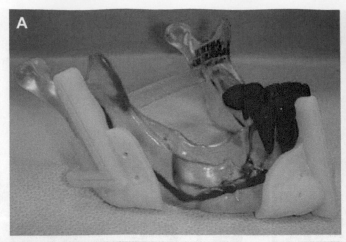

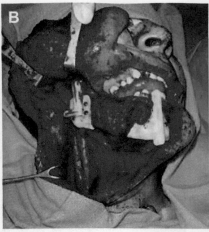

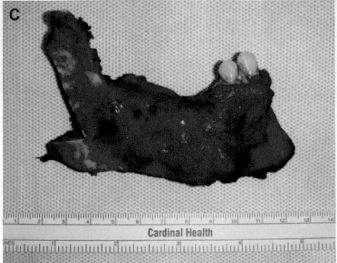

Fig. 35. (A–C) Extirpation of the mandibular mass using preplanned cutting guides.

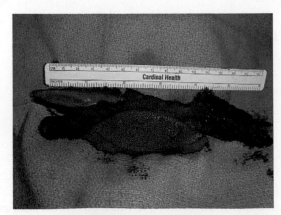

Fig. 36. Osteocutaneous fibula flap after osteotomies.

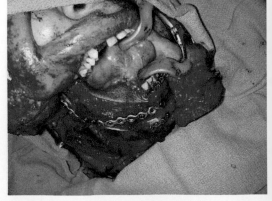

Fig. 37. Insetting of double-barreled fibula with intraoral positioning of skin paddle.

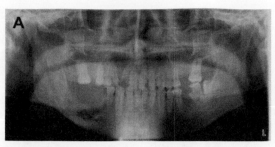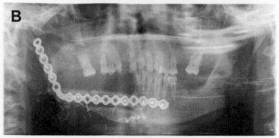

Fig. 38. (*A*) Preoperative and (*B*) postoperative orthopantomogram showing adequate mandibular reconstruction.

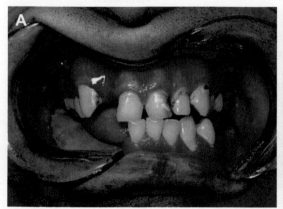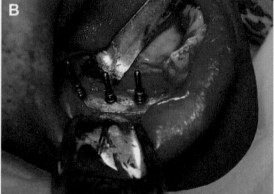

Fig. 39. (*A*) Postoperative intraoral view with skin paddle visible. (*B*) Placement of osteointegrated implants.

CASE 7. MANDIBULAR RECONSTRUCTION WITH IMMEDIATE ENDOSSEOUS IMPLANTS

A 36-year-old woman with ameloblastoma presented for resection and reconstruction. She had an obvious deformity on her left mandible (**Fig. 40**A), which correlated with her preoperative CT scan (see **Fig. 40**B).

Preoperative planning determined that after resection there would be a left hemimandible defect, with preservation of the condyle. Using 3D planning, the defect was reconstructed with 2 fibular osteotomies, and the immediate placement on endosseous implants. A dental splint with guides for the implants was created (**Fig. 41**).

Postoperative results revealed excellent cosmetic outcome, with restoration of normal occlusion and oral rehabilitation (**Fig. 42**).

3D planning of mandible reconstruction seems to be an efficient and methodical way to perform these complex surgeries; however, the plan is only relevant if it can be accurately implemented. A review of the last 33 mandibular reconstructions performed at New York University, and followed with postoperative CT scans, identified average differences from the preoperative scans of 4.75 mm at the gonions, 3 mm at the condyles, 1.41 mm at the mandibular osteotomies, and 2.21 mm in the fibula segments (**Fig. 43**). These differences are negligible, which indicates that the virtual surgical plan designed on a computer can be readily implemented in the clinical setting, with reproducible results.

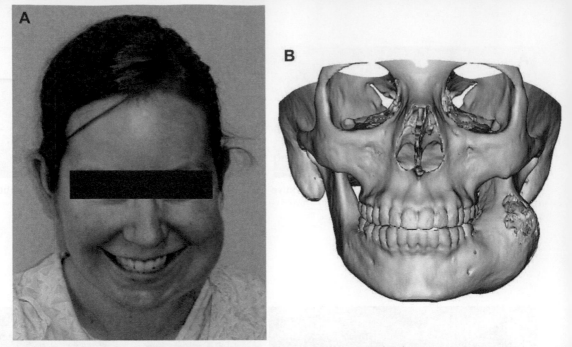

Fig. 40. (*A*) Deformity of left mandible. (*B*) Computed tomography scan of deformity.

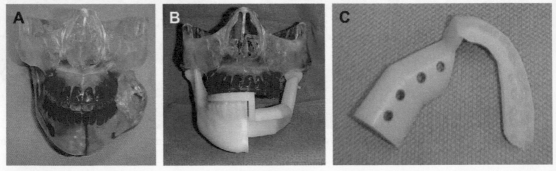

Fig. 41. (*A*) Preoperative model. (*B*) Planned reconstruction with endosseous implant guide. (*C*) Endosseous implant guide.

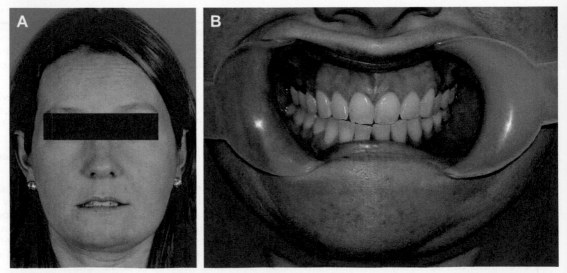

Fig. 42. (*A*) Postoperative result. (*B*) Full oral rehabilitation.

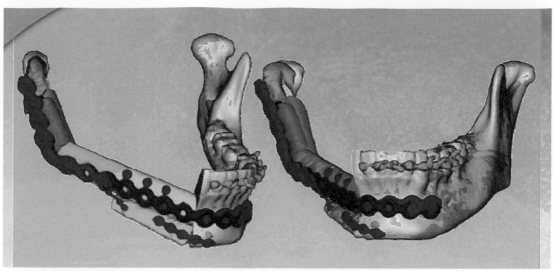

Fig. 43. Differences between postoperative computed tomography scan and preoperative virtual plan. Postoperative segments are in green, preoperative planned segments are in blue.

planning decreases operative time and overall morbidity to the patient while providing an overall more consistent result.

This reconstruction section focuses on mandible reconstruction with vascularized fibula flaps. Although other osteomyocutaneous flaps can be used in head and neck reconstruction, the tenets outlined here can be easily applied to any donor site. The following case reports outline how the authors perform these surgeries, and their considerations for special situations such as immediate placement of implants and double barreling of fibula segments.

SUMMARY AND FUTURE DIRECTIONS

These select cases not only illustrate the ease, cost effectiveness, and reliability of preoperative 3D virtual planning in facial bone surgery, but show potential for more complex planning by application of the volumetric analysis software engine to simulate soft-tissue changes and dynamic occlusal and TMJ simulation. Based on the authors' experiences and results, virtual planning for correction of congenital craniofacial deformities and facial syndromes can be of great benefit and will produce more desirable results than traditional methods.

REFERENCES

1. Ellis E 3rd. Accuracy of model surgery: evaluation of an old technique and introduction of a new one. J Oral Maxillofac Surg 1990;48(11):1161–7.
2. Cevidanes LH, Tucker S, Styner M, et al. Three-dimensional surgical simulation. Am J Orthod Dentofacial Orthop 2010;138(3):361–71.
3. Tepper OM, Sorice S, Hershman GN, et al. Use of virtual 3-dimensional surgery in post-traumatic craniomaxillofacial reconstruction. J Oral Maxillofac Surg 2011;69(3):733–41.
4. Bell RB. Computer planning and intraoperative navigation in cranio-maxillofacial surgery. Oral Maxillofac Surg Clin North Am 2010;22(1):135–56.

This page intentionally left blank

Assessment of Rhinoplasty Techniques by Overlay of Before-and-After 3D Images

Dean M. Toriumi, MD, Tatiana K. Dixon, MD*

KEYWORDS

- 3D imaging • Stereophotogrammetry • Rhinoplasty
- Postoperative results • Objective measurements

Assessment of facial plastic surgery outcomes is predominantly qualitative in the current literature. Results are analyzed by quantifying physician opinion, as well as patient quality of life and satisfaction. Although the surveys used are standardized and validated, the results are still highly subjective.

Emphasis has therefore shifted to a more objective evaluation of outcomes. Facial measurements provide a quantitative assessment of operative results. Originally, these were performed with craniofacial anthropometry, the direct measurement of the patient in the clinical setting using calipers and measuring tape. Because of the time commitment this caused for the patient, direct measurements were replaced by the measurement of photographs, which are quickly obtained and can be archived for analysis without causing any inconvenience to the patient.

TWO-DIMENSIONAL IMAGING ASSESSMENT OF RHINOPLASTY TECHNIQUES IN LITERATURE

Frontal, lateral, oblique, and base views of the nose are among the standardized images that allow comparison of surgical techniques and results from different surgeons. In the rhinoplasty literature, two-dimensional (2D) photographs have been used to show the effect of cephalic trim, columellar strut, lateral crural steal, and lateral crural overlay on tip rotation and projection.[1,2] Relative measurements of frontal pictures have also been used to show the change in nasal width after spreader grafts.[3]

SHORTCOMINGS OF 2D IMAGING OF THE NOSE

When dealing with 2D digital photographs, there are certain limitations. The face and nose are three-dimensional (3D) structures, and subtleties can be lost when they are portrayed in 2 dimensions. Particularly in the frontal view, it can be difficult to appreciate small irregularities of the nose. Patient positioning is important because slight changes in the Frankfort plane can cause apparent changes in tip rotation and nasal length on the frontal view. In addition, the lens used by the photographer should be chosen to produce the least distortion while maximizing the depth of field to ensure that the whole face is in focus (typically met by lenses between 90 and 105 mm). Lenses with shorter focal lengths provide a better depth of field (so the whole face is in focus) but cause obvious facial distortion.[4] Another pitfall of 2D photography is the lighting. When the angle between the subject-camera axis and the flash is more than 45°, tip-defining points seem wider apart (and vice versa). Measurement errors can also be introduced by magnification, parallax, and differences in subject-to-camera distances.[5]

Financial disclosures: Dr Toriumi is not employed or paid by 3dMD.
Department of Otolaryngology-Head & Neck Surgery, University of Illinois at Chicago, 1855 West Taylor, Chicago, IL 60611, USA
* Corresponding author.
E-mail address: tfeuer1@uic.edu

Facial Plast Surg Clin N Am 19 (2011) 711–723
doi:10.1016/j.fsc.2011.07.011

Even changing the photographer can cause changes in comparative measurements because of differences in technique and interpretation of the parameters of standardized photography.

3D IMAGING TECHNIQUES

3D imaging has been developed to overcome some of these obstacles and enable more precise evaluation of changes of the nose after rhinoplasty. In addition to angle, distance, and area measurements, 3-D imaging allows calculations of volumes and topographic distances.

Several forms of 3-D imaging modalities have been developed and tested. Computed tomography, 3D ultrasonography, moiré topography, laser scanning, and stereophotogrammetry are just a few of these techniques. Stereophotogrammetry involves taking multiple synchronous photographs from different angles, which are then digitally melded to generate a 3D image. This modality has gained popularity because it does not expose patients to radiation, as in computed tomography.

Our institution uses the 3dMD system (3dMD Inc, Atlanta, GA), which consists of 6 digital cameras, 3 on each side of the patient. A random light pattern is then projected onto the patient's face, and the cameras, which are set in an optimum configuration, capture simultaneous images. The images are captured in 2 milliseconds rather than the 20 seconds necessary for laser scanning, decreasing error from patient movement, and increasing patient convenience.[6] The system is connected to a computer, where the captured dataset is saved. We then use 3dMD Vultus software to upload and manipulate the images. The 6 captured images are merged to produce a single 3D polygon surface mesh, with a resolution of up to 40,000 polygons per 6.45 cm^2. The wire frame is then layered with soft tissue color and features.[7] This results in a 3D image that can be rotated in space and viewed from any angle. The software has an intuitive interface and requires basic computer skills to navigate. The images are dragged and rotated with a point and click of the mouse and the different capabilities of the system are showcased on the toolbar with picture icons. The 3dMD system is one of a few 3D imaging systems currently on the market. **Table 1** shows a list of equipment and software currently available.

VALIDATION AND RELIABILITY

In addition to acquiring data rapidly and noninvasively, stereophotogrammetry has proved to have excellent precision and reproducibility. Lübbers and colleagues[8] (2010) compared 201 direct measurements of a mannequin head with measurements of the 3D images captured by the 3dMD device. Measurements were performed by 3 observers, and repeated 5 times. There were no statistically significant differences between the direct measurements and the measurements of the images. The operator error (error resulting from inaccuracies in placing landmarks) was noted to be 0.1 mm without use of a zoom to magnify the images, and 0.04 mm with a zoom. Weinberg and colleagues[9] (2006) compared 2 photogrammetric systems (Genex and 3dMD) with each other and with direct anthropometry. On a sample of 18 mannequin heads, 12 linear distances were measured twice by each of the 3 methods. Statistically significant differences were observed for 9 of the measurements, but these were consistently on the submillimeter level. It was therefore concluded that the 2 systems produce interchangeable results. Wong and colleagues[10] (2008) measured 18 standard craniofacial distances twice, directly on 20 normal adults. The craniofacial surfaces of the 20 adults were imaged using the 3dMD device and the same distances were measured digitally, twice for each subject. Seventeen of the 18 measurements were found to be within 1 mm of the digital distances. Littlefield and colleagues (2004) tested the imaging system against a high-precision coordinate-measuring device and found the error to be 0.236 mm. Aldridge and colleagues[11] (2005) acquired 2 images of 15 subjects

Table 1		
3D Imaging equipment and software (listed alphabetically)		
Company	**Equipment**	**Software**
3dMD (Atlanta, GA)	3dMDface System	3dMD Vultus
Canfield Scientific Inc. (Fairfield, NJ)	Vectra 3D Imaging System	Mirror Imaging Vectra 3D Sculptor
Genex Technologies	3D Facecam Capture System	3D Surgeon

and mapped 20 standard anthropometric landmarks on each image. The landmark data were collected twice for each image by a single investigator with a minimum of 24 hours between measurement trials to prevent memory-biased placement of the landmarks. The grand mean of the precision calculated across subjects along all axes (x, y, z) was 0.827 mm. The repeatability was found to be 95% for 181 of the 190 landmarks. In all of these studies, 3D stereophotogrammetry was found to be an objective, accurate, and reliable system for quantifying the dimension of the soft tissues of the face.

ASSESSMENT OF DIFFERENT RHINOPLASTY TECHNIQUES WITH 3D IMAGING

By overlaying preoperative and postoperative 3-dimensional stereophotogrammetric imaging, it is possible to assess the resulting changes in every plane. In the literature, this technique has been used to measure the changes in volume of the nose after rhinoplasty for patients with unilateral clefts. Van Loon and colleagues[12] (2010) evaluated the results of 12 patients with unilateral clefts who received 3D imaging before and 3 months after rhinoplasty. The images were superimposed to generate a topographic distance map of preoperative and postoperative tissue changes. The volumes of the right and left half of the nose were also calculated and the preoperative and postoperative results were compared. A similar technique was used to evaluate the results of rhinoplasty with hump reduction. Van Heerbeek and colleagues[13] (2009) studied the results of 12 patients undergoing hump reduction. 3D imaging was performed 1 day before surgery and 6 months after surgery. The images were superimposed using 4 landmarks that did not change during surgery. A distance was then calculated between both surfaces, which resulted in a color-based image indicating unchanged (white areas), decreased (red discoloration), and increased (green discoloration) facial volumes. A higher intensity of discoloration corresponded with a larger volume change. To calculate the amount of maximal reduction, the distance between the preoperative and postoperative images was calculated at the point of maximal discoloration. Honrado and colleagues[7] (2006) compared the preoperative and postoperative imaging of 32 patients who received maxillary advancement surgery. A similar technique to the 2 previously mentioned studies was used to generate color-based histograms of soft tissue volume differences. Changes in nasal measurements such as nasal tip projection, columellar length, and nasolabial angle were also

compared in this study by placing landmarks and measuring the distances and angles between them.

At our institution, every patient receives preoperative imaging, as well as postoperative imaging at designated time intervals. This system allows us to track the 3D changes in the postoperative nose with time. The patient is seated in a chair a set distance from the cameras and positioned with the Frankfort horizontal plane parallel to the floor (**Fig. 1**). This position gains maximum light exposure to the face. The patient is photographed with all facial muscles relaxed, to ensure that there are no distortions of the nose. It is also important that patients loosely pull back their hair away from their faces; this prevents facial distortion from pulling of the hair and prevents landmarks and registration surfaces such as the forehead from being covered.

ASSESSMENT EXAMPLE 1: NASAL DORSAL AUGMENTATION

A deficient nasal dorsum of congenital, iatrogenic, or traumatic cause is corrected with dorsal augmentation. Autologous cartilage grafts are most commonly used and remain the gold standard for dorsal augmentation.[14] Dorsal augmentation can produce other changes in the nose such as nasal lengthening from augmenting the radix and raising the nasal starting point, decreasing the depth of the nasofrontal angle, and increasing dorsal projection. It is important to be aware of these changes when performing a complete evaluation of the results of nasal dorsal augmentation.

As a first step, the change of shape of the nasal dorsum can be evaluated by extracting the profile in the midsagittal plane from preoperative and postoperative 3D images. The profile lines are

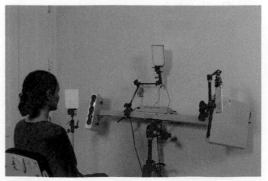

Fig. 1. Camera setup. The patient is seated a set distance from the camera with their chin positioned with the Frankfort plane horizontal to the floor.

Patient A

Patient B – chin augmentation also performed

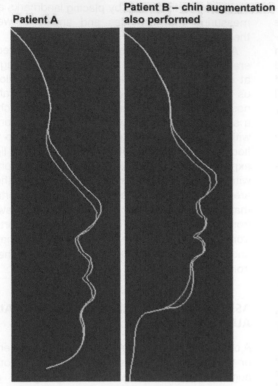

Fig. 2. Superimposed midsagittal plane profile extractions. The changes in nasal length and dorsal height are easily seen.

registered together to ensure that the areas of the face that did not change match precisely. The areas of the face that are to be superimposed are chosen to exclude operative fields, hair, and skin blemishes that change with time (**Fig. 3**). A root mean square (RMS) error is calculated at this time to assess the variation of the 2 surfaces that were selected. An RMS of less than 0.5 is desirable. If this is not achieved, the images are re-registered with different area selections. To check alignment and fully conceptualize the operative changes, the transparency of one of the images can be increased, or one of the images can be converted to a wire mesh so that both images can be seen simultaneously (**Fig. 4**).

The volume of the preoperative image is then subtracted from that of the postoperative image, and the changes in volume are reflected as color changes on the face, resulting in a topographic image that maps the changes in volume by color coding (**Fig. 5**). The areas of largest color volume increase are red, and the areas of volume decrease are green. This color coding then allows the observer to easily see the areas of largest volume change, whether augmentation or reduction. In the literature, this has been used to pinpoint the area of largest volume change, so that a distance measurement could be made at the point of largest change.[11]

Although the topographic image maps the relative changes in volume, the absolute values of the volume of the preoperative and postoperative nose can be obtained for any part of the nose. To see the nasal volume changes with dorsal augmentation, a surface area is manually selected over the nasal dorsum. The volume overlying the selected surface is then calculated (**Fig. 6**). To ensure that the same surface is selected for the preoperative and postoperative images, the images are registered as described earlier.

then superimposed to highlight the differences in dorsal height and nasal length (**Fig. 2**). The figures show examples of each type of assessment for 2 patients, patient A and patient B.

The relative changes in volume over the area of the nasal dorsum are best visualized with a difference histogram. Preoperative and postoperative images are first superimposed on each other and

Patient A

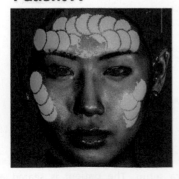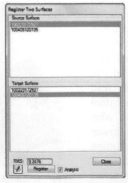

Patient B

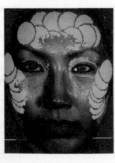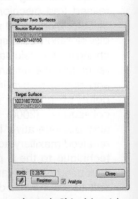

Fig. 3. Area selection. The software superimposes the pictures based on the surfaces selected. Skin blemishes, hair, and operated surfaces are excluded to allow more precise alignment.

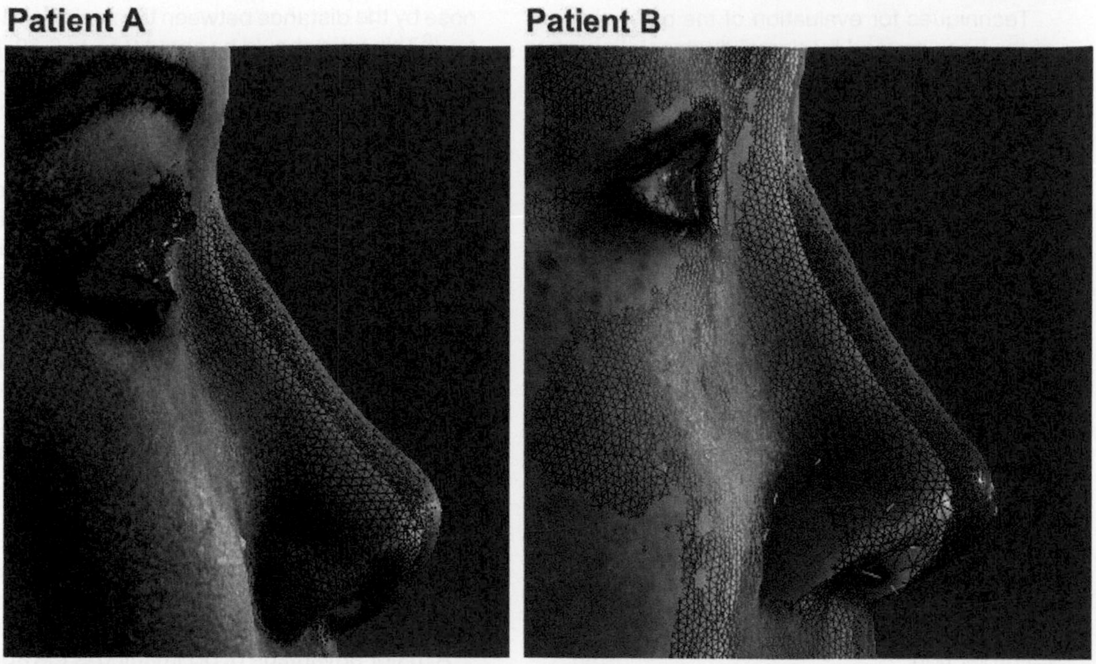

Patient A   # Patient B

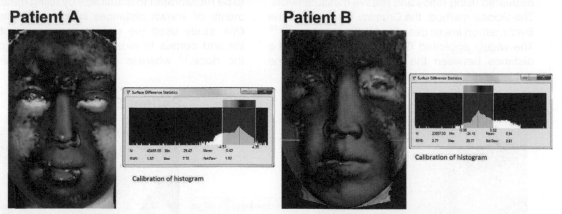

Fig. 4. Superimposed images after registration. The postoperative image is in mesh, allowing the extent of dorsal augmentation to be visualized.

Patient A   # Patient B

Calibration of histogram   Calibration of histogram

Fig. 5. Volume histogram. A topographic map is projected on the preoperative image. Areas of volume increase are red and areas of volume decrease are green. Blue areas are unchanged.

Patient A   # Patient B

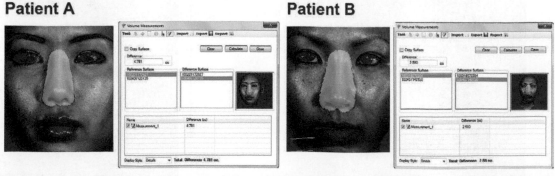

Fig. 6. Selection and calculation of volume change. The area wanted is selected with a paintbrush and the software calculates the difference in volume between the preoperative and postoperative images.

Techniques for evaluation of the other changes of the nose caused by dorsal augmentation, such as changes in nasal length, tip projection, and nasolabial angle, are described later.

ASSESSMENT EXAMPLE 2: INCREASING TIP PROJECTION

Controlling tip projection is an important aspect of rhinoplasty. Altering the tripod complex of the nose (the paired lateral crura and the combined medial crura), the use of extended columellar struts, setting back the medial crura onto the caudal septum, placement of tip grafts, and placement of dome binding sutures are all examples of techniques that affect tip projection and the stability of the projection with time.[15] 3D imaging provides an invaluable tool to objectively assess the effects of each of these techniques. Because increasing tip projection narrows the nasal base and opens the nasolabial angle,[15] assessment of these factors should be included to fully assess tip projection.

Tip projection is the anterior protrusion of the nasal tip from the face, and has historically been evaluated using ratios and relative measurements. The Goode method, the Crumley triangle, and the Byrd method are all described in the literature.[16–18] The widely accepted Goode method divides the distance between the alar root and tip of the nose by the distance between the nasion and nasal tip.[18] This ratio should be about 0.55 to 0.60. Using the 3D imaging landmark, points can be placed at the nasion and the nasal tip (**Fig. 7**). The x, y, z coordinates are recorded and the direct distance between these points is calculated by the software. To obtain the distance between the alar root and the nasal tip, the distance between a point on a plane and any place where that plane cuts the nose can be measured. First, an axial plane is rotated and transposed so that it cuts through the nasal tip. A point on that plane is then selected at the level of the alar base of the nose in the midline. Any distance from the point chosen to where the axial plane meets the face can be calculated. For tip projection, the distance calculated is from the chosen point at the base of the nose to where the axial plane cuts the nose at the nasal tip (**Fig. 8**). The projection of the nose can be either used as an absolute measurement from nasal base to nasal tip, or it can be divided by the previously calculated nasal length to obtain the Goode ratio.

A major advantage of 3D imaging is the ability to perform absolute measurements. In the past, absolute measurements from photographs had to be recalibrated to actual size by using measurements of known distances in the photographs. One study used the expected diameter of the iris and cornea to recalculate the true length of the nose,[19] whereas with 3D imaging, simple

Patient A

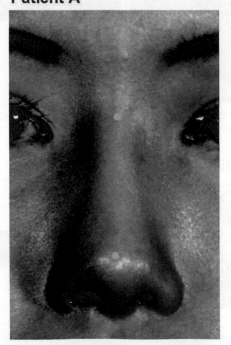

Patient B

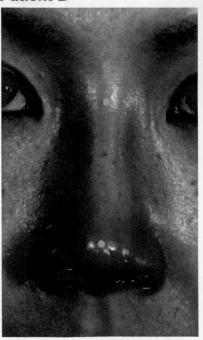

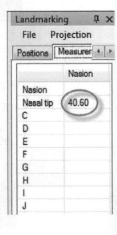

Fig. 7. Nasion to nasal tip measurement. The software calculates the distance between manually selected points.

Patient A

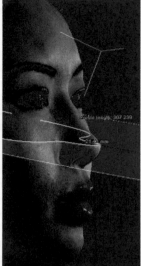

Patient B

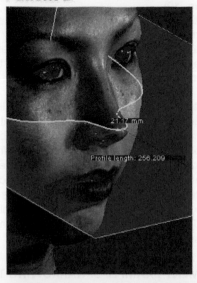

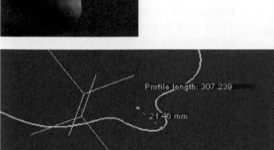

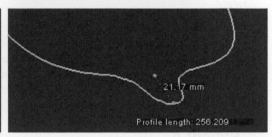

Fig. 8. Measurement of tip projection. An axial plane is positioned so that it cuts the nose at the nasal tip. A point on the plane is chosen at the level of the alar base in the midline. The distance between the nasal tip and the chosen point is calculated by the software.

point-to-point measurements reflect the actual difference and do not need to be recalibrated. Therefore, nasal projection measurement can be as easy as measuring the distance from the plane of the nasal base to the nasal tip, as described earlier. Honrado and colleagues[7] (2006) made

this even more straightforward, and measured the distance from the subnasale to the nasal tip by simply placing 2 landmarks (**Fig. 9**).

Nasal base width is easily calculated by placing landmark points at the widest portion of the alar base on each side of the nose. The software

Patient A   **Patient B**

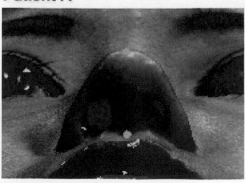
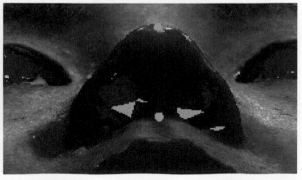

Fig. 9. Subnasale to tip measurement. The points are manually selected and direct distance between the points is calculated.

calculates the distance between the selected points (**Fig. 10**).

Tip rotation is measured with the nasolabial angle, and can be further characterized by the columellar/lobular angle. To calculate angles, 3 points need to be selected and the angle is then calculated from the x, y, z coordinates. In the case of the nasolabial angle, landmarks are placed at the vermillion border of the upper lip in the midline, the subnasale, and the nasal tip (**Fig. 11**). For calculating the columellar/lobular angle, points are placed at the subnasale, infratip lobule, and the tip-defining point. The columellar/lobular angle is then calculated by subtracting the resultant angle from 180° (**Fig. 12**). The nasofacial angle, or any other angle, can also be obtained by selecting the 3 appropriate points representing the intersecting lines tangential to the face.

ASSESSMENT EXAMPLE 3: NARROWING THE NOSE

Narrowing the upper and middle third of the nose is a frequently desired aesthetic outcome of rhinoplasty. This narrowing is typically achieved with dorsal hump removal combined with osteotomies, or by placing a narrow dorsal graft to raise the dorsum and increase lateral wall shadowing. 3D imaging has the advantage compared with 2D imaging of rotating the image in space and observing the full shape of the nose, so that measurements are not distorted by shadowing.

To visualize the change in overall shape of the nasal vault, the axial profile can be extracted. Superimposing preoperative and postoperative profile extractions allows us to evaluate whether the changes in width are ventral or dorsal, or whether the base has been untouched and a narrow dorsal graft has been added (**Fig. 13**).

When measuring the width of the nose, landmark points are placed on either side of the nose and distance is calculated from the chosen perspective x, y, z coordinates. By registering subsequent postoperative photographs together, the chosen points can be superimposed onto the subsequent photographs to measure change in width with time. It is important that the images be rotated to view the profile view (perpendicular to the x axis) when transferring the points to keep the chosen point at the same height and length of the nose (y and z coordinates) while the change in width (x axis) is measured. Since the landmarks are chosen by pointing and clicking on the images, using the zoom function and

Patient A

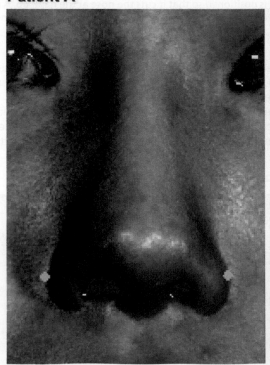

Patient B

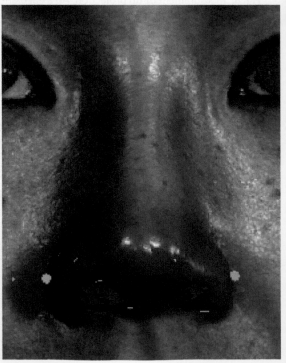

Fig. 10. Alar base width measurement. The points are manually placed at the widest points of the alar base and the distance between the points is determined.

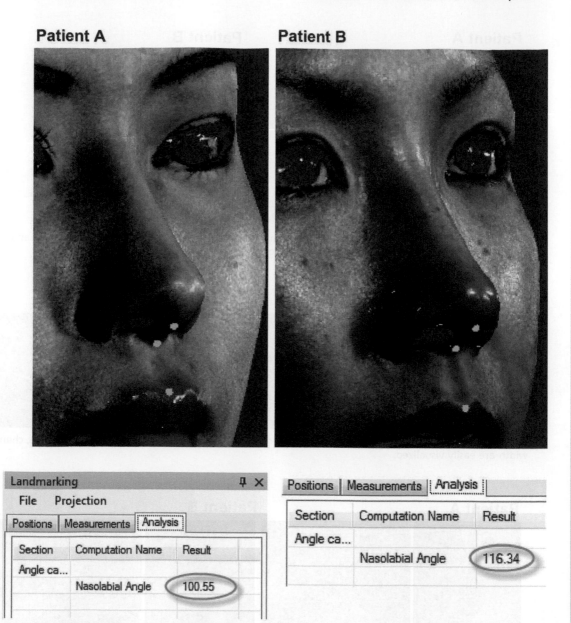

Fig. 11. Nasolabial angle calculation. Landmarks are placed at the vermillion border of the upper lip in the midline, the subnasale, and the nasal tip.

increasing the size of the nose on the screen increases the accuracy of the point transference, because it is easier to click on the same area of the nose. The 3dMD software also has the option of superimposing a grid over the face. When the image is rotated in the y-z plane (perpendicular to the x axis) the position of the point on the y-z grid is noted and this same point is chosen in the next image (**Fig. 14**). Registering the photographs and superimposing landmarks ensures that the same area of the nose is measured. This process

allows us to quantify change in width of the nose as the edema resolves and scar contracture occurs.

3D imaging also calculates topographic distances between points. Rather than measuring straight point-to-point distances, which can be performed with 2D photographs, the distance from point to point can be measured along the contour of the nose (**Fig. 15**). If a narrow dorsal graft has been placed over a stable wide nasal base, the point-to-point distance will not change,

Patient A

Patient B

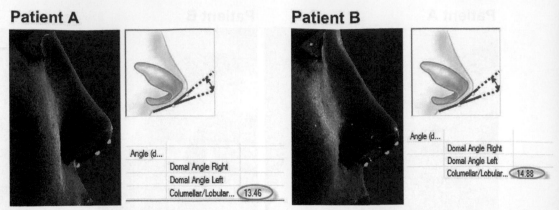

Angle (d...

Domal Angle Right	
Domal Angle Left	
Columellar/Lobular...	13.46

Angle (d...

Domal Angle Right	
Domal Angle Left	
Columellar/Lobular...	14.88

Fig. 12. Columellar/lobular angle calculation. Landmarks are placed at the subnasale, infratip lobule, and the tip-defining point. The resultant angle is subtracted from 180°.

Patient A

Patient B

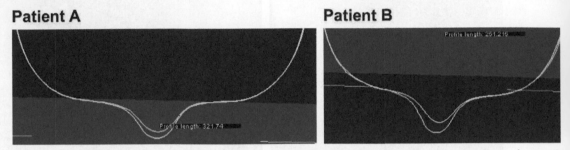

Profile length: 261.216

Profile length: 321.74

Fig. 13. Axial profile extraction. By superimposing preoperative and postoperative profile extractions, changes in width are easily visualized.

Patient A

Patient B

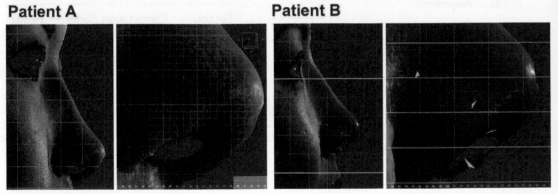

Fig. 14. Superimposed grid. The grid becomes smaller as the zoom function is used, allowing point placement to be more precise.

but the topographic distance will. When measuring topographic distances, it is important that extraneous points, which could cause error in measurement, do not create calculation errors. It is therefore sometimes necessary to crop the images and remove unnecessary hairlines and the neck before registering the photographs (**Fig. 16**).

ASSESSMENT EXAMPLE 4: NASAL LENGTHENING

There are several techniques of nasal lengthening, including caudal extension grafts or extended columellar strut grafts combined with extended spreader grafts, repositioning of the lower lateral cartilages, shield graft with lateral crural grafts, or

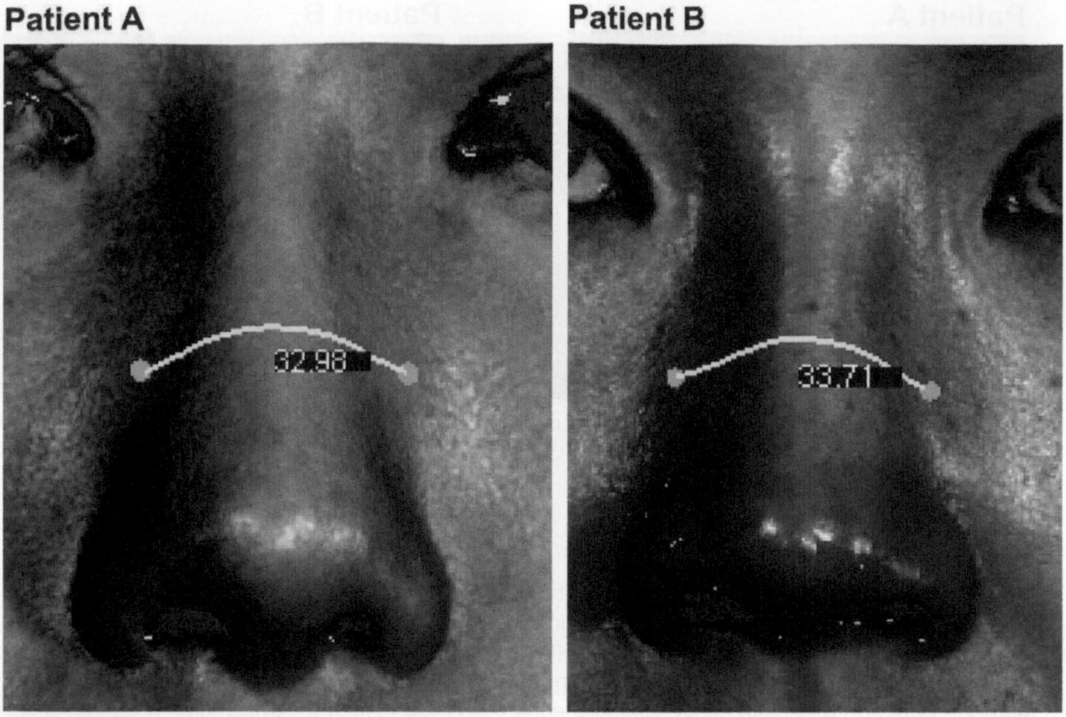

Patient A

Patient B

Fig. 15. Measurement of topographic distance. The distance between 2 manually selected points is measured along the contour of the face.

placement of a cartilage graft in the radix to elevate the nasal starting point. Common structural changes introduced as a consequence of nasal lengthening are widening of the alar base, retraction of the ala, and loss of tip projection or dorsal augmentation.[20] These structural changes must be corrected to provide an ideal outcome.

Therefore, measurements of these parameters should be considered while evaluating the nasal length.

Sagittal profile extraction, as described earlier, is a good first step to help the investigator fully appreciate the change in the shape of the nose (see **Fig. 2**).

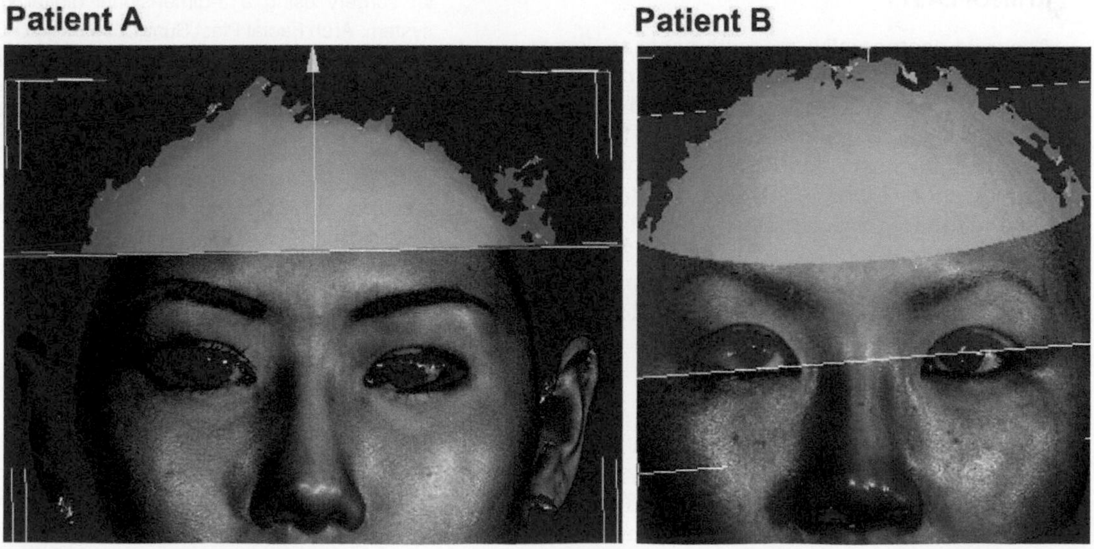

Patient A

Patient B

Fig. 16. Cropping images removes extraneous points that could cause error in measurement. The portion highlighted in green will be erased from the dataset.

Patient A

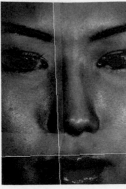
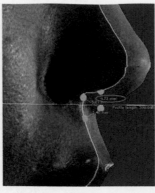

Patient B

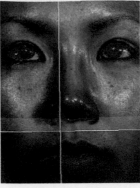
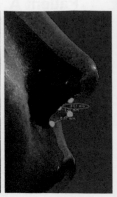

Fig. 17. Measuring alar retraction/columellar show. The distances from the axial plane at the level of the columella and the points where the sagittal plane cuts the ala are calculated. The columellar show is the distance perpendicular to the axial plane highlighted by the green circle.

Nasal length can be defined by the distance from the glabella to the subnasale,[21] or, as in the Goode ratio, from the nasion to the tip-defining point.[18] Placing landmarks and measuring the distance between them can easily measure either of these distances.

To measure alar retraction, an axial plane is rotated and transposed so that it is parallel to the columella, and going through the subnasale. A sagittal plane perpendicular to this axial plane is then moved so that it cuts through the ala. The perpendicular distance from the axial plane to the point of the bisection of the sagittal plane through the ala is then measured (**Fig. 17**).

SUMMARY OF 3D EVALUATION FOR RHINOPLASTY

Accurate postoperative measurements are important for objective evaluations of surgical outcomes. 3D stereophotogrammetry has proved to be an objective, accurate, and reliable system for quantifying the dimension of the soft tissues of the face. This article provides a description of techniques used to assess rhinoplasty results with the overlay of before-and-after 3D images. Use of 3D stereophotogrammetry provides the clinical investigator with a reliable objective means of reporting clinical data in the patient requiring rhinoplasty.

REFERENCES

1. Foda HM, Kridel RW. Lateral crural steal and lateral crural overlay: an objective evaluation. Arch Otolaryngol Head Neck Surg 1999;125(12):1365–70.
2. Ingels K, Orhan KS. Measurement of preoperative and postoperative nasal tip projection and rotation. Arch Facial Plast Surg 2006;8(6):411–5.
3. Ingels KJ, Orhan KS, van Heerbeek N. The effect of spreader grafts on nasal dorsal width in patients with nasal valve insufficiency. Arch Facial Plast Surg 2008;10(5):354–6.
4. Swamy RS, Sykes JM, Most SP. Principles of photography in rhinoplasty for the digital photographer. Clin Plast Surg 2010;37(2):213–21.
5. Farkas LG, Bryson W, Klotz J. Is photogrammetry of the face reliable? Plast Reconstr Surg 1980;66(3):346–55.
6. Honrado CP, Larabee WF Jr. Update in three-dimensional imaging in facial plastic surgery. Curr Opin Otolaryngol Head Neck Surg 2004;12(4):327–31.
7. Honrado CP, Lee S, Bloomquist DS, et al. Quantitative assessment of nasal changes after maxillomandibular surgery using a 3-dimensional digital imaging system. Arch Facial Plast Surg 2006;8(1):26–35.
8. Lübbers HT, Medinger L, Kruse A, et al. Precision and accuracy of the 3dMD photogrammetric system in craniomaxillofacial application. J Craniofac Surg 2010;21(3):763–7.
9. Weinberg SM, Naidoo S, Govier DP, et al. Anthropometric precision and accuracy of digital three-dimensional photogrammetry: comparing the Genex and 3dMD image systems with one another and with direct anthropometry. J Craniofac Surg 2006;17(3):477–83.
10. Wong JY, Oh AK, Ohta E, et al. Validity and reliability of craniofacial anthropometric measurement of 3D digital photogrammetric images. Cleft Palate Craniofac J 2008;45(3):232–9.
11. Aldridge K, Boyadjiev SA, Capone GT, et al. Precision and error of three-dimensional phenotypic measures acquired from 3dMD photogrammetric images. Am J Med Genet A 2005;138(3):247–53.
12. Van Loon B, Maal TJ, Plooij JM, et al. 3D stereophotogrammetric assessment of pre- and postoperative

volumetric changes in the cleft lip and palate nose. Int J Oral Maxillofac Surg 2010;39(6):534–40.

13. Van Heerbeek N, Ingels K, Van Loon B, et al. Three dimensional measurement of rhinoplasty results. Rhinology 2009;47(2):121–5.

14. Dresner HS, Hilger PA. An overview of nasal dorsal augmentation. Semin Plast Surg 2008;22(2): 65–73.

15. Toriumi DM. Structure approach in rhinoplasty. Facial Plast Surg Clin North Am 2002;10(1):1–22.

16. Crumley RL, Lanser M. Quantitative analysis of nasal tip projection. Laryngoscope 1988;98(2):202–8.

17. Byrd HS, Hobar PC. Rhinoplasty: a practical guide for surgical planning. Plast Reconstr Surg 1993; 91(4):642–54.

18. Goode RL. A method of tip projection measurement. In: Powell N, Humphrey B, editors. Proportions of the aesthetic face. New York: Thieme-Stratton; 1984. p. 15–39.

19. Sporri S, Simmen D, Briner HR, et al. Objective assessment of tip projection and the nasolabial angle in rhinoplasty. Arch Facial Plast Surg 2004; 6(5):295–8.

20. Toriumi DM, Patel AB, DeRosa J. Correcting the short nose in revision rhinoplasty. Facial Plast Surg Clin North Am 2006;14(4):343–55.

21. Powell N, Humphreys B. Considerations and components of the aesthetic face. In: Smith JD, editor. Proportions of the aesthetic face. New York: Thieme-Stratton; 1984. p. 20–6.

This page intentionally left blank

3D Photography in the Objective Analysis of Volume Augmentation Including Fat Augmentation and Dermal Fillers

Jason D. Meier, MD[a],*, Robert A. Glasgold, MD[b],
Mark J. Glasgold, MD[b]

KEYWORDS

- Three-dimensional imaging • Volume • Hyaluronic acid
- Autologous fat • Photography

THREE-DIMENSIONAL PHOTOGRAPHY

Three-dimensional (3D) photography provides a means for objective evaluation of both pretreatment facial volume loss and the results of volume replacement therapy in treatment of the aging face. In recent years there has been an increasing appreciation of the role of facial volume changes in the aging process and the benefits of implementing volume augmentation as part of the facial rejuvenation armamentarium. One of the challenges leading to this change was making patients and physicians aware of the volume changes that occur with aging and providing a means of showing the results of addressing these. Standard two-dimensional (2D) photography has limitations in providing this information, providing limited information on volume changes and thus being inadequate in evaluating the success of facial augmentation techniques. Before the development of 3D photography, there was no reliable or in-office method to quantitatively measure and assess volume replacement treatment using either injectable fillers or autologous fat grafting. Analysis of standard 2D photographs with subjective rating systems of improvement was the only methods used in measuring outcomes of facial augmentation. The subjectivity of these techniques was an inherent weakness that led to debates regarding the adequacy of study results.

CANFIELD VECTRA-CR 3D CAMERA SYSTEM

Our experience with 3D photography technology has been limited to the Canfield Vectra-CR 3D camera system (Canfield Imaging Systems, Fairfield, New Jersey). It provides excellent 3D detail as well as the ability to quantitatively measure

Funding support: No funding was provided for this study.
Disclosures: The Vectra imaging system used in these studies was supplied by Canfield Imaging Systems, Fairfield, New Jersey. No financial support was provided by any corporation and the synthetic filler products were not provided on a discounted or complementary basis for the study.
a University of Florida, 11701-32 San Jose Boulevard, Suite 211, Jacksonville, FL 32223, USA
b Robert Wood Johnson Medical School, University of Medicine and Dentistry of New Jersey, 31 River Road, New Brunswick, NJ 08904, USA
* Corresponding author.
E-mail address: jmeier.md@gmail.com

Facial Plast Surg Clin N Am 19 (2011) 725–735
doi:10.1016/j.fsc.2011.07.012

volume changes and provide a colorimetric graphic analysis of such volume changes. These colorimetric photographs can be easily shown in both research papers and to patients. The Canfield Vectra 3D photographic system has been an excellent objective tool for evaluating volume changes because it has been shown to have an accuracy of 5 to 20 μm in testing by the National Institute of Standards and Technology.

This camera is compact and can fit in a corner of a small photographic studio that may have already been set up in the office for 2D photography. Lighting does not have an effect on the results because highlights on the skin from various sources of light can be removed by the software during the analysis. The level of computer expertise required to use the system and efficiently obtain 3D photographs is minimal. However, obtaining quantitative data for evaluation requires some expertise in software use but can be easily acquired after a few hours of training and use. Overall, the software is intuitive and user-friendly. The retail cost of the Canfield Vectra M3 Face and Neck 3D photography system is $27,500. The Vectra X3 Face and Body system retails for $39,500. In either case, it is a turnkey system that includes camera system and computer, Mirror 3D Image Management and Analysis tools, Sculptor 3D simulation tools, on-site installation and training, and 1-year upgrades and warranty.

STUDIES IN THE LITERATURE QUANTIFYING FAT TRANSFER: AUGMENTATION OUTCOMES
2009 Initial Study: Midface Fat Graft Survivability

The first study in the literature to clinically quantify autologous fat transfer and volume replacement or augmentation was performed using the Canfield Vectra 3D camera in 2009.[1] This study was undertaken because of the lack of clinical objective data in the literature regarding longevity, predictability, and survivability of the fat grafts. There were conflicting results from numerous studies each recommending various techniques to improve the survivability of transplanted autologous fat.[2] Autologous fat grafting has been incorporated more recently in treatment of the aging face because of a better understanding of the aging process and facial volume loss as well as to achieve a natural rejuvenated appearance.

Before this study, there was great disparity in the literature regarding the results of fat grafting in terms of survivability and long-term outcomes. Studies that evaluated the durability of transplanted fat have reported volume retention between 20% and 90%. However, most of these

data are based on subjective analysis of 2D photographs or anecdotal assessment based on the physician's experience. Most studies claimed to use objective analysis but, in reviewing their methodology, their data came from evaluation based on subjective interpretation of results from 2D photographs.[3-6] In the few truly objective studies attempted, magnetic resonance imaging (MRI) or ultrasonography was used to measure fat survivability and longevity. Both of these showed quantified volume retention at 1 year.[7-9] However, using measurements with MRI or ultrasound requires significant cost and inconvenience to the patient compared with the 3D photography system that can be performed in an office.

After obtaining institutional review board approval, analysis of all patients who underwent autologous fat transfer to the midface region at our private practice during a 12-month period was completed. Written informed consent was obtained before any procedures and patients were followed prospectively for at least 1 year. Patients who did not complete preoperative or postoperative 3D imaging were excluded.

Standard atraumatic harvesting and injecting techniques with blunt cannulas were used. Autologous fat grafting was frequently combined with other facial procedures, such as rhytidectomy and blepharoplasty (**Table 1**). Care was taken to inject fat into a plane that was not surgically interrupted during the combined procedures.

Thirty-three patients (accounting for 66 hemifacial regions) were included in the autologous fat transfer study and were prospectively followed for at least 1 year and analyzed with the Canfield scientific Vectra camera and software.[1] Care was taken to ensure

Table 1
Ancillary procedures

Ancillary Procedures	Number
Upper lid blepharoplasty	14
Lower lid (transconjunctival) blepharoplasty	11
Deep plane rhytidectomy	10
Touch-up fat grafting	8
Browlift	3
Septorhinoplasty	2
Submental liposuction	2
Mentoplasty	1
Canthopexy	1

Data from Meier JD, Glasgold RA, Glasgold MJ. Autologous fat grafting: long-term evidence of its efficacy in midfacial rejuvenation. Arch Facial Plast Surg 2009;11(1):24–8.

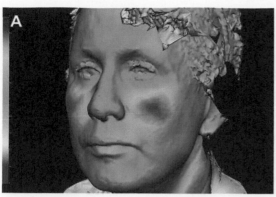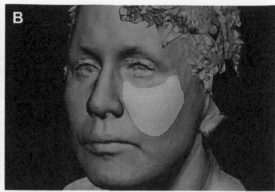

Fig. 1. (*A*) 3D colorimetric analysis of patient 9 showing areas of volume change (*blue*) at 18-month follow-up. Volume retention 68% on left side, 55% on right side. Increasing depth of blue color represents increased volume. (*B*) 3D midface area of patient 9 (*blue*) measured at 18-month follow-up visit. (*From* Meier JD, Glasgold RA, Glasgold MJ. Autologous fat grafting: long-term evidence of its efficacy in midfacial rejuvenation. Arch Facial Plast Surg 2009;11(1):24–8; with permission. Copyright © American Medical Association. All rights reserved.)

similar nonsmiling facial tone in both preoperative and postoperative photographs. 3D color schematic representation of volume changes between preoperative and postoperative photographs was first obtained (**Fig. 1**A). The midface region that was defined and measured included the inferior orbital rim, the nasojugal groove, the anterior cheek, and the lateral cheek. The midface region as defined was selected and highlighted as the area of volume measurement (see **Fig. 1**B). Quantitative volume measurements were then made using the Canfield Vectra imaging software, which compares the volume differences between preoperative and postoperative images in this midface region. All volume measurements were recorded in milliliters (mL).

The mean amount injected into each midface region was 10.1 mL. All but 3 patients had equal amounts injected into each side in the midface. At a mean follow-up of 16 months, the amount of augmentation was recorded in milliliters and compared as a percentage with the total amount injected into the midface region at the initial procedure. There was some variability between patients in the absolute amount and percentage of volume retention (**Table 2**). Overall, the mean absolute volume augmentation that was present at the last follow-up examination was 3.3 mL. The mean percentage of volume that was present at the last follow-up examination was 31.8%, which was statistically significant (*P*<.05).

Touch-up or secondary procedures were performed in 8 patients. These patients had a lower overall percentage of volume retention (29.6%). A statistical analysis of our data showed that neither patient age nor concurrent surgical procedures (blepharoplasty or rhytidectomy) had a significant effect on the amount of volume that remained in long-term follow-up.

Others have stressed the need for standardized and meticulous photography to evaluate postoperative fat grafting results.[6] The importance of photographic evaluation of results cannot be overemphasized because it guides the surgeon and analyzes the efficacy of fat grafting (ie, what volume amounts to use) as well as effectively showing the postoperative results to patients. Despite efforts to control consistency of photographic technique, documenting volume replacement including fat grafting results for these purposes with 2D photography is difficult. 2D photography is limited in its ability to document volume changes because these changes in facial shape and contour are often reflected as changes in shadowing. Even with standardized lighting techniques, determination of volume changes with 2D photography is inherently variable. Using 3D photography and software, the volume change that occurs with time can predictably and reliably be followed. We strongly advocate the use of 3D photography for surgeons who are using fat transfer or fillers in their practices. We have found that a decrease in volume occurs in the first 2 to 3 months after fat transfer, after which an increase of volume occurs in the next year to a stabilized volume (**Figs. 2–4**).

2010 Study: Tear Trough Fat Graft Survivability

A second study that was performed with the 3D imaging quantification of volume augmentation was published in 2010 regarding volume augmentation in the tear trough with filler based on hyaluronic acid.[10] Volume loss in the tear trough and infraorbital rim areas is one of the first signs of aging and imparts a tired appearance to the face. In addition to proper

Table 2
Patient data

Patient	Side	Follow-up (mo)	Amount Injected (mL)	Final Volume (mL)	% Volume Retained	Age (y)
1	Right	17	6	0.7496	12.5	50
	Left		6	0.7829	13	
2	Right	20	6.8	0.8029	11.8	51
	Left		6.8	0.9432	13.9	
3	Right	15	14.5	8.256	56.9	53
	Left		14.5	7.749	53.4	
4	Right	14	13	2.108	16.2	63
	Left		13	2.436	18.7	
5	Right	18	13.5	2.218	16.4	60
	Left		13.5	1.615	12	
6	Right	17	11.5	2.014	17.5	43
	Left		11.5	3.789	32.9	
7	Right	17	7	1.258	17.9	39
	Left		7	1.308	18.7	
8	Right	16	13	5.57	42.8	53
	Left		13	2.174	16.7	
9	Right	14	12	6.549	54.6	61
	Left		12	8.186	68.2	
10	Right	18	20	7.329	36.6	46
	Left		20	5.637	28.2	
11	Right	20	9.5	1.433	15.1	53
	Left		9.5	3.412	35.9	
12	Right	19	10.5	3.073	29.3	56
	Left		10.5	6.092	58	
13	Right	16	8	3.384	42.3	52
	Left		8	3.175	39.7	
14	Right	21	11.5	1.308	11.4	70
	Left		8.5	3.524	41.5	
15	Right	17	10.5	2.494	23.8	58
	Left		11	5.949	54.1	
16	Right	17	10.5	2.661	25.3	45
	Left		10.5	3.22	30.7	
17	Right	19	10	4.099	41	39
	Left		10	4.125	41.3	
18	Right	17	5.5	0.4935	9	55
	Left		5.5	1.396	25.4	
19	Right	18	10.5	3.611	34.4	50
	Left		10.5	4.234	40.3	
20	Right	17	3.5	3.109	88.8	54
	Left		3.5	2.624	75	
21	Right	14	22.5	8.492	37.7	56
	Left		22.5	12.91	57.4	
22	Right	17	6.5	0.6243	9.6	64
	Left		6.5	0.0622	1	

(continued on next page)

Table 2
(continued)

Patient	Side	Follow-up (mo)	Amount Injected (mL)	Final Volume (mL)	% Volume Retained	Age (y)
23	Right	15	13	1.697	13.1	43
	Left		13	3.527	27.1	
24	Right	16	3	0.117	3.9	63
	Left		3	0.554	18.5	
25	Right	13	13	2.495	19.2	54
	Left		13	2.551	19.6	
26	Right	12	11	1.145	10.4	64
	Left		11	2.622	23.8	
27	Right	15	16	3.606	22.5	59
	Left		16	6.501	40.6	
28	Right	15	4	0.6819	17	44
	Left		3	0.5722	19.1	
29	Right	12	6	2.581	43	66
	Left		6	3.583	59.7	
30	Right	15	8.5	6.377	75	50
	Left		8.5	7.153	84.2	
31	Right	16	8	2.343	29.3	51
	Left		8	3.746	46.8	
32	Right	13	11	4.169	37.9	69
	Left		11	5.183	47.1	
33	Right	14	8	0.257	3.2	58
	Left		8	0.832	10.4	

Data from Meier JD, Glasgold RA, Glasgold MJ. Autologous fat grafting: long-term evidence of its efficacy in midfacial rejuvenation. Arch Facial Plast Surg 2009;11(1):24–8.

placement and technique, correction of the tear trough requires precise volume augmentation because even a slight overcorrection is noticeable and unacceptable. There is an increased risk of bruising when injecting this area, which is why this technique requires excellent skill and technique because it is less forgiving than other facial areas.

The authors anecdotally noted in their clinical practice that patients treated with hyaluronic acid filler in the tear trough were showing continued correction well beyond a year after initial injection. The persistence of volume in this region, and especially an accurate measurement of the volume that is retained, were difficult to obtain with standard lighting and 2D photography. 3D photography eliminates these lighting differences and allows for measurement of exact volume changes that have occurred after injection. This study used Restylane (Medicis Aesthetics, Scottsdale, AZ). Medicis Aesthetics reports a general duration of effect of approximately 6 months in the nasolabial folds, which is the on-the-label location for most hyaluronic acid filler injections.[11] Few studies in

the literature exist regarding the durability of Restylane or other hyaluronic acid injectables in other regions such as the tear trough.[12] Most of the studies on the durability of hyaluronic acids in various facial locations used direct physician observation of the results or observations made from 2D photographs. There were no previous studies with quantitative analysis of hyaluronic acid fillers in any region.[13–19]

In this study, patients that presented to the cosmetic surgery practice for rejuvenation of the periorbital region were evaluated for volume augmentation in the tear trough region using hyaluronic acid filler injection. Any patient with a history of hyaluronic acid injections performed in this region or in the infraorbital region in the preceding 2 years was excluded. Any patient with a history of surgery in this area was also excluded. Twelve patients were identified as candidates and patients were asked to refrain from using aspirin or nonsteroidal antiinflammatory medications for at least 10 days before the procedure. Informed consent was obtained for

A   B

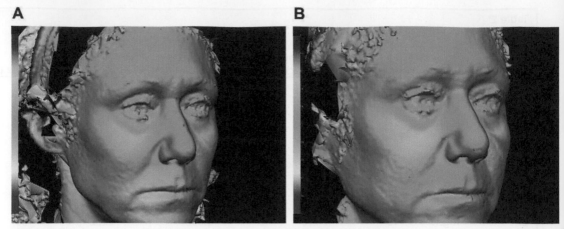

Fig. 2. (A) Patient 19: 3-D colorimetric analysis 2 months after surgery. (B) Patient 19: 3-D colorimetric analysis at 18 months after surgery. Increased amount of volume shown by increased blue color change in midface. (From Meier JD, Glasgold RA, Glasgold MJ. Autologous fat grafting: long-term evidence of its efficacy in midfacial rejuvenation. Arch Facial Plast Surg 2009;11(1):24–8; with permission. Copyright © American Medical Association. All rights reserved.)

the off-label use of the hyaluronic acid filler in the tear trough. Both 2D and 3D images were obtained following the removal of any makeup in the treatment area and before topical anesthesia was applied. Topical anesthesia was applied and standard serial puncture technique in a submuscular plane was performed. No patients in the study required greater than 0.5 mL of hyaluronic acid per tear trough. Patients returned in 4 weeks for reevaluation and 2D and 3D images were taken at that time. At that follow-up visit, the need for touch-up injections was determined and, if needed, performed that day with the same hyaluronic acid material. The patient was then followed up again in another 4 weeks after touch-up for repeated photographic imaging.

3D imaging was performed at the following time points: baseline (week 0), 1 month following treatment (week 4), and at the final long-term follow-up

appointment (minimum of 8 months after treatment). If the patient received a touch-up treatment at week 4, they were required to have a third follow-up visit 1 month after the touch-up treatment for measurement of final posttreatment volume. Images were obtained using the Canfield Vectra 3D camera system and software. Measurements of volume at each of these time points were performed in a blinded fashion (**Table 3**). 3D colorimetric analysis provided identification of the areas of volume change (**Fig. 5**). To decrease the variability, each calculation of volume was performed twice and results were averaged.

Twelve patients were initially enrolled in the study, after which 2 were lost to follow-up. Ten patients were studied long-term, with each patient having bilateral injection for a total of 20 sites for evaluation. All patients achieved satisfactory augmentation and rejuvenation by both the patient

A   B

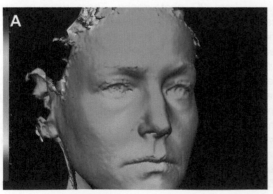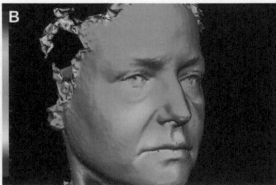

Fig. 3. Patient 16: 3-D colorimetric analysis at 3 months (A) and 17 months (B) after surgery. (From Meier JD, Glasgold RA, Glasgold MJ. Autologous fat grafting: long-term evidence of its efficacy in midfacial rejuvenation. Arch Facial Plast Surg 2009;11(1):24–8; with permission. Copyright © American Medical Association. All rights reserved.)

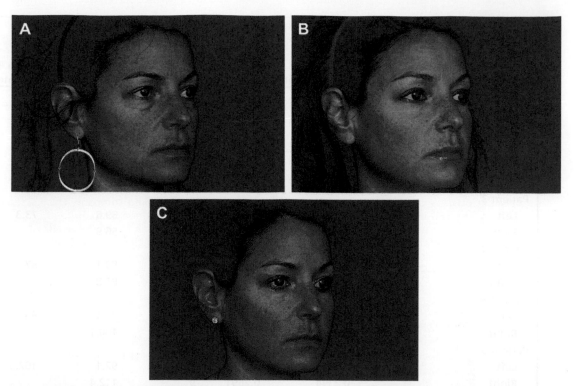

Fig. 4. Patient 16. Corresponding 2D photographs taken before surgery (*A*), and 3 months (*B*) and 17 months (*C*) after surgery. (*From* Meier JD, Glasgold RA, Glasgold MJ. Autologous fat grafting: long-term evidence of its efficacy in midfacial rejuvenation. Arch Facial Plast Surg 2009;11(1):24–8; with permission. Copyright © American Medical Association. All rights reserved.)

and physician evaluation at the 1-month follow-up. Five patients required touch-up at the 4-week visit. The average length of follow-up was 14.4 months, with a range of 8.5 to 22.8 months. Median follow-up was 14.1 months. 3D images obtained at each follow-up visit were compared with the patient's pretreatment images. The differences in the volume in the tear trough regions between pretreatment and posttreatment images were calculated to determine the exact amount of volume augmentation as well as residual volume. Maintenance of volume was determined as a percentage that remained at the final follow-up visit in comparison with the volume at the initial 4-week visit.

The average calculated volume augmentation achieved, as measured at the 4 week follow-up visit after initial treatment or touch-up treatment, was 0.21 mL per site. The range was 0.09 to 0.36 mL per site. At the final follow-up visit, the average maintenance of volume for all sites was 85%. The mean of volume augmentation and maintenance of long-term follow-up is depicted in **Fig. 6**. Of the 10 patients treated, 9 patients showed maintenance of greater than half of their augmentation volume and all patients achieved greater than 45% overall maintenance of their volume (**Fig. 7**).

As expected, there were some mild treatment-associated adverse events, including redness, swelling, and ecchymosis, which were transient and typically did not last longer than 1 week. All patients reported satisfaction with the final results. Subjective diminishment of their injected volume corresponded with the objective 3D data.

This study was the first long-term quantitative evaluation of the persistence of hyaluronic acid fillers for facial augmentation in any area including the tear trough. A specific advantage of using 3Dphotography is that multiple injectable materials for facial augmentation can rapidly and quantitatively be measured, which is especially important with the number and rapidly increasing variety of injectable dermal fillers that are available. Poorly substantiated manufacturer's claims regarding longevity of these materials are prevalent, and subjective analysis, not quantitative measurement, primarily exists in the literature as the data to support these claims.

The finding that 85% of the volume remained at long-term follow-up at an average of 15 months after injection is consistent with the authors' clinical observations. The patient with the longest follow-up at 23 months retained approximately 73% of the volume that was originally injected. The greater durability of hyaluronic acids injected

Table 3
Patient data

Patient	After Injection (mL)	Final F/U (mL)	F/U Length (mo)	% Retained	Mean % Retained
Patient 1					
Left	0.2001	0.1078	21.75	53.9	45.6
Right	0.1249	0.0466	21.75	37.3	
Patient 2					
Left	0.2337	0.1516	17	64.9	53.7
Right	0.2316	0.0984	17	42.5	
Patient 3					
Left	0.2152	0.1929	22.75	89.6	73.3
Right	0.2089	0.1189	22.75	56.9	
Patient 4					
Left	0.1257	0.1108	11.5	88.1	87
Right	0.2262	0.1941	11.5	85.8	
Patient 5					
Left	0.1823	0.131	8.5	71.9	86
Right	0.1667	0.1668	8.5	100.1	
Patient 6					
Left	0.2745	0.2528	9	92.1	102.3
Right	0.2394	0.2691	9	112.4	
Patient 7					
Left	0.0942	0.0645	15.75	68.5	87.5
Right	0.1114	0.1185	15.75	106.4	
Patient 8					
Left	0.1302	0.1823	13.5	140	115.2
Right	0.1155	0.1044	13.5	90.4	
Patient 9					
Left	0.3574	0.3965	9.75	110.9	101.6
Right	0.3567	0.3287	9.75	92.2	
Patient 10					
Left	0.2504	0.2985	14.75	119.2	99.1
Right	0.2695	0.2128	14.75	79	
Total postinjection volume	4.11				
Mean postinjection volume change (mL)	0.2055				
Mean volume retention (mL)		0.1774			
Mean follow-up (mo)			14.43		
Mean percent volume retention				85.1	

Abbreviation: F/U, follow-up.

Data from Donath AS, Glasgold RA, Meier JD, et al. Quantitative evaluation of volume augmentation in the tear trough with a hyaluronic acid based filler: a 3-dimensional analysis. Plast Reconstr Surg 2010;125(5):1515–22.

into this region may be explained by the limited soft tissue movement of the area and the depth of placement, compared with the manufacturers' results from studying the nasolabial fold where hyaluronic acid is injected into the dermis of a more dynamic facial region.

3D Photography: effect on clinical practice

3D photography allows for a better and quantitative analysis of volume replacement in both in-office procedure and surgical results. In our practice, it has enhanced patient care through research analyses as well as helping patients understand the

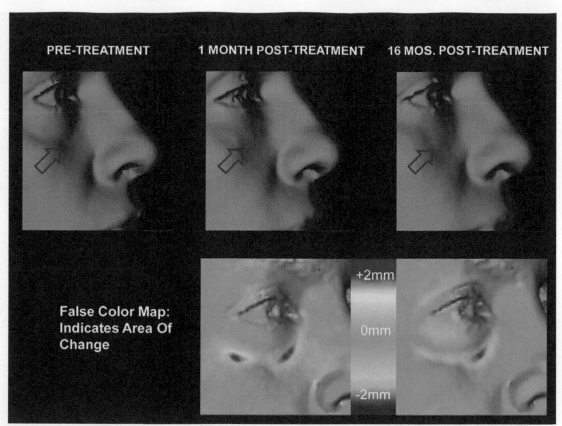

Fig. 5. 3D imaging showing pretreatment (*left*), 1-month posttreatment (*center*), and long-term posttreatment (*right*) visualization of the tear trough using monochromatic (*above*) and false color mapping (*below*) techniques to identify the areas of augmentation. (*From* Donath AS, Glasgold RA, Meier JD, et al. Quantitative evaluation of volume augmentation in the tear trough with a hyaluronic acid based filler: a three-dimensional analysis. Plast Reconstr Surg 2010;125(5):1515–22; with permission © Wolters Kluwer Health.)

goals of treatment, setting appropriating expectations, and in showing to them the results of treatment. 3D imaging is helpful in the analysis of results when speaking with patients regarding their treatment, and increases the satisfaction level of each patient who undergoes treatment. This benefit is particularly true of hyaluronic acid filler injections that are performed in the office. Much smaller volumes are used compared with autologous fat transfer when performing filler injections in the office. Small differences in lighting or skin pigmentation often affect 2D photographic analysis. This problem is eliminated with 3D photography because lighting is standardized and skin pigmentation can be removed for complete and better analysis of volume changes alone. In addition, 3D photography allows precise evaluation of images in the same 3D plane by having the ability to rotate images on all axes. This ability to rotate the images represents an additional advance in providing objective results even without quantification of the

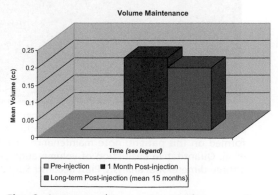

Fig. 6. Average volume augmentation per site at pretreatment, short-term posttreatment (1 month), and long-term posttreatment imaging sessions. (*From* Donath AS, Glasgold RA, Meier JD, et al. Quantitative evaluation of volume augmentation in the tear trough with a hyaluronic acid based filler: a three-dimensional analysis. Plast Reconstr Surg 2010; 125(5):1515–22; with permission © Wolters Kluwer Health.)

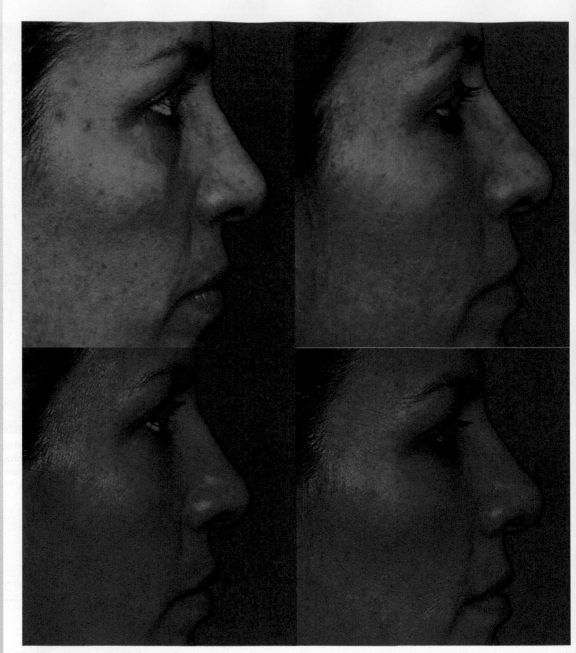

Fig. 7. 2D images of patient before treatment (*above, left*), 1 month after treatment (*above, right*), 16 months after treatment (*below, left*), and 24 months after treatment (*below, right*). No touch-up injections were performed on this patient; note maintenance of effect at 24 months. (*From* Donath AS, Glasgold RA, Meier JD, et al. Quantitative evaluation of volume augmentation in the tear trough with a hyaluronic acid based filler: a three-dimensional analysis. Plast Reconstr Surg 2010;125(5):1515–22; with permission © Wolters Kluwer Health.)

volume retention. In clinical practice, there are many patients who could not appreciate their results of small-volume filler enhancement with 2D photography. However, they could easily appreciate the results with the 3D imaging system, which improved their overall satisfaction level.

3D photography: effect on surgical procedures
The results and use of 3D photography do not necessarily make the surgical or in-office procedure smoother or faster. However, this technology allows the individual surgeon to determine the volume to be used based on scientific data

through analysis of their techniques and individual results. The autologous fat transfer study results, with an average of 32% of the initial volume injected remaining at approximately 1.5 years of follow-up, is routinely used by the surgeon in planning the initial injection amounts as well as in establishing appropriate patient expectations before surgery. Autologous fat transfer can have variable results that are well documented in the literature. Therefore, it is especially important to have quantitative measurements of one's own techniques to more reliably and precisely obtain a specific amount of volume augmentation as well as to determine which patients would benefit from a touch-up procedure.

SUMMARY

3D imaging provides an objective and quantitative analysis for both research applications and clinical practice. It allows for a better and more accurate assessment of both small and large volume augmentation in the midface region. Further studies are necessary to determine whether 3D photography is as useful in assessing more dynamic areas such as the nasolabial folds and lips.

REFERENCES

1. Meier JD, Glasgold RA, Glasgold MJ. Autologous fat grafting: long-term evidence of its efficacy in midfacial rejuvenation. Arch Facial Plast Surg 2009;11(1): 24–8.
2. Calabria R. Fat grafting: fact or fiction? Aesthetic Surg 2005;25:55.
3. Ersek RA. Transplantation of purified autologous fat: a three year follow-up is disappointing. Plast Reconstr Surg 1991;87:219.
4. Fulton JE, Suarez M, Silverton K, et al. Small volume fat transfer. Dermatol Surg 1998;24:857–65.
5. Fournier PF. Fat grafting: my technique. Dermatol Surg 2000;26:1117–28.
6. Coleman SR. Long-term survival of fat transplants: controlled demonstrations. Aesthetic Plast Surg 1995;19:421.
7. Horl HW, Feller AM, Biemer E. Technique for liposuction fat reimplantation and long-term volume evaluation by magnetic resonance imaging. Ann Plast Surg 1991;26:248.
8. Goldman R, Carmargo CP, Goldman B. Fat transplantation and facial contour. Am J Cosmet Surg 1998;15: 41–4.
9. Glogau RG. Microlipoinjection. Arch Dermatol 1988; 124:1340.
10. Donath AS, Glasgold RA, Meier JD, et al. Quantitative evaluation of volume augmentation in the tear trough with a hyaluronic acid based filler: a three-dimensional analysis. Plast Reconstr Surg 2010; 125(5):1515–22.
11. Hirmand H. The tear trough and hyaluronic acid/Restylane: is it a happy union? Presented at: Annual Meeting of the American Society for Aesthetic Plastic Surgery and the Aesthetic Surgery Education and Research Foundation. New Orleans, April 30–May 4, 2005.
12. Kane MA. Treatment of tear trough deformity and lower lid knowing with injectable hyaluronic acid. Aesthetic Plast Surg 2005;29:363–7.
13. Lambros VS. Hyaluronic acid injections for correction of the tear trough deformity. Plast Reconstr Surg 2007;120(Suppl 6):74S–80S.
14. PubMed (web site). PubMed search using terms "hyaluronic acid," "face," "facial," and "filler." Available at: http://www.ncbi.nlm.nih.gov. Accessed June 18, 2008.
15. Matarasso SL, Carruthers JD, Jewell ML, Restylane Consensus Group. Consensus recommendations for soft tissue augmentation with non-animal stabilized hyaluronic acid (Restylane). Plast Reconstr Surg 2006;117(Suppl 3):3S–34S.
16. Andre P. Evaluation of the safety of a non-animal stabilized hyaluronic acid (NASHA – Q-Medical, Sweden) in European countries: a retrospective study from 1997-2001. J Eur Acad Dermatol Venereol 2004;18: 422–5.
17. Narins RS, Brandt R, Leyden J, et al. A randomized, double-blind, multicenter comparison of the efficacy of and tolerability of Restylane versus Zyplast for the correction of nasolabial folds. Dermatol Surg 2003; 29:588–95.
18. Carruthers J, Klein AW, Carruthers A, et al. Safety and efficacy of nonanimal stabilized hyaluronic acid for improvement of mouth corners. Dermatol Surg 2005;31:276–80.
19. Airan LE, Born TM. Nonsurgical lower eyelid lift. Plast Reconstr Surg 2005;116:1785–92.

This page intentionally left blank

3D In Vivo Optical Skin Imaging for Intense Pulsed Light and Fractional Ablative Resurfacing of Photodamaged Skin

Matteo Tretti Clementoni, MD[a],*,
Rosalia Lavagno, MD[a], Maximilian Catenacci, MD[b],
Roman Kantor, PhD[c], Guido Mariotto, PhD[c],
Igor Shvets, PhD[d]

KEYWORDS

- 3D • Photoaging • Photodamaged skin
- Fractional laser treatment • Skin topography

Topography of the skin surface as well as melanin and hemoglobin concentration and distribution are a mirror of the functional skin status. Changes in these features not only are a tool for early-stage diagnosis of diseases but also give an indication of the response to medical and cosmetic treatment. Therefore, their evaluation is of great interest for dermatologic research. However, although physicians can apply classification rules to visual diagnosis, the overall clinical approach is subjective and qualitative, with a critical dependence on training and experience. Over the past 20 years, several noninvasive techniques for measuring the skin's properties have been developed and tested to extend the accuracy of visual assessment alone. Many of them were not only very precise but also very complicated; others were very simple but approximations.

In this article, a new optical, precise, user-friendly measuring system is presented to demonstrate the effectiveness of the most common laser treatments on photodamaged skin. Many of the skin changes commonly associated with aging, changes in pigmentation, telangiectasia, sallowness, and wrinkling are actually the result of sun exposure. Changes in pigmentation (blotchy brown freckles and age spots), dryness, areas of redness, thinning of the dermis, loss of elasticity, fine lines, and deep wrinkles are all signs of chronic UV exposure. Excluding injectables, surgery, and peelings, the most common procedures to improve these changes in the skin appearance are the IPL treatments and, more recently, the fractional resurfacings. Preoperative and postoperative images of patients treated with these procedures and analyzed using this new three-dimensional (D) in vivo optical skin imaging system are shown.

[a] Istituto Dermatologico Europeo, Milano, Italy
[b] Skindermolaser, Roma, Italy
[c] Miravex Ltd, Trinity Research and Innovation, O'Reilly Institute, Trinity College Dublin, Dublin, Ireland
[d] School of Physics, Trinity College Dublin, Dublin, Ireland
* Corresponding author.
E-mail address: mtretti@laserplast.org

Facial Plast Surg Clin N Am 19 (2011) 737–757
doi:10.1016/j.fsc.2011.07.014
1064-7406/11/$ – see front matter © 2011 Elsevier Inc. All rights reserved.

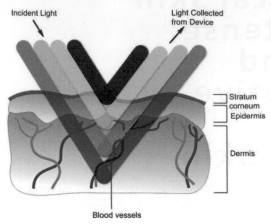

Fig. 1. Several light-emitting diodes with different wavelengths illuminate the skin. The reflected lights generate different images that are used by the system to generate the 3D image.

THE SKIN IMAGING DEVICE

The Antera 3D (Miravex, Ireland) imaging system consists of a handheld imaging device connected through a long firewire cable to a computer. The system is completed by proprietary software running on a Windows-based standard laptop or desktop personal computer. The imaging technique of

Antera 3D is based on the acquisition of a number of images under varying but strictly controlled illumination conditions. Several light-emitting diodes are used to illuminate the skin with different colors and different illumination directions (**Fig. 1**). The acquired image data are then used for spatial and spectral analysis for reconstruction of the texture of the skin and analysis of skin constituents.

Skin texture reconstruction is achieved using a technique based on shape from shading,[1] substantially modified to eliminate skin glare and vastly improve the accuracy of measured data.[2] The texture reconstructed in this way is then used for quantitative skin analysis, such as depth and width of wrinkles, lesions of the skin, and overall skin roughness.

The acquired spectral data are used to map the distribution and concentration of melanin and hemoglobin. Unlike traditional imaging techniques, in which only 3 color channels (red, green, and blue) are used, the Antera 3D uses reflectance mapping of 7 different light wavelengths spanning the entire visible spectrum. This mapping allows for a much more precise analysis of the skin colorimetric properties, which are mostly determined by 2 dominant chromophores: melanin and hemoglobin. Acquired spectral images are transformed into skin spectral reflectance maps, and the skin surface shape is used to compensate for light

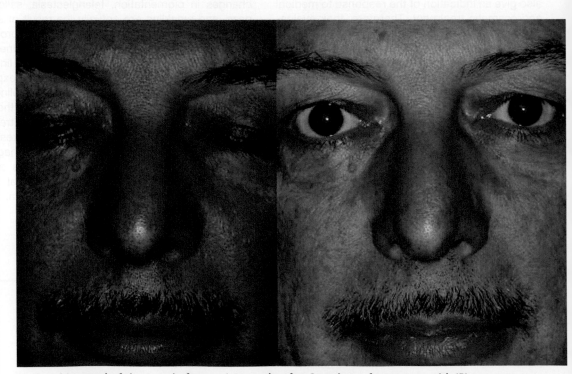

Fig. 2. A big vessel of the nose before and 6 months after 2 sessions of treatment with IPL.

intensity variation due to the varying direction of incident illumination. The reflectance data are transformed into skin absorption coefficients and used to quantify melanin and hemoglobin concentrations using mathematical correlation with known spectral absorption data of these chromophores.[3]

The images acquired with the Antera 3D can be visualized in several different modes: standard color skin, texture elevation map, and melanin and hemoglobin concentration maps with 2D and 3D perspective representation. The clinician can select specific skin areas for quantitative analysis and carry out before and after analyses with previously acquired images. Spot-On, the automatic matching technique that registers two or more images to one another is used to compensate for relative shifts and rotations between images, ensuring accurate data analysis. The measurement data can be presented by quickly creating a report that shows the analyzed images together with the measured values and comparison charts. Data can be stored on the computer or included in other document processing applications such as Microsoft Word or Microsoft PowerPoint.

Numeric data collected from one image must not be considered as absolute values but 2 or more images must be compared. The percentage modification of these data (data on melanin distribution, hemoglobin distribution, and surface topography) is very useful to demonstrate the effectiveness of a treatment.

INTENSE PULSED LIGHT TREATMENT OF FACIAL AGING SKIN

Current trends in aesthetic treatment of facial skin call for an effective adjunct to injectables or surgery. Patients look for treatment that offers a return to a more youthful appearance through restoration of even color and smoothness, relief from pigmentary sun damage, and the redness associated with ectatic vessels. In addition, this patient group requires treatments that are short and pain free and allow immediate return to all social activities.

Following more than 20 years of treatment of vascular lesions using the pulsed dye laser, new laserlike intense pulsed light (IPL) devices were

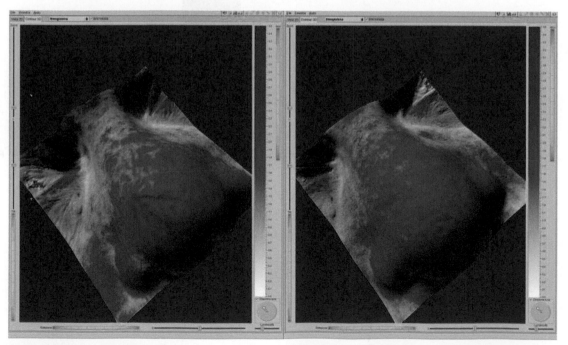

Fig. 3. The Antera 3D image of the patient in **Fig. 2** before and after the treatment. Darker the color (*blue-purple*), higher the hemoglobin concentration.

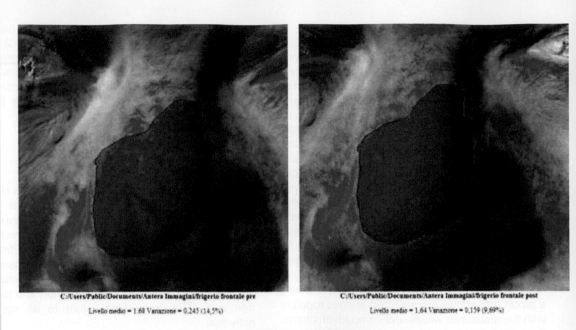

C:\Users\Public\Documents\Antera Immagini\Trigerio frontale pre

Livello medio = 1.68 Variazione = 0.245 (14,5%)

C:\Users\Public\Documents\Antera Immagini\Trigerio frontale post

Livello medio = 1.64 Variazione = 0.159 (9,69%)

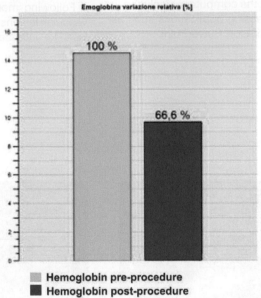

Emoglobina variazione relativa [%]

100 %

66,6 %

Hemoglobin pre-procedure
Hemoglobin post-procedure

Fig. 4. The mathematical hemoglobin variation analysis of the area of the tip of the nose of the patient in **Fig. 2** clarifies an improvement of more than 33%.

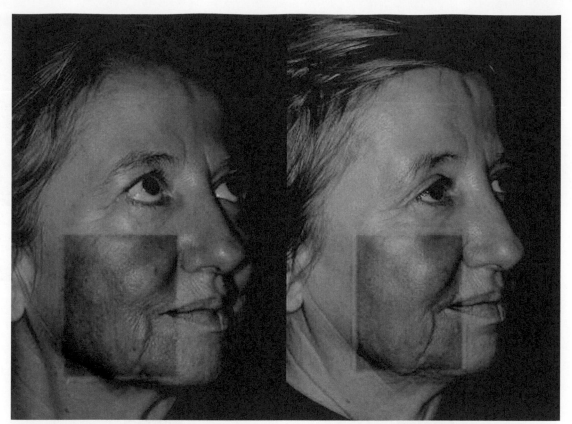

Fig. 5. A 56-year-old patient before and after 4 sessions of IPL treatment. The coloured square shows the area subjected to the 3D analysis.

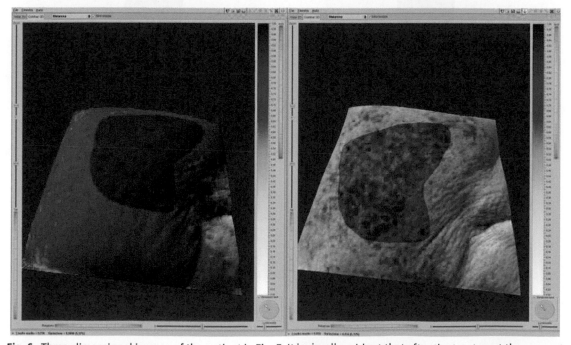

Fig. 6. Three-dimensional images of the patient in **Fig. 5**. It is visually evident that after the treatment the amount of melanin and its variation are improved.

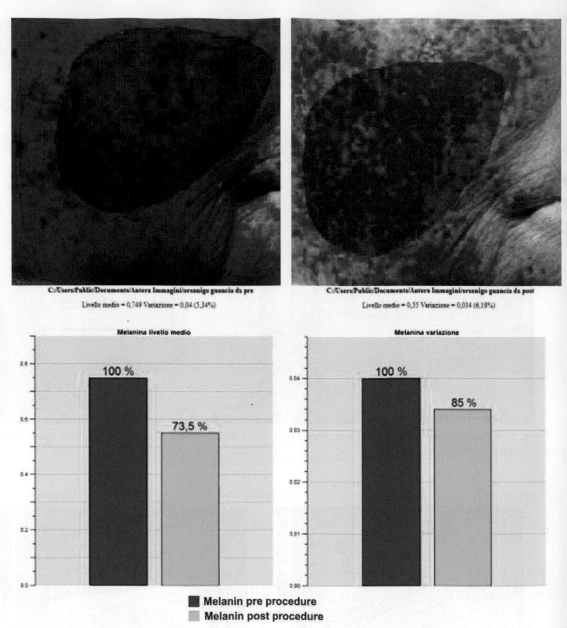

C:\Users\Public\Documents\Antera Immagini\orsanigo guancia dx pre
Livello medio = 0,749 Variazione = 0,04 (5,34%)

C:\Users\Public\Documents\Antera Immagini\orsanigo guancia dx post
Livello medio = 0,55 Variazione = 0,034 (6,18%)

Melanina livello medio

100 %

73,5 %

Melanina variazione

100 %

85 %

Melanin pre procedure
Melanin post procedure

Fig. 7. The mathematical analysis of the result implies that the melanin level is reduced by more than 25% and that its variation is improved by 15%.

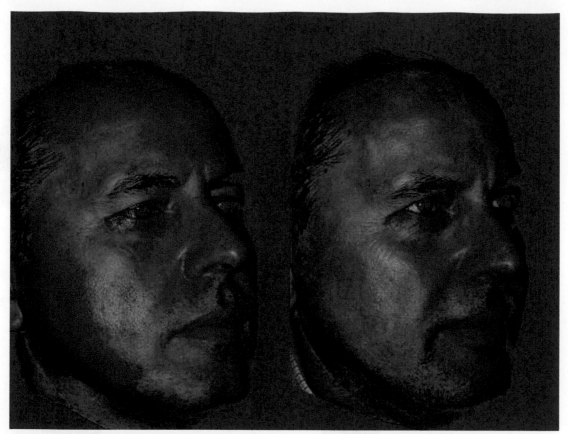

Fig. 8. A 52-year-old man with a facial photoaging with prevalent vascular component. On the right, the outcome obtained after 4 sessions of treatment with IPL.

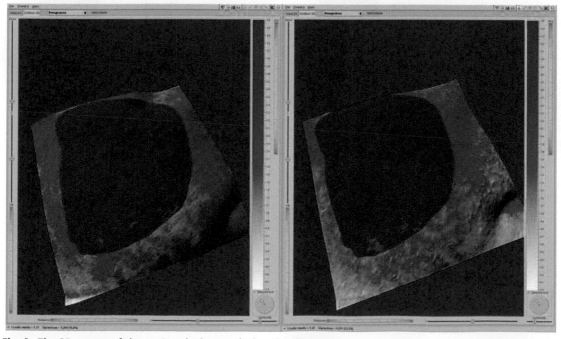

Fig. 9. The 3D aspect of the patient before and after the IPL treatment.

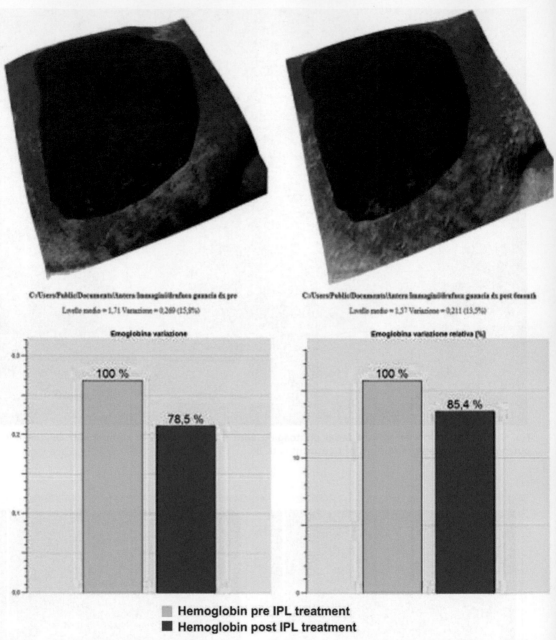

C:/Users/Public/Documents/Antera Immagini/ilrafsea geancia dx pre

Lvelle medio = 1,71 Variazione = 0,269 (15,8%)

C:/Users/Public/Documents/Antera Immagini/ilrafsea geancia dx post 6ennth

Lvelle medio = 1,57 Variazione = 0,211 (13,5%)

Emoglobina variazione

100 %

78,5 %

Emoglobina variazione relativa (%)

100 %

85,4 %

■ Hemoglobin pre IPL treatment
■ Hemoglobin post IPL treatment

Fig. 10. The mathematical analysis of the hemoglobin implies that the improvement after the IPL treatment is not around 15%.

developed at the end of the last century. These IPL devices treat these UV exposure–correlated conditions with success and provide a solution for the essential lifestyle criteria when used in a carefully administered program. This new IPL skin rejuvenation technique now has a clinical history of more than 300,000 treatments with excellent patient acceptance. IPL differs from laser light in that, rather than monochromatic single wavelength, IPL emits a noncoherent broad-spectrum light. The IPL devices used in the rejuvenation procedure emit a spectrum extending from 500 nm to 1200 nm. To customize the light energy delivery for a given procedure, the operator uses a cutoff filter, or light guide, of designated wavelength, below which the spectrum is selectively eliminated. The IPL system conforms to the principle of selective photothermolysis. For dilated vessels, as seen in patients with sun damage and rosacea, the light energy with high absorption by hemoglobin and oxyhemoglobin reaches the dermal capillary bed and selectively destroys the abnormal vessels. For sun spots and lentigos, as

seen in patients with sun damage, the light crumbles the granules of melanin distributed at the dermoepidermal junction. Macrophages can then therefore remove these smaller granules of melanin.[4] The operator controls all aspects of the light pulse, including cutoff wavelength (nm), energy level (J/cm^2), pulse duration (milliseconds), pulse pattern (single, double, or triple), and delay time between pulses (milliseconds). This allows for precise control of light energy, which in this procedure is used for customization for skin type, procedure progress, and other variables.

Big vessels of the nose can be treated (**Fig. 2**) with few sessions of treatment combining different cutoff (590and 560 nm), different energy (22 and 19 J/cm2), and different pulse duration and delay time. The 3D images (**Fig. 3**) visually clarify the effectiveness of the treatment while the report that mathematically analyses the prepictures and postpictures presents the percentage of improvement (**Fig. 4**).

Sunspots and irregularities of the skin color can be treated with a few sessions of treatment (**Fig. 5**)

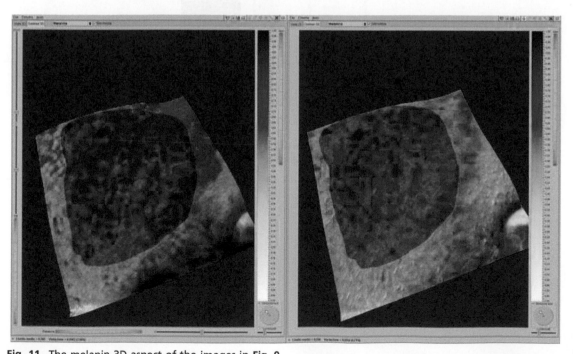

Fig. 11. The melanin 3D aspect of the images in **Fig. 9**.

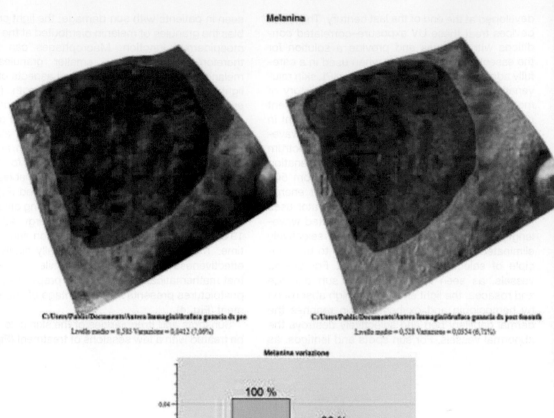

Melanina

C:\Users\Public\Documents\Astera Immagini\Grafica guancia ds pre
Livello medio = 0,585 Variazione = 0,0412 (7,06%)

C:\Users\Public\Documents\Astera Immagini\Grafica guancia ds post fluodt
Livello medio = 0,528 Variazione = 0,0354 (6,71%)

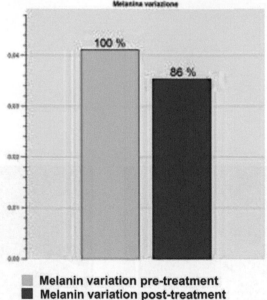

Melanina variazione

100 %

86 %

■ Melanin variation pre-treatment
■ Melanin variation post-treatment

Fig. 12. The mathematical analysis of the melanin variation of the patient in **Figs. 8** and **11**. The improvement of melanin variation was 14%.

crumbling the pigment granules at different depth. Clinical images show a change that is less easy to discern, while using the 3D system, the improvement can be better appreciated (**Fig. 6**) and quantified (**Fig. 7**).

A complete IPL treatment should result in an improvement of telangiectasia, a global reduction of the melanin amount, fewer irregularities in melanin distribution, and a smoother skin. The vascular improvement is often clinically evident (**Fig. 8**), whereas other features are usually not so noticeable. The 3D system can highlight the vascular improvement as well as calculate the percentage change (**Figs. 9** and **10**), but more benefits can be seen from the device on melanin variation (**Figs. 11** and **12**) and skin surface analysis (**Figs. 13** and **14**).

FRACTIONAL ABLATIVE RESURFACING

The drive to attain cosmetic facial improvement with rapid recovery and minimal risk has galvanized laser skin rejuvenation. Although traditional ablative carbon dioxide (CO_2) laser resurfacing was widely considered, since its emergence in the marketplace in the mid-1990s, as the gold standard,[5–13] the increased risk of prolonged wound healing, infection, and pigmentary alteration spurred researchers to look for better options.[14–18] As a result, the market for nonablative techniques grew fast, and many devices claimed to be efficient for wrinkle reduction and photodamaged skin improvement. However, after a critical review of recent literature, it seems clear that none of these nonablative methods are comparable with ablative skin resurfacing in terms of efficacy.[19–22] At the beginning of 2000, the question was how to bring together good results, low downtime, and low risks of adverse effects. In 2004, Manstein and colleagues[23] proposed to deliver energy, leaving intact skin bridges between one shot and another. The laser effect is located in the exposed tissue column while the healing processes start from these intact skin bridges. Through delivery of microscopic noncontiguous zones of thermal damage, it was observed that nonexposed epidermal cells and dermal tissue facilitated rapid healing. The concept of fractional

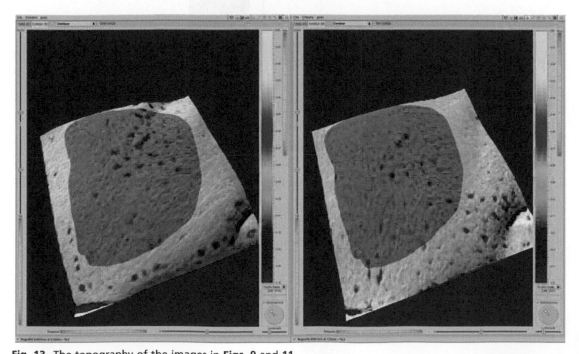

Fig. 13. The topography of the images in **Figs. 9** and **11**.

Contour

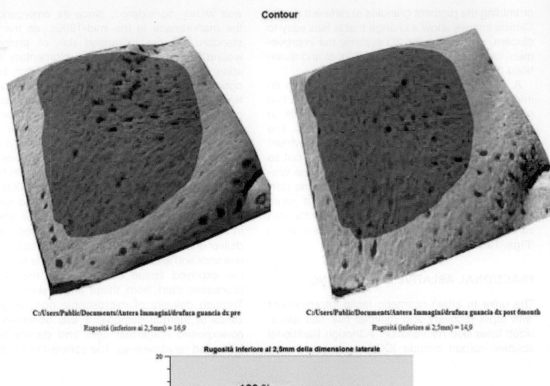

C:\Users\Public\Documents\Antera Immagini\drufuca guancia dx pre

Rugosità (inferiore ai 2,5mm) = 16,9

C:\Users\Public\Documents\Antera Immagini\drufuca guancia dx post 6month

Rugosità (inferiore ai 2,5mm) = 14,9

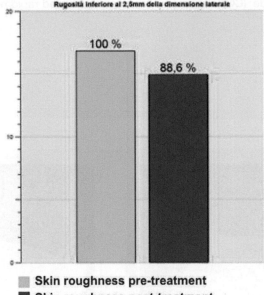

Rugosità inferiore al 2,5mm della dimensione laterale

100 %

88,6 %

- Skin roughness pre-treatment
- Skin roughness post-treatment

Fig. 14. The mathematical analysis of the skin roughness implies that the patient obtained an improvement of 12%.

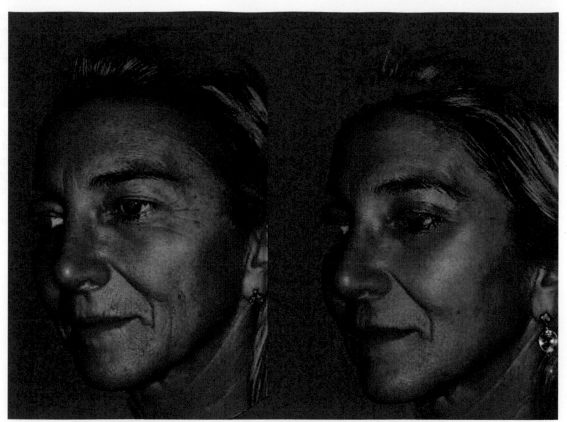

Fig. 15. A 57-year-old woman before and 9 months after an ablative ultrapulsed fractional CO_2 resurfacing.

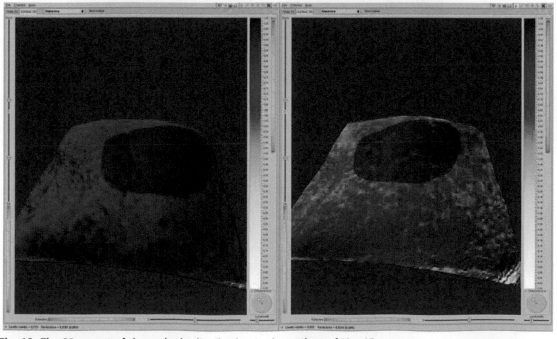

Fig. 16. The 3D aspect of the melanin distribution in the patient of **Fig. 15**.

delivery of energy was originally proposed for a nonablative wavelength but very quickly also applied to the ablative lasers. The idea was to incorporate the well-known results of ablative lasers while maintaining a short recovery time and a low incidence of adverse side effects.

Fractional ablative CO_2 resurfacing performed with an ultrapulsed device can yield good outcomes with only one session of treatment and a recovery time of 5 days. The overall appearance of the patient can be appreciated with clinical images (**Fig. 15**), but, using the Antera 3D device, the improvement of melanin distribution is much more clear. A report of a quantified melanin distribution modification can be easily generated (**Figs. 16 and 17**).

The analysis of the skin topography is exciting. The device allows not only calculation of the modification of a wide skin area (**Fig. 18**) but also evaluation of the degree of individual deep wrinkles before and after treatment (**Figs. 19 and 20**).

The device is also very helpful when a limited anatomic region is treated (**Fig. 21**). On lower eyelids, for example, not only can the modification of melanin distribution be evaluated and calculated (**Figs. 22 and 23**) but also the modification of skin topography can give precise indications of wrinkle improvement (**Fig. 24**). In this case, the hemoglobin concentration analysis can give a correct indication of neovascularization, which means, new collagen production in the case of higher hemoglobin presence after treatment (**Fig. 25**).

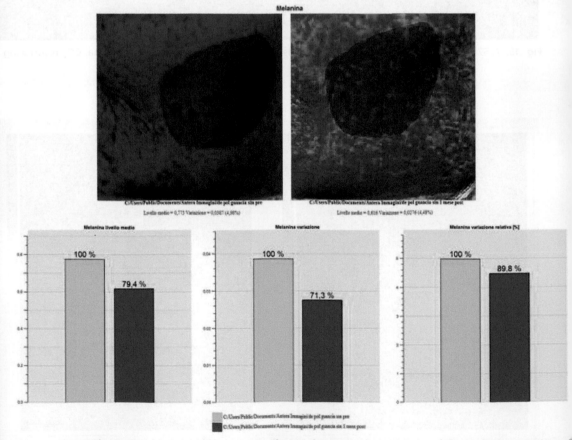

Fig. 17. The mathematical analysis of the area in **Fig. 16** shows an improvement of the melanin variation of around 30%.

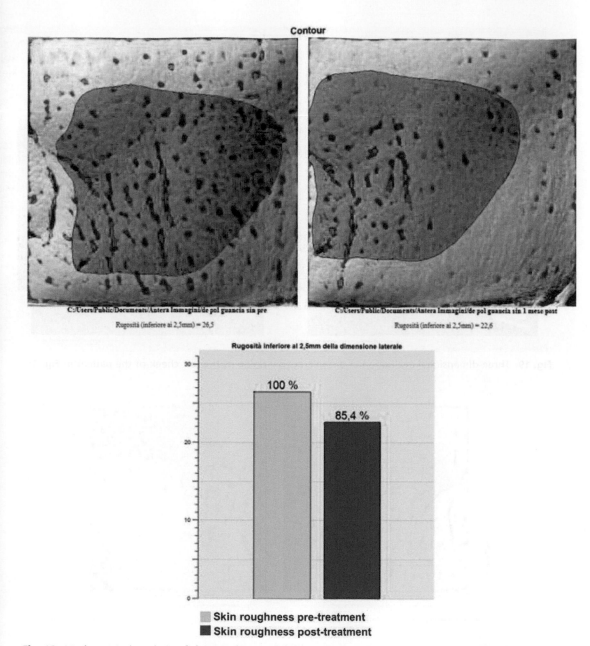

Contour

C:/Users/Public/Documents/Antera Immagini/de pol guancia sin pre

Rugosità (inferiore ai 2,5mm) = 26,5

C:/Users/Public/Documents/Antera Immagini/de pol guancia sin 1 mese post

Rugosità (inferiore ai 2,5mm) = 22,6

Rugosità inferiore al 2,5mm della dimensione laterale

100 %

85,4 %

■ Skin roughness pre-treatment
■ Skin roughness post-treatment

Fig. 18. Mathematical analysis of the roughness of the area in **Fig. 16**. The improvement was 15%.

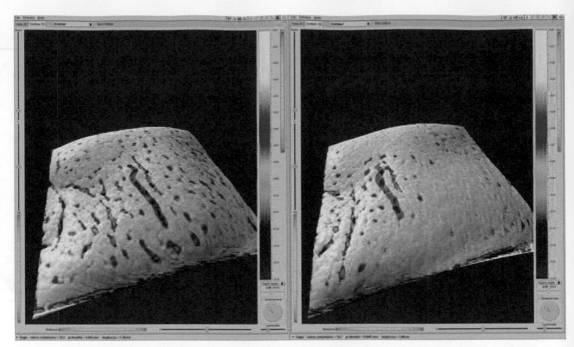

Fig. 19. Three-dimensional evaluation of a single deep wrinkle of the left cheek of the patient in **Fig. 15**.

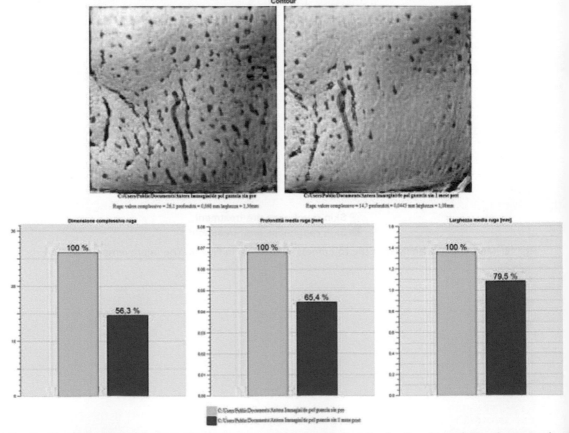

Fig. 20. The mathematical analysis of a single deep wrinkle implies that the fractional resurfacing determined an improvement of length, width, and depth of an average of 33%.

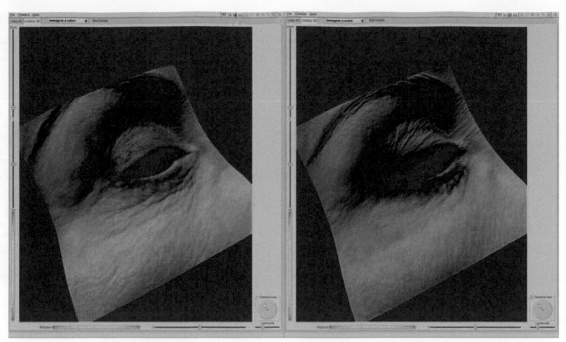

Fig. 21. Before and after 3D images of a lower eyelid treated with an ablative ultrapulsed fractional CO_2 resurfacing.

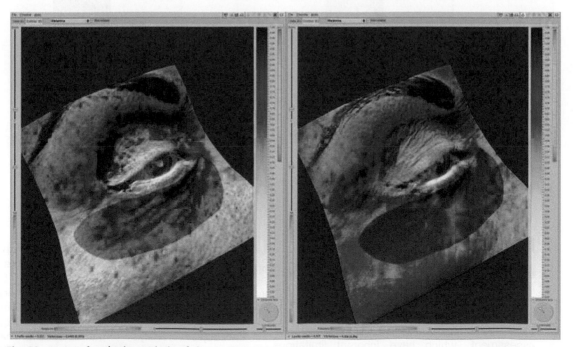

Fig. 22. Areas of melanin analysis of the previous patient.

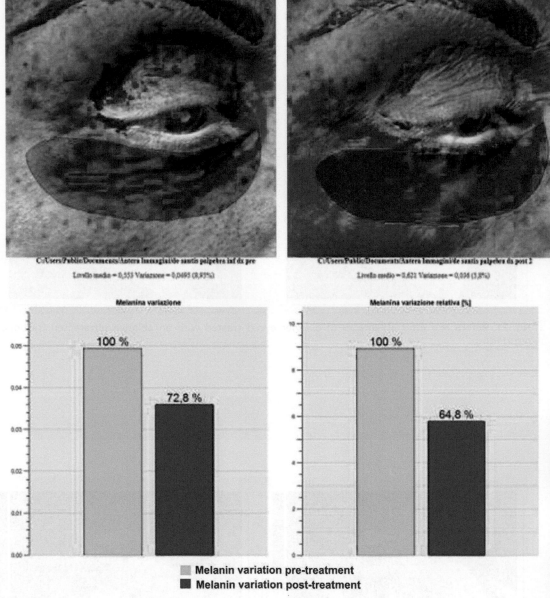

C:\Users\Public\Documents\Antera Immagini\de santis palpebra inf dx pre
Livello medio = 0,555 Variazione = 0,0495 (8,93%)

C:\Users\Public\Documents\Antera Immagini\de santis palpebra dx post 2
Livello medio = 0,621 Variazione = 0,036 (3,8%)

Melanina variazione

Melanina variazione relativa [%]

100 %

72,8 %

100 %

64,8 %

■ Melanin variation pre-treatment
■ Melanin variation post-treatment

Fig. 23. Mathematical analysis of the melanin variation implies that the improvement was higher than 35%.

DISCUSSION

All aesthetic procedures need an objective evaluation method. Simple visual analog score scales can be used, but their reliability depends on evaluators' experience. Conventional methods of evaluation have included photographic and clinical assessment, which have inherent limitations.

Computerized image analysis of silicone replicas has been shown to be a reproducible objective technique for measuring skin topography, but it is complex and cannot be used during everyday activities.[24] The 3D in vivo imaging system we are using provides a real-time, precise, quick, and objective analysis of patient-specific characteristics potentially enabling clinicians to predict

Contour

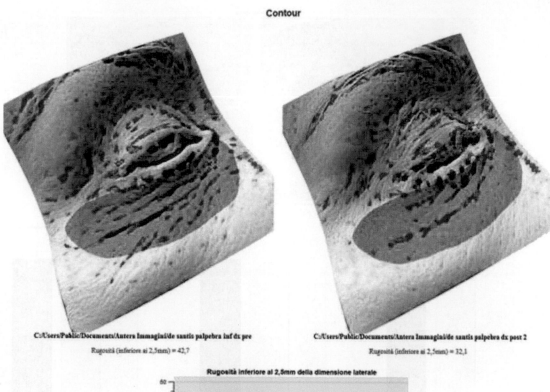

C:\Users\Public\Documents\Antera Immagini\de santis palpebra inf dx pre

Rugosità (inferiore ai 2,5mm) = 42,7

C:\Users\Public\Documents\Antera Immagini\de santis palpebra dx post 2

Rugosità (inferiore ai 2,5mm) = 32,1

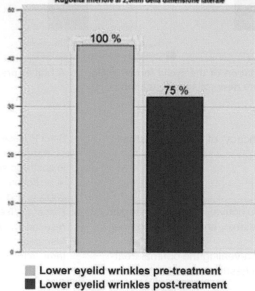

■ Lower eyelid wrinkles pre-treatment
■ Lower eyelid wrinkles post-treatment

Fig. 24. Wrinkles of the lower eyelid improved by 25%.

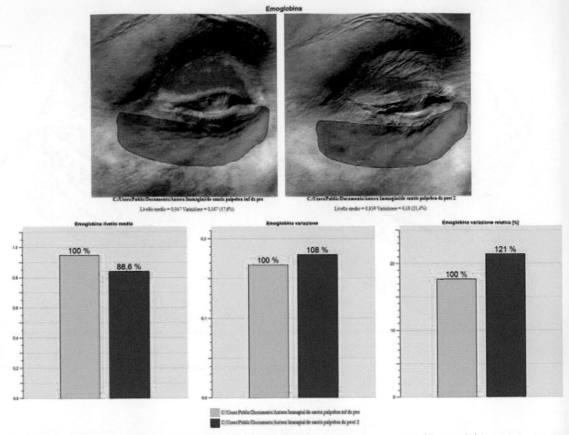

Fig. 25. Hemoglobin variation of the eyelid shown in **Fig. 21**. A higher presence of hemoglobin means neovascularization and therefore new collagen formation.

the limitations and efficacy of various aesthetic procedures.

SUMMARY

It is now possible to objectively quantify changes in skin hemoglobin, melanin, and surface contour in 3D.

This tool is useful for revealing the optimal treatment of skin surface in aesthetic facial surgery.

REFERENCES

1. Horn BKP. Obtaining Shape from Shading Information. In: Winston PH, editor. The Psychology of Computer Vision. McGraw-Hill (NY): 1975; p. 115–55.
2. Method and apparatus for imaging tissue topography. PCT patent application PCT/EP2010/001168, Irish Patent No. S85695. US application serial number, 13/203,005. EP patent application number, 10711832.5.
3. Anderson RR, Parrish JA. The optics of human skin. J Invest Dermatol 1981;77:13–9.
4. Bitter P, Nase GP. Skin rejuvenation for sun damage aging and rosacea using intense pulsed light. Lasers in aesthetic surgery. In: Keller G, Lacombe V, Lee P, et al, editors. New York: Thieme Medical Publishers 2000. p. 351–7.
5. Ratner D, Tse Y, Marchell N, et al. Cutaneous laser resurfacing. J Am Acad Dermatol 1999;41:365–89.
6. Manuskiatti W, Fitzpatrick RE, Goldman MP. Long-term effectiveness and side effects of carbon dioxide laser resurfacing for photoaged facial skin. J Am Acad Dermatol 1999;40:401–11.
7. Fitzpatrick RE, Goldman MP, Satur NM, et al. Pulsed carbon dioxide laser resurfacing of photoaged facial skin. Arch Dermatol 1996;132:395–402.
8. Schwartz RJ, Burns AJ, Rohrich RJ, et al. Long term assessment of CO_2 facial laser resurfacing: aesthetic results and complications. Plast Reconstr Surg 1999;103:592–601.
9. Hamilton MM. Carbon dioxide laser resurfacing. Facial Plast Surg Clin North Am 2004;12(3):289–95.
10. Lent WM, David LM. Laser resurfacing: a safe and predictable method of skin resurfacing. J Cutan Laser Ther 1999;1(2):87–94.

11. Airan LE, Hruza G. Current lasers in skin resurfacing. Facial Plast Surg Clin North Am 2002;10(1):87–101.

12. Fitzpatrick RE. CO_2 laser resurfacing. Dermatol Clin 2001;19(3):443–51.

13. Fitzpatrick RE. Maximizing benefits and minimizing risk with CO_2 laser resurfacing. Dermatol Clin 2002;20(1):77–86.

14. Bernstein LJ, Kauvar AN, Grossman MC, et al. The short- and long-term side effects of carbon dioxide laser resurfacing. Dermatol Surg 1997;23:519–25.

15. Nanni CA, Alster TS. Complications of carbon dioxide laser resurfacing. An evaluation of 500 patients. Dermatol Surg 1998;24:315–20.

16. Sriprachya-Anunt S, Fitzpatrick RE, Goldman MP, et al. Infections complicating pulsed carbon dioxide laser resurfacing for photoaged facial skin. Dermatol Surg 1997;23:527–36.

17. Berwald C, Levy JL, Magalon G. Complications of the resurfacing laser: retrospective study of 749 patients. Ann Chir Plast Esthet 2004;49(4):360–5.

18. Sullivan SA, Dailey RA. Complications of laser resurfacing and their management. Ophthal Plast Reconstr Surg 2000;16(6):417–26.

19. Sadick NS. Update on non-ablative light therapy for rejuvenation: a review. Lasers Surg Med 2003;32:120–8.

20. Williams EF III, Dahiya R. Review of nonablative laser resurfacing modalities. Facial Plast Surg Clin North Am 2004;12(3):305–10.

21. Grema H, Greve B, Raulin C. Facial rhytides—subsurfacing or resurfacing? A review. Lasers Surg Med 2003;32(5):405–12.

22. Bjerring P. Photorejuvenation—an overview. Med Laser Appl 2004;19:186–95.

23. Manstein D, Herron GS, Sink RK, et al. Fractional photothermolysis: a new concept for cutaneous remodeling using microscopic patterns of thermal injury. Lasers Surg Med 2004;34(5):426–38.

24. Grove GL, Grove MJ, Leyden JJ, et al. Skin replica analysis of photodamaged skin after therapy with tretinoin emollient cream. J Am Acad Dermatol 1991;25:231–7.

This page intentionally left blank

3D Analysis of Tissue Expanders

Kate McCarn, MD*, Peter A. Hilger, MD

KEYWORDS

- Facial reconstruction • Tissue expanders
- 3-dimensional imaging • Paramedian forehead flap

Three-dimensional imaging technology has only recently been described in the literature as a means to plan and better understand tissue expansion. This application is a logical use of the technology as the volume changes achieved with tissue expansion are controlled and often dramatic. This article reviews some of the phenomena associated with tissue expansion that are amenable to study with 3-dimensional imaging and reviews selected cases from the literature where the technology has been used to answer clinical questions and plan procedures. The future directions and limitations of the use of this technology in the head and neck will also be described.

TISSUE EXPANSION

Tissue expansion in a form near its modern evolution was first described as a means of head and neck reconstruction in 1957,[1] and it has been proven a safe and effective means of reconstructing many defects in the head and neck. Although expanded tissue undergoes histologic changes, it provides a better color and texture match for many areas of the head and neck than tissue obtained from distant donor sites. Important changes related to tissue expansion include decreased density of hair follicles, increased vasculariity of the tissue, and the formation of a fibrous capsule around the expander.[2]

IMPLANT SELECTION

Various tissue expanders are available commercially. The choice of implant is dependent upon the surgeon's assessment of the defect to be reconstructed. Rectangular implants provide the greatest increase in surface area for the volume added,[3] and oval implants have been shown to give a greater increase in surface area with a lower amount of pressure as compared with round implants.[4] A greater surface area of tissue is obtained from a single oval tissue expander than 2 spherical expanders with a combined volume equal to the oval expander; however, multiple expanders are frequently used in the head and neck because of the complex nature of the anatomy.[4] Overfilling expanders is a safe practice but increases the risk of leak at the injection port.[5]

An accurate assessment of the size of the defect and the amount of skin required to reconstruct the defect is critical to implant selection. This is often based upon 2-dimensional measurements of the defect and adjacent skin. Specifically within the head and neck, linear measurements between points of static bony anatomy (ie, the nasion, angle of mandible, and midpoint of the clavicle) on the side of the defect may be compared with the contralateral normal side in determining the amount of skin required for a given reconstruction.[6] Two-dimensional measurements of complex 3-dimensional defects can be misleading and often underestimate the surface area that will be required to fill a given defect.

The authors have nothing to disclose.
No funding support.
Division of Facial Plastic and Reconstructive Surgery, Department of Otolaryngology Head and Neck Surgery, University of Minnesota, 420 Delaware Street MMC 396, Minneapolis, MN 55455, USA
* Corresponding author.
E-mail address: drmccarn@gmail.com

Facial Plast Surg Clin N Am 19 (2011) 759–765
doi:10.1016/j.fsc.2011.07.013
1064-7406/11/$ – see front matter © 2011 Elsevier Inc. All rights reserved.

POSTERIOR EXPANSION VOLUME AND BONY REMODELING

Tissue expanders can cause significant changes to the tissues underlying the implant that cannot be appreciated while the implant is in place. This phenomenon has been described as posterior expansion volume by Tepper and colleagues[7] as it relates to breast reconstruction. The expander remodels the chest wall; thus some of the volume injected into the expander does not contribute to an increased surface area of skin available for the reconstruction. In this situation, there is a discrepancy between the volume change measured and the volume injected. This phenomenon is seen in the head and neck as well; expanders cause bony remodeling of the calvarium, with bone resorption in the center of the implant and reactive bone formation at the periphery.[8]

CONTRACTION

Once a tissue expander is removed, significant contraction of the expanded tissue is noted in the ensuing weeks and months. Some surgeons will remove all or part of the capsule around the expander, with the thought that the capsule with its increased density of fibroblasts is contributing to this phenomenon. Three-dimensional imaging has proven to be useful in analyzing contraction; a 20% decrease in expanded volume was noted over the 12 months subsequent to reconstruction of a patient with hemifacial microsomia using 3-dimensional photogrammetry.[9,10]

THREE-DIMENSIONAL ANALYSIS

Several means of obtaining 3-dimensional surface images are presently available[9] and are discussed more extensively elsewhere in this issue. Computed tomography (CT)-assisted 3-dimensional imaging generates a 3-dimensional surface image by superimposing photographs onto the surface generated by a CT scan, which is time-consuming and requires radiation exposure.

Three-dimensional laser scanners have been in use for some time and use a beam or stripe of laser light to capture multiple data points in space and generate a 3-dimensional image. Scanners are becoming faster and more portable. Stereophotogrammetry uses two or more cameras of a known focal length at different angles to the subject. The computer is able to generate a 3-dimensional rendering of the subject to within a millimeter. The Canfield VECTRA M3 3-D (Canfield Imaging Systems, A Division of Canfield Scientific Inc, Fairfield, ND, USA) camera and accompanying Mirror software were used to analyze data for the case presented in this article.

THREE-DIMENSIONAL ANALYSIS OF TISSUE EXPANDERS

Reconstructive surgeons have begun to adopt 3-dimensional surface analysis of tissue expansion over the past decade. Initial reports analyzing cleft patients[11] were among the first in using 3-dimensional facial imaging to understand a specific clinical entity and demonstrated the promise that this modality holds for improved understanding of complex facial structures.

Tissue expansion is a logical use for 3-dimensional imaging in that it allows surgeons to follow serial injections of a known volume and observe the effects on surface area over time.

Ying and colleagues[12] first described the use of 3-dimensional analysis of tissue expansion using a laser scanner in a burn patient. Images were taken preoperatively to compare the normal side with the side to be reconstructed, and the difference in surface area was calculated to determine the area of expanded tissue that would be necessary for the repair. This calculation agreed closely with the actual measured size of the cheek defect. Subsequent imaging was performed on postoperative day 12 showing a 44% reduction in the surface area of the flap.

Tepper and colleauges described the use of 3-dimensional analysis of tissue expanders in 12 patients undergoing unilateral breast reconstruction.[7] In the course of their study they used a 3-dimensional laser scanner to analyze patients before mastectomy, during tissue expansion, and postoperatively. The images were used to guide expansion volume, implant selection, and contralateral augmentation or reduction procedures. Overall they found improved breast symmetry when comparing pre- and post-reconstructive photographs. They also noted a discrepancy between injected and observed volume, which they attributed to remodeling of the chest wall and termed posterior expansion volume.

Jayaratne and colleagues described the use of 3-dimensional photogrammetry to determine the volume needed in the reconstruction of a patient with hemifacial microsomia by measuring the difference in volume between the 2 sides to be 16 cm³. A tissue expander was placed over the mandible, and serial expansions were performed until the expander had increased the volume to twice the required volume to allow for contraction. The expander was removed; a scapula free flap was used to correct the bony deficiency, and then serial 3-dimensional photographs were taken, showing that the majority of contraction occurred over the first 3 months. However, over the course of a year, 20% of the total volume gained by expansion was lost. This report was the first in using 3-dimensional photogrammetry to analyze tissue expanders in the head and neck.

Case Presentation

The Canfield VECTRA 3-D camera (Canfield Imaging Systems, A Division of Canfield Scientific Inc, Fairfield, ND, USA) was used to take photos during and after expansion in a patient undergoing an expanded paramedian forehead flap for reconstruction of a post-traumatic nasal defect. This case highlights some of the important uses, limitations, and questions that can be answered using this technology.

The patient was a young male who sustained severe facial injuries including a total nasal avulsion with soft tissue loss involving the upper lip. He had undergone multiple reconstructive procedures including a prior nasal reconstruction with a paramedian forehead flap. This reconstruction was complicated by a postoperative infection that caused loss of the structural grafts and partial loss of the paramedian forehead flap (**Fig. 1**). Due to the scarring from the prior procedure and the large quantity of tissue required for coverage, reconstruction using an expanded paramedian forehead flap was planned.[13]

A tissue expander was placed, and serial expansion was performed twice weekly in the clinic with 10 cc of saline until a sufficient amount of nonhair-

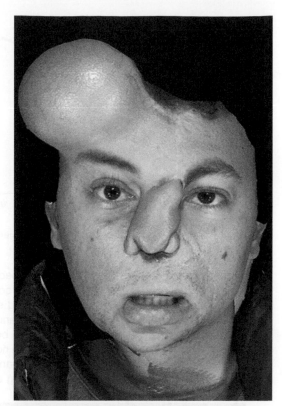

Fig. 2. Patient at conclusion of tissue expansion.

bearing skin was available for the reconstruction (**Fig. 2**). Due to the fact that half of the expander was buried deep to the scalp, a precise volumetric analysis of the tissue expansion was not possible. The Canfield VECTRA 3D camera and software were used to obtain photographs during expansion and after the nasal reconstruction.

The total surface area of skin anterior to the hairline on the expanded side was 113 cm^2 versus 38 cm^2 on the nonexpanded side. As the expander was partially buried under the scalp, an accurate measure of the volume before and after expansion was not possible. The surface area increased with expansion more rapidly at first and slowed as the total volume of the expander increased (**Fig. 3**). Volume changes were demonstrated by coregistering images using fixed points on the photographs (ie, medial and lateral canthi, the apex of the previous paramedian forehead flap, and a nevus on the left cheek). Accurate coregistration was confirmed by creating a color map comparing the volumetric differences between the 2 images as seen in **Fig. 4**.

After expansion was completed, the patient underwent division and inset of his previous forehead flap pedicle; the skin from the previous forehead flap was used as turn-in flaps to create an internal lining inferiorly. Costal cartilage was used

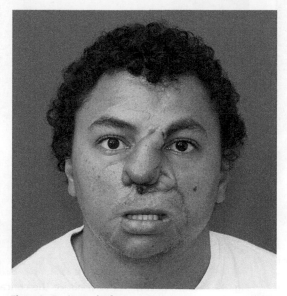

Fig. 1. Patient before implantation of a tissue expander.

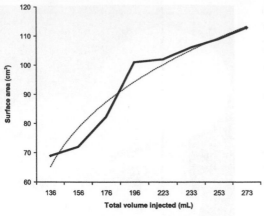

Fig. 3. Change in surface area as total volume injected increases.

to construct dorsal and alar struts as described by Weng and colleagues, and the entire outer cover was reconstructed using expanded forehead skin (**Fig. 5**). The flap was raised over the expander, and the capsule was excised. Significant bony remodeling of the calvarium was noted with a ridge of reactive bone at the margins of the expander and a depression at the center. After raising and

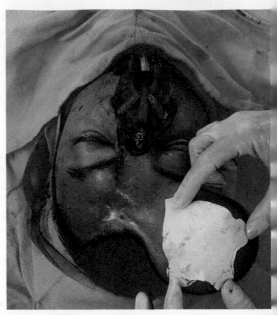

Fig. 5. Template for expanded paramedian forehead flap. Costal cartilage was used for structural support, and turn-in flaps were used for internal lining inferiorly.

rotating the flap, the forehead was closed primarily with minimal distortion of the hairline.

The patient returned to the clinic 2 weeks later for a postoperative visit. His incisions were well healed; there was minimal distortion of his hairline (**Fig. 6**). The patient returned 1 month later for

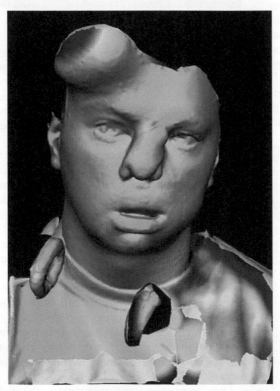

Fig. 4. Colorimetric mapping of the volume difference between baseline and follow-up images showing the total amount of change in volume over the course of expansion. Green areas show no change in volume, and red is 20 mm of expansion.

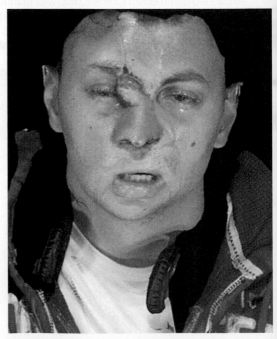

Fig. 6. 2 weeks postoperatively, notice the concavity over the right frontal bone where the expander caused significant expansion.

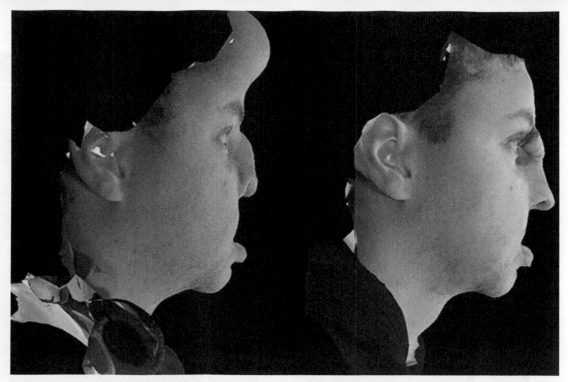

Fig. 7. Pre- and postoperative profile views, note the improved nasal projection.

follow-up imaging, continuing to heal well. His nasal projection was improved by 8 mm, yielding a much-improved profile (**Fig. 7**). Analysis of the 2- and 10-week postoperative views showed a 5 mm difference in the projection of the bony rim around the expander, and a 5 mm decrease in the size of the vascular pedicle, consistent with the observed decrease in soft tissue edema. Overall, the volume of the bony defect in the forehead decreased by 7.5 cm^3, consistent with decreased edema but also potentially with some bony remodeling, as the contour of the defect from the tissue expander was visibly improved (**Fig. 8**). The surface area of the defect decreased from 61.9 cm^2 to 54.9 cm^2. The projection of the nasal tip was reduced by less than 1 mm. The surface area of the paramedian forehead flap decreased from 24.6 cm^2 to 22.2 cm^2, contraction of 9.8%.

FUTURE DIRECTIONS

Application of 3-dimensional technology to tissue expanders is in its infancy. 3-dimensional imaging has the potential to help reconstructive surgeons improve surgical planning[710] by allowing the precise measurement of surface area and volume. Morphing software was used in this case retrospectively to generate a model with improved nasal projection and dorsal height (**Fig. 9**). Based upon this model, the actual surface area of tissue required to cover the new nose calculated as 25.8 cm^2. This compares to 22 cm^2 for the actual

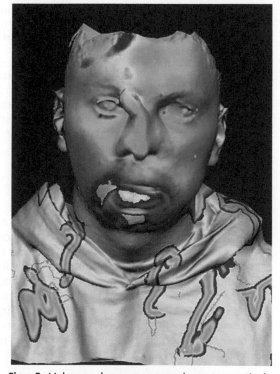

Fig. 8. Volume changes mapped postoperatively; green indicates no volume change. Note the change in volume over the lower third of the face; this is an artifact created by the patient having his jaw slightly open in 1 photo and not the other. The volume changes in the upper third of the face reflect an improvement in postoperative edema.

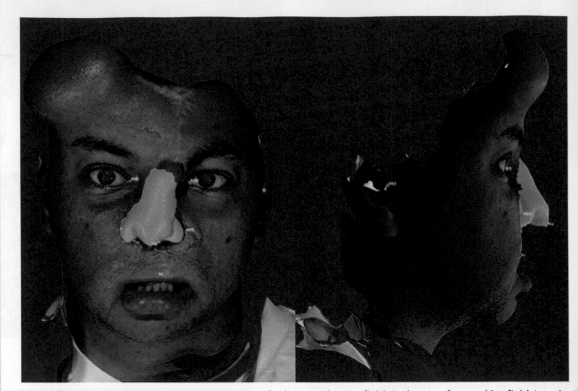

Fig. 9. The patient's preoperative nose was morphed using the Canfield Sculptor software (Canfield Imaging Systems, A Division of Canfield Scientific Inc, Fairfield, ND, USA), and the resulting image was measured to determine the size of the flap that would be required to create a new soft tissue cover for the nose.

flap that was used. The requirement of overexpansion to counteract postoperative contraction and the effect of capsulectomy on postoperative contraction are also future directions of study that may help improve understanding of the behavior of expanded tissue.

LIMITATIONS

The use of 3-dimensional laser scanning and photogrammetry is limited in the head and neck by several factors. Hair-bearing areas cannot be accurately imaged unless shaved. The lower third of the face is constantly in motion and minor differences in the jaw and tongue position can account for several millimeters difference or cubic centimeters of volumetric difference, as seen in **Fig. 8**. Using a chin rest or even a customized mouth guard in conjunction with a chin rest can be used to overcome this factor if necessary.

SUMMARY

Three-dimensional imaging technology is becoming more readily available and commonly used by reconstructive surgeons. The application of this technology to tissue expansion holds the

potential to answer many questions about the planning, expansion, and postoperative phases of reconstruction. Improved understanding of the need for overexpansion, the effect of capsulectomy on contraction, posterior expansion volume, and the bony remodeling that occurs beneath expanders may result from the application of 3-dimensional imaging technology. 3-dimensional morphing and analysis can be used to determine the amount of tissue that will be required to reconstruct a given defect. This area is just now beginning to be explored by clinicians, but holds the promise of allowing reconstructive surgeons to plan and execute complex procedures in the head and neck.

REFERENCES

1. Neumann C. The expansion of an area of skin by progressive distension of a subcutaneous balloon. Plast Reconstr Surg 1957;19(2):124–30.
2. Swenson RW. Controlled tissue expansion in facial reconstruction. In: Baker SR, editor. Local flaps in facial reconstruction. Philadelphia: Elsevier-Mosby; 2007. p. 667–89.
3. van Rappard JH, Sonneveld GJ, Borghouts JM. Geometric planning and the shape of the expander. Facial Plast Surg 1988;5:287.

4. Brobmann GF, Huber J. Effects of different-shaped tissue expanders on transluminal pressure, oxygen tension, histopathalogic changes and skin expansion in pigs. Plast Reconstr Surg 1985;76(5):731–6.

5. Baker SR, Swanson NA. Clinical applications of tissue expansion in head and neck surgery. Laryngoscope 1990;3:100.

6. Hsiao C, Hsiao G, Chang L. Accurate assessment of tissue expansion in the lower face and anterior neck by a simple measurement technique. Br J Plast Surg 1999;52:339–42.

7. Tepper O, Karp N, Small K, et al. Three-dimensional imaging provides valuable clinical data to aid in unilateral tissue expander–implant breast reconstruction. Breast J 2008;14(6):543–50.

8. Moelleken B, Mathes S, Cann C, et al. Long-term effects of tissue expansion on cranial and skeletal bone development in neonatal miniature swine: clinical findings and histomorphometric correlates. Plast Reconstr Surg 1990;86(5):825–34.

9. Honrado C, Larrabee WF. Update in three-dimensional imaging in facial plastic surgery. Curr Opin Otolaryngol Head Neck Surg 2004;12: 327–31.

10. Jayaratne YS, Lo J, Zwahlen RA, et al. Three-dimensional photogrammetry for surgical planning of tissue expansion in hemifacial microsomia. Head Neck 2010;32(12):1728–35.

11. Ferrario V, Sforza C, Dellavia C, et al. A quantitative three-dimensional assessment of soft tissue facial asymmetry of cleft lip and palate adult patients. J Craniofac Surg 2003;14(5):739–46.

12. Ying J, Zhang F, Schwartz J, et al. Assessment of facial tissue expansion with three dimensional digitizer scanning. J Craniofac Surg 2002;13(5): 687–92.

13. Weng R, Li Q, Gu B, et al. Extended forehead skin expansion and single-stage nasal subunit plasty for nasal reconstruction. Plast Reconstr Surg 2010; 124(4):1119–28.

This page intentionally left blank

3D Analysis of Dentofacial Deformities: A New Model for Clinical Application

Jonathan M. Sykes, MD[a],*, S.H. Amin, MD[b],
D.C. Hatcher, DC, DDS, MSc, MRCD(c)[c], J. Kim, MD[a]

KEYWORDS

• Midface deformities • Soft tissue changes • Le Fort
• Three-dimensional imaging

Accurate facial analysis is the cornerstone of aesthetic and functional surgery of the face. Its importance is defined by the necessity to define preoperative and postoperative goals, as a function of both surgical objectives and meeting patient desires and expectations. Simulating and defining the augmentation of soft tissue position after surgery has been a paramount objective of surgeons for more than a century, yet current methods of attaining this objective remain dated. This article discusses the use of advanced imaging technology and software analysis to objectify midface soft tissue movement in a three-dimensional (3D) model after Le Fort osteotomies and maxillary advancement. Although discussed here in the context of a single procedure, the potential applications of this method of analysis are countless.

Facial analysis is rooted in antiquity, with coordinate measurement systems being adopted in Egypt, India, Greece, and Byzantium.[1] The renaissance brought about a more technical system of analysis, notably Leonardo da Vinci's facial proportions. The current aesthetic ideal is a combination of patient desires, contemporary concepts of beauty, and the surgeon's concept of beauty.

Measurement systems, based on two-dimensional (2D) analysis have been created to capture these ideals. These techniques include cephalometrics and clinical photography. The 2D model uses multiple coordinates in an attempt to capture the third dimension, which is depth. Although useful, this model limits analysis to mostly linear surgical vectors (eg, anterior-posterior dimension). Current measurements depend on soft tissue coordinates relative to fixed bony landmarks.

Present technology allows only limited analysis in 2 dimensions. For example, analysis of midface soft tissue following Le Fort osteotomies is generally performed using lateral views, which is a limited measurement technique. After midfacial advancement, the upper lip is changed in size, position, and shape. Limited 2D analysis allows us to measure the change in projection, or length of the lip in a given plane. However, the observer sees the changes in the lip in 3 dimensions, not on a single plane. Just as the human eye analyzes the entire midface after Le Fort osteotomies, so should the analysis.

3D imaging protocols have been studied for more than a decade. However, broad

[a] Division of Facial Plastic Surgery and Reconstructive Surgery, UC Davis Health System, UC Davis Medical Group, 2521 Stockton Boulevard, Suite 6206, Sacramento, CA 95817, USA
[b] Kaiser Northern California Otolaryngology Residency Program, 280 West MacArthur Boulevard, Oakland, CA 94611, USA
[c] Private Practice at Diagnostic Digital Imaging, 99 Scripts Drive, Suite 101, Sacramento, CA 95825, USA
* Corresponding author.
E-mail address: jonathan.sykes@ucdmc.ucdavis.edu

Facial Plast Surg Clin N Am 19 (2011) 767–771
doi:10.1016/j.fsc.2011.08.001
1064-7406/11/$ – see front matter © 2011 Elsevier Inc. All rights reserved.

advancements in imaging techniques and analytical software are beginning to transfer these tools from research to clinical application. 3D imaging has the potential to largely replace standard cephalometry, in which the head film is a 2D representation of a 3D object. Cone beam computed tomography (CBCT) in combination with surface scanning allows the creation of the electronic patient,[2–8] allowing the ability to create, modify, and predict surgical outcomes. This situation not only provides an opportunity for surgical planning but also creates a powerful communication interface between treating physicians and patients. This article proposes the use of 3D imaging protocols to accurately assess surgical treatment goals before and after orthognathic surgery.

Global goals in plastic surgery include visualization and measurement of presurgical simulation and outcomes of surgery. This process needs to be simple and accurate. Presurgical simulation should create a surgical objective and a blueprint for surgery. Outcomes assessment creates the opportunity to measure cause-and-effect relationships between skeletal manipulations or soft tissue augmentations and the final soft tissue results. Outcomes analyses can be used to refine the simulation and outcomes predictions.

3D MODELING TECHNIQUE

An example of current 2D analysis is shown by lip analysis. The boundaries of the lip reside in the lower third of the face. The vertical boundaries of the upper lip are the subnasale (superiorly) and stomion superius (inferiorly), and those of the lower lip are the stomion inferius (superiorly) and menton (inferiorly). The upper lip/lower lip height ratio ($Sn-Stm_s/Stm_i-Me'$) is approximately 1:2. Holdaway[9,10] describes 11 techniques for measuring soft tissue balance, which include facial angle, upper lip curvature, skeletal convexity at point A, upper lip strain and thickness, and lower sulcus depth. These parameters are measured with 2D imaging techniques, including standard 6-view photography and cephalograms. Current measurement parameters measure the change in lip position as a function of upper lip thickness and position in relation to fixed bony points.

Schendel and Lane[2] have described image fusion techniques and their application to surgical craniofacial and dental anatomy. This article furthers this application to the evaluation of soft tissue anatomy. Image fusion is a combination of CBCT and 3D facial surface imaging (stereo photogrammetry). Stereo photogrammetry is an advanced software system applied to the fundamental technique of taking 2 or more pictures of the same object using single reflex

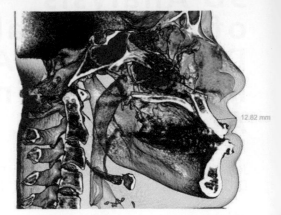

Fig. 1. Preoperative skeletal radiograph demonstrating the soft tissue and skeletal relationship of the maxilla, mandible, nose, and lips.

lenses, at a distance differential similar to the distance between a pair of eyes. This process creates a composite 3D model using complex triangulation algorithms to identify and match unique surface markers. After a 3D geometric shape has been formed, the software maps color texture onto the model. Each color represents the amount the soft tissue has moved anteriorly or posteriorly in relation to a fixed bony landmark. This surface image is overlaid on the skeletal framework obtained from the CBCT scan, with the skull base used as an anchoring point. The clinician is able to use the color mapping to quickly analyze postsurgical changes. The result is the most accurate electronic representation of surgical changes to craniofacial anatomy available to date.

As presented in this article, a 3D model was created showing presurgical and postsurgical midface movement in relation to fixed bony

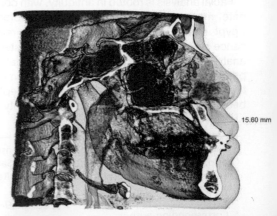

Fig. 2. Postoperative skeletal radiograph showing the skin and bony changes of the face following a Le Fort I osteotomy.

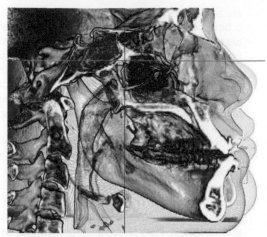

Fig. 3. Pre and postoperative images following Le Fort I osteotomy are superimposed to illustrate changes in lip position.

structures. The presurgical and postsurgical CBCT volumes were imported into InVivo 5.1 (Anatomage, San Jose, CA). The 2 scans were superimposed onto a common Cartesian coordinate system using the skull bases as registration targets. The skull bases were outside the operative areas and expected to be morphometrically stable

during the study period. The software used a voxel intensity minimization algorithm to register the 2 skull base volumes. The registered volumes could be viewed simultaneously and measured using digital calipers. This method allows for visualization and analysis of the hard and soft tissue changes. The analysis of a surgical patient was performed, with a primary focus on upper lip changes before and after Le Fort I osteotomy. Soft tissue measurements were taken from 3 points: subnasale, the most anterior lip projection (**Figs. 1** and **2**), and stomion, on an arc taken from the odontoid process to the nasolabial fold. An example of a lip movement change at the vermilion border incorporating vertical change is shown after the patient's Le Fort osteostomy (**Fig. 3**), measured to be 7.84 mm.

In addition, a color map of the face was created showing presurgical and postsurgical soft tissue movement in relation to fixed bony structures. The user is able to scan the postoperative image with crosshairs returning movement changes based on the superimposed coordinate systems. For example, in the right midcheek, our patient had movement anteriorly of 3 mm after surgery, quantified by dragging crosshairs over the region of interest. For the physician, the color system allows for an instant global view of postoperative changes.

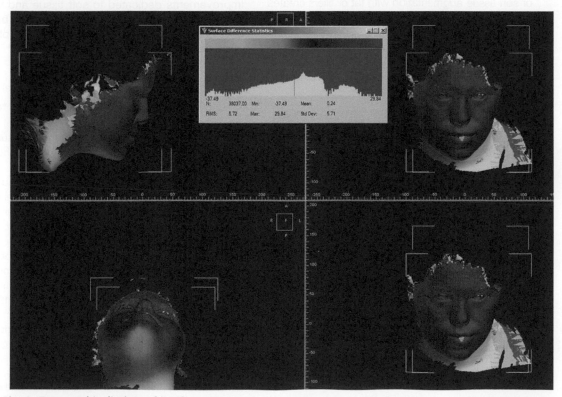

Fig. 4. Topographic displays of lip changes.

Topographic displays of lip changes are displayed in **Fig. 4**. 3D surface changes after surgery are shown in **Fig. 5**.

FUTURE APPLICATIONS

3D modeling is the next stage in the evolution of surgical planning. There has been much advancement in bony 3D modeling, but little in the way of soft tissue analysis. This article shows how soft tissue changes can be measured with 3D software. Multiple 2D planes were easily quantified using a 3D coordinate system. Future studies will demonstrate volume measurements, which can be applied to analysis of any region of the face, with emphasis on the cheeks and chin.

The multiobject software platform (InVivo) combines all points onto a common coordinate system volume rendering to simultaneously visualize the hard and soft tissues from any point of view. This process allows the user to make measurements: linear, angular, curved, volumetric, and cross-sectional. The software also allows the user to superimpose before and after 3D volumes, and register volumes over stable anatomic sites.

Our specialty uses 2D photography to analyze horizontal movements, which occur after an implant is placed or another surgical procedure is performed. However, placement of an implant, bony movement, or soft tissue augmentation with fat or fillers creates 3D changes, which previously were inadequately quantified. The goal of improved 3D software and techniques is to accurately quantify the entire change or movement, not just the 2D soft tissue change. If these techniques can be refined, the applications are significant, with far-reaching consequences. First, a better communication tool could more accurately show to our patients what their posttreatment outcome could be. Second, it would enable the physician to correctly understand and plan individual treatments. Third, surgeons would more clearly understand the 3D changes of a given treatment and its limitations, and make modifications to improve future therapy.

An example of the restrictions of current 2D technology and analysis is illustrated with bony genioplasty and advancement. Currently, the preoperative to postoperative change is analyzed on 2D lateral photographs looking at the position of the soft tissue pogonion before and after surgery. However, some genioplasty procedures that adequately enhance the pogonion in the midline (the present measured end point) create deficiency lateral to midline in the area where the oblique osteotomy has been performed. An advantage of the application of 3D technology would be to specifically evaluate volume deficiencies in the area of the osteotomies. Our eventual goal is to quantify the entire volumetric changes associated with bony movement, prosthetic implantation, and fat transplantation.

The study reported in this article uses 3D technology, but primarily uses 2D fixed reference points. In the future, the current software with improvements dedicated to soft tissue and volumetric studies will enable the practitioner to better understand the 3D changes created by implants and orthognathic surgery.

REFERENCES

1. Jacobsen A. Radiographic cephalometry. Carol Stream (IL): Quintessence; 1995.
2. Schendel SA, Lane C. 3D orthognathic surgery simulation using image fusion. Semin Orthodont 2009;15(1):48–56.
3. Gossett CB, Preston CB, Dunford R, et al. Prediction accuracy of computer assisted surgical visual treatment objectives as compared with conventional visual treatment objectives. J Oral Maxillofac Surg 2005;63:609–17.
4. Adams GL, Gansky SA, Miller AJ, et al. Comparison between traditional 2-dimensional cephalometry and a 3-dimensional approach on human dry skulls. Am J Orthod Dentofacial Orthop 2004;126(4):397–409.
5. Stratemann S, Huang J, Maki K, et al. Comparison of cone beam computed tomography imaging with physical measures. Dentomaxillofac Radiol 2008;37(2):80–93.
6. Swatsty D, Lee JS, Huang JC, et al. Anthropometric analysis of the human mandibular cortical

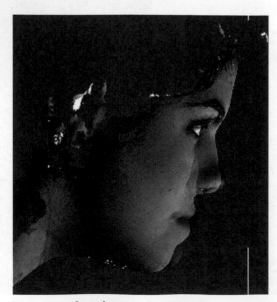

Fig. 5. 3D surface changes after surgery.

bone as assessed by cone-beam computed tomography. J Oral Maxillofac Surg 2009;67(3): 491–500.

7. Hatcher DC, Dial C. 3D surface imaging of the face. J Calif Dent Assoc 2009;37(3):193–7.

8. Swasty D, Lee J, Huang J, et al. Cross-sectional human mandibular morphology as assessed in vivo by cone beam computed tomography in patients with different facial dimensions. Am J Orthod Dentofacial Orthop 2011;139(Suppl 4): e377–89.

9. Holdaway RA. A soft-tissue cephalometric analysis and its use in orthodontic treatment planning. Part I. American Journal of Orthodontics 1983;84:1–28.

10. Holdaway RA. A soft-tissue cephalometric analysis and its use in orthodontic treatment planning. Part II. American Journal of Orthodontics 1984; 85:279–93.

This page intentionally left blank

Index

Facial Plast Surg Clin N Am 19 (2011) 773–789
doi:10.1016/S1064-7406(11)00135-0
1064-7406/11/$ – see front matter © 2011 Elsevier Inc. All rights reserved.

This page intentionally left blank

United States Postal Service

Statement of Ownership, Management, and Circulation
(All Periodicals Publications Except Requester Publications)

1. Publication Title	2. Publication Number								3. Filing Date
Facial Plastic Surgery Clinics of North America	0	1	3	-	1	2	2		9/16/11

4. Issue Frequency	5. Number of Issues Published Annually	6. Annual Subscription Price
Feb, May, Aug, Nov	4	$339.00

7. Complete Mailing Address of Known Office of Publication (Not printer) (Street, city, county, state, and ZIP+4®)

Elsevier Inc.
360 Park Avenue South
New York, NY 10010-1710

Contact Person
Stephen Bushing

Telephone (Include area code)
215-239-3688

8. Complete Mailing Address of Headquarters or General Business Office of Publisher (Not printer)

Elsevier Inc., 360 Park Avenue South, New York, NY 10010-1710

9. Full Names and Complete Mailing Addresses of Publisher, Editor, and Managing Editor (Do not leave blank)

Publisher (Name and complete mailing address)

Kim Murphy, Elsevier, Inc., 1600 John F. Kennedy Blvd. Suite 1800, Philadelphia, PA 19103-2899

Editor (Name and complete mailing address)

Joanne Husovski, Elsevier, Inc., 1600 John F. Kennedy Blvd. Suite 1800, Philadelphia, PA 19103-2899

Managing Editor (Name and complete mailing address)

Barton Dudlick, Elsevier, Inc., 1600 John F. Kennedy Blvd. Suite 1800, Philadelphia, PA 19103-2899

10. Owner (Do not leave blank. If the publication is owned by a corporation, give the name and address of the corporation immediately followed by the names and addresses of all stockholders owning or holding 1 percent or more of the total amount of stock. If not owned by a corporation, give the names and addresses of the individual owners. If owned by a partnership or other unincorporated firm, give its name and address as well as those of each individual owner. If the publication is published by a nonprofit organization, give its name and address.)

Full Name	Complete Mailing Address
Wholly owned subsidiary of	4520 East-West Highway
Reed/Elsevier, US holdings	Bethesda, MD 20814

11. Known Bondholders, Mortgagees, and Other Security Holders Owning or Holding 1 Percent or More of Total Amount of Bonds, Mortgages, or Other Securities. If none, check box → ☐ None

Full Name	Complete Mailing Address
N/A	

12. Tax Status (For completion by nonprofit organizations authorized to mail at nonprofit rates) (Check one)
The purpose, function, and nonprofit status of this organization and the exempt status for federal income tax purposes:
☐ Has Not Changed During Preceding 12 Months
☐ Has Changed During Preceding 12 Months (Publisher must submit explanation of change with this statement)

PS Form 3526, September 2007 (Page 1 of 3) (Instructions Page 3)) PSN 7530-01-000-9931 **PRIVACY NOTICE:** See our Privacy policy in www.usps.com

13. Publication Title	14. Issue Date for Circulation Data Below
Facial Plastic Surgery Clinics of North America	August 2011

15. Extent and Nature of Circulation		Average No. Copies Each Issue During Preceding 12 Months	No. Copies of Single Issue Published Nearest to Filing Date
a. Total Number of Copies (Net press run)		1051	1000
b. Paid Circulation (By Mail and Outside the Mail)	(1) Mailed Outside-County Paid Subscriptions Stated on PS Form 3541. (Include paid distribution above nominal rate, advertiser's proof copies, and exchange copies)	435	408
	(2) Mailed In-County Paid Subscriptions Stated on PS Form 3541 (Include paid distribution above nominal rate, advertiser's proof copies, and exchange copies)		
	(3) Paid Distribution Outside the Mails Including Sales Through Dealers and Carriers, Street Vendors, Counter Sales, and Other Paid Distribution Outside USPS®	78	86
	(4) Paid Distribution by Other Classes Mailed Through the USPS (e.g. First-Class Mail®)		
c. Total Paid Distribution (Sum of 15b (1), (2), (3), and (4))	►	513	494
d. Free or Nominal Rate Distribution (By Mail and Outside the Mail)	(1) Free or Nominal Rate Outside-County Copies Included on PS Form 3541	70	71
	(2) Free or Nominal Rate In-County Copies Included on PS Form 3541		
	(3) Free or Nominal Rate Copies Mailed at Other Classes Through the USPS (e.g. First-Class Mail)		
	(4) Free or Nominal Rate Distribution Outside the Mail (Carriers or other means)		
e. Total Free or Nominal Rate Distribution (Sum of 15d (1), (2), (3) and (4))	►	70	71
f. Total Distribution (Sum of 15c and 15e)	►	583	565
g. Copies not Distributed (See instructions to publishers #4 (page #3))	►	468	435
h. Total (Sum of 15f and g)	►	1051	1000
i. Percent Paid (15c divided by 15f times 100)	►	87.99%	87.43%

16. Publication of Statement of Ownership
☐ If the publication is a general publication, publication of this statement is required. Will be printed in the **November 2011** issue of this publication. — Publication not required

17. Signature and Title of Editor, Publisher, Business Manager, or Owner

Stephen R. Bushing
Stephen R. Bushing –Inventory/Distribution Coordinator

Date
September 16, 2011

I certify that all information furnished on this form is true and complete. I understand that anyone who furnishes false or misleading information on this form or who omits material or information requested on the form may be subject to criminal sanctions (including fines and imprisonment) and/or civil sanctions (including civil penalties).

PS Form 3526, September 2007 (Page 2 of 3)

Moving?

Make sure your subscription moves with you!

To notify us of your new address, find your **Clinics Account Number** (located on your mailing label above your name), and contact customer service at:

Email: journalscustomerservice-usa@elsevier.com

800-654-2452 (subscribers in the U.S. & Canada)
314-447-8871 (subscribers outside of the U.S. & Canada)

Fax number: 314-447-8029

Elsevier Health Sciences Division
Subscription Customer Service
3251 Riverport Lane
Maryland Heights, MO 63043

*To ensure uninterrupted delivery of your subscription, please notify us at least 4 weeks in advance of move.

Printed and bound by CPI Group (UK) Ltd, Croydon, CR0 4YY

03/10/2024

01040359-0002